Oxford Medical Publications

Reproductive Health Care for Women and Babies

AF740247

Reproductive Health Care for Women and Babies

Edited by

Benjamin P. Sachs
Obstetrician–Gynecologist-in-Chief
Beth Israel Hospital
Harvard Medical School/Harvard School of Public Health
Boston, USA

Richard Beard
Head of Department of Obstetrics and Gynecology
St Mary's Hospital Medical School
London, England

Emile Papiernik
Chief, Department of Obstetrics and Gynecology
Hospital Baudeloque
Paris, France

Cristine Russell
Special Health Correspondent,
Washington Post
Freelance Writer
Darien, CT, USA

New York Oxford Tokyo
OXFORD UNIVERSITY PRESS
1995

DE MONTFORT UNIVERSITY LIBRARY
18.7.97
Loc./Form
Class 362.1982 REP

Oxford University Press, Walton Street, Oxford OX2 6DP
Oxford New York
Athens Auckland Bangkok Bombay
Calcutta Cape Town Dar es Salaam Delhi
Florence Hong Kong Istanbul Karachi
Kuala Lumpur Madras Madrid Melbourne
Mexico City Nairobi Paris Singapore
Taipei Tokyo Toronto
and associated companies in
Berlin Ibadan

Oxford is a trade mark of Oxford University Press

Published in the United States
by Oxford University Press Inc., New York

© Benjamin P. Sachs, Richard Beard, Emile Papiernik,
Cristine Russell, and the contributors listed on pp. xiii–xv, 1995

All rights reserved. No part of this publication may be reproduced, stored in a retrieval system, or transmitted, in any form or by any means, without the prior permission in writing of Oxford University Press. Within the UK, exceptions are allowed in respect of any fair dealing for the purpose of research or private study, or criticism or review, as permitted under the Copyright, Designs and Patents Act, 1988, or in the case of reprographic reproduction in accordance with the terms of licences issued by the Copyright Licensing Agency. Enquiries concerning reproduction outside those terms and in other countries should be sent to the Rights Department, Oxford University Press, at the address above.

This book is sold subject to the condition that it shall not, by way of trade or otherwise, be lent, re-sold, hired out, or otherwise circulated without the publisher's prior consent in any form of binding or cover other than that in which it is published and without a similar condition including this condition being imposed on the subsequent purchaser.

A catalogue record for this book is available from the British Library

Library of Congress Cataloging in Publication Data
Reproductive health care for women and babies / edited by Benjamin P. Sachs . . . [et al.].
(Oxford medical publications)
1. Maternal health services–Government policy. 2. Women's health services–Government policy. I. Sachs, Benjamin P. II. Series.
[DNLM: 1. Women's Health Services. 2. Child Health Services. 3. Maternal Health Services. 4. Family Planning. 5. Fertility.
WA 310 R4242 1995]
RG940.R48 1995 362.1'982–dc20 94–31076

ISBN 0 19 262530 6

Typeset by
Electronic Book Factory Ltd., Fife
Printed in Great Britain by
Bookcraft Ltd., Midsomer Norton, Avon

Preface

We were motivated to edit a book on health-care policy because the well-being of women and children in our society today is so intimately tied to policy. However, health policies are often formulated in a haphazard fashion. They result from a process of political compromise that reflects the strengths of various interest groups. These include women and children, the physicians who care for them, health managers, insurance companies, consumer groups, legislators, and the media. This book strives to appeal to all of these groups by having the issues laid out by experts in the field, but written with a view to the broader audience.

Our objective is deceptively simple: to educate and interest our audience by illustrating the intricate links between medical research, clinical medicine, public policy, and health communication. Improvements in all four components are essential if patients are to receive medically sound, compassionate, and cost-effective care. In editing this book, we have ambitious hopes that better understanding of such information will in turn have an indirect impact on future policy development and political action.

Through better communication of the issues – from reproductive problems to cancer screening – we hope to empower women to take preventive steps toward health improvement, to participate in medical decision making, and to play a greater political role in the formation of health policy. We hope to stretch physicians beyond their traditional training in the diagnosis and treatment of disease into a broader role in thinking about crucial societal issues. If physicians are to have a central role in the formation of health policy, they need to reorient themselves to the broader picture and voice their individual and collective views. Patient and physician views should share a common vision of improved health for women and children.

For those who pay for health care, whether in the public or private sector, these issues are crucial if they are to support effective care. Also, the task faced by the legislators who seek to play an informed role in the formation of national health policy is often made more difficult by the failure to be fully aware of issues confronting women and children in our global society. Hopefully, our text will fill this gap by giving all of these constituencies a clearer road map to follow.

This book was written in a turbulent time for health services in the USA, the UK, and France. The USA is faced with the daunting task of beginning the reformation of its health care system. Even without new national legislation, market forces are drastically changing the way that health care is provided. The UK is pondering on the wisdom of some of the changes brought about by the creation of an internal market system. The political motivation for change has come from the high cost of health care, which most countries believe that they can no longer afford. These countries, plagued by spiralling costs in health care,

are grappling with the issue of the almost unlimited potential demand for care and the cost of new technologies. Those that already provide comprehensive health care coverage to their citizens are also coping with ethical conflicts involving the rationing of services.

We have defined universal health policy issues related to women and children that cross national borders because many of the issues are the same. We have included authors from both sides of the Atlantic in order to take advantage of different experiences and to understand different approaches that have been taken. For example, the much higher rates of infant mortality, teenage pregnancies, and unwanted pregnancies in the USA compared to western Europe indicates that the USA has a lot to learn from Europe. If one considers the ongoing debate in the USA regarding the introduction of new technologies and the re-evaluation that is occurring, then this perhaps is an example of Yankee ingenuity. The agressive stand taken by the United States Food and Drug Administration towards evaluation of new technologies is one such example.

But, what do women want? When it comes to health, they want – and need – much more: more preventive services, more access to medical care, more humane care, and more information about what they can do to live longer, healthier lives. They want a balance between nature and overly intrusive medicine, with care that ensures, for example, that the childbirth process will proceed as naturally as the mother wants unless complications warrant medical intervention to assure the health of mother and child or that the treatment of diseases such as breast cancer will balance the need to treat aggressively against the preservation of a woman's breast. Overtreatment can often be worse than undertreatment.

In short, women are demanding that their personal wishes receive far more attention from those who provide and pay for women's health services.

A recent comprehensive survey of the health of American women was conducted for the Commonwealth Fund, a United States philanthropy located in New York City, by a well-known polling firm, Louis Harris and Associates. The findings, from interviews in early 1993 with a national cross-section of more than 2500 women and 1000 men, were striking. They revealed the gaping holes in the current system and the growing dissatisfaction of women patients.

1. In the past 12 months, more than one-third of women did not have a Pap smear, a clinical breast examination, a pelvic examination, or a complete physical examination. Forty-four per cent of women over age 50 did not have a mammogram. The figures are worse for women over age 65 – at least half said that they had not had a Pap smear or a mammogram in the past year. Poor women are twice as likely not to get annual Pap smears.

2. Thirteen per cent of women reported that they failed to receive the care they need in a given year, compared with 9 per cent of men. Among uninsured women, more than one-third failed to receive needed care. The poor, less educated, and women of color are more likely to be uninsured. Women are more likely than men to be poor and to seek government-funded health benefits.

3. The health habits of women continue to put them at risk of serious diseases. Nearly seven out of ten women reported being overweight and one out of three women said they never engaged in vigorous exercise. One out of four women smokes. Seventy per cent of women are not taking daily calcium supplements to help prevent osteoporosis; a similar number are not very familiar with this bone-weakening disease.

4. Women report more communication problems with doctors than men and are more likely to change doctors because of their dissatisfaction. One out of four women said that they had been 'talked down to' or treated like a child by a physician. Nearly one out of five women had been told that a reported medical problem was 'all in your head'.

5. Depression and low self-esteem are also greater problems for women. Forty per cent of the women surveyed reported being severely depressed in the past week, compared with 26 per cent of men. Younger women, under age 45, reported more depression than older women.

6. Nearly one in five women aged 18–44 reported having had an abortion. Women with dependent children who are either single, widowed, divorced, or separated had the highest rate – 29 per cent – followed by women who are married with dependent children (15 per cent).

Such issues, long ignored or underappreciated in medical research and public policy circles, are increasingly receiving attention not only from medical and public health experts, but from politicians, insurance companies, and the media.

Urged on by media interest, those who study and provide health care to women and children are increasingly expected to explain their work and its relevance to the public. The ensuing coverage has elevated women's health to a high-profile issue that often reaches news pages or the evening television news. This attention, however, has created a challenge for newsmakers and the media alike, particularly when new findings provide contradictory or confusing information that urgently needs to be put into context. Improving health communication, by focusing on the most important risks women face and what can be done about them, may be as crucial to improving women's health as new medical discoveries and better health care delivery.

It is too soon to see what impact the spotlight on women's health care issues will have on the health of women and their children in the USA and Europe. The rights of women and the status of their health care are also important issues, with many European countries far ahead of the USA in terms of political will and support for translating women's right into basic health protection for them and their children. The decade of the 1990s will test whether the current international focus on women's rights, which include health, will stand the test of time.

Boston, USA B. P. S.
London, UK R. B.
Paris, France E. P.
Darien, CT, USA C. R.
October 1994

Contents

V. Impact of adverse infant outcomes

VI. Obstetrics and public policy

Contributors

Sir Donald Acheson, Department of Health, Richmond House, 79 Whitehall, London SW1A 2NS, UK

Mary Ellen Avery, Harvard Medical School, Children's Hospital, Newborn Medicine, 221 Longwood Avenue, Room A423, Boston, MA 02115, USA

Richard W. Beard, Department of Obstetrics and Gynaecology, St Mary's Hospital Medical School, Norfolk Place, London, W2 1PG, UK

Willard Cates, Jr, Family Health International, Research Triangle Park, NC 27709, USA

Jocelyn Chamberlain, DH Cancer Screening Evaluation Unit, The Institute of Cancer Research, Section of Epidemiology, 15 Cotswold Road, Sutton, Surrey SM2 5NG, UK

David Chapin, Department of Obstetrics and Gynecology, Beth Israel Hospital/Harvard Medical School, Kirstein 308, 330 Brookline Avenue, Boston, MA 02215, USA

Jean Chapple, Department of Obstetrics and Gynaecology, St Mary's Hospital Medical School, Norfolk Place, London W2 1PG, UK

Wendy Chavkin, Chemical Dependency Institute, Beth Israel Medical Center, First Ave and 16th St, New York, NY 10003, USA

Deborah Cotton, Infectious Disease Unit, Gray 5, Massachusetts General Hospital, Fruit Street, Boston, MA 02114, USA

Karen Dawson, Monash University and Medical Centre, Centre for Early Human Development, Level 5, 246 Clayton Road, Clayton, Melbourne, Victoria 3168, Australia

Roger K. Freeman, Memorial Medical Center of Long Beach, Department of Obstetrics and Gynecology, 2801 Atlantic Avenue, PO Box 1428, Long Beach, CA 90801–1426, USA

Roxane Gardner, Department of Obstetrics and Gynecology, Beth Israel Hospital/Harvard Medical School, Kirstein 231, 330 Brookline Ave, Boston, MA 02215, USA

Rachel Benson Gold, The Alan Guttmacher Institute, 1120 Connecticut Avenue NW, Washington DC 20036, USA

Robert L. Goldenberg, Department of Obstetrics and Gynecology, Division of Maternal-Fetal Medicine, University of Alabama at Birmingham, University Station, Birmingham, AL 35233–7333, USA

Stanley Henshaw, Alan Guttmacher Institute, 120 Wall Street, New York, NY 10005, USA

Howard Hiatt, Division of General Medicine, Brigham and Women's Hospital/Harvard Medical School, 75 Francis Street, Boston, MA 02115, USA

Bruce Kessel, Department of Obstetrics and Gynecology, Division of Reproductive Endocrinology, Beth Israel Hospital/Harvard Medical School, 330 Brookline Avenue, Dana 851, Boston, MA 02215, USA

Lorraine V. Klerman, Department of Maternal and Child Health, School of Public Health, University of Alabama at Birmingham, 112 Mortimer Jordan Hall, Birmingham, AL 35294–2010, USA

Bruce Korf, Department of Clinical Genetics, Children's Hospital/Beth Israel Hospital, Harvard Medical School, 300 Longwood Avenue, Boston, MA 02215, USA

Shoo K. Lee, Neonatal Intensive Care Unit, Beth Israel Hospital/Harvard Medical School, 330 Brookline Avenue, Boston, MA 02215, USA

Luigi Mastroianni, Jr, Department of Obstetrics and Gynecology, Hospital of the University of Pennsylvania, 3400 Spruce St, 106 Dulles, Philadelphia, PA 19104, USA

Irwin R Merkatz, Department of Obstetrics and Gynecology, Rm B 502 Albert Einstein College of Medicine, 1300 Morris Park Ave, Bronx, NY 10461, USA

Karin B. Nelson, National Institute of Neurological Disorders and Stroke, Federal Building, Rm 714, 7550 Wisconsin Avenue, Bethesda, MD 20892, USA

Thorkild F. Nielsen, Department of Obstetrics and Gynecology, Central Hospital, Boras, Sweden

Jonathan Niloff, Department of Obstetrics and Gynecology, Division of Gynecologic Oncology, Beth Israel Hospital/Harvard Medical School, 330 Brookline Avenue, Boston, MA 02215, USA

Emile Papiernik, Department of Obstetrics and Gynaecology, Hospital Baudeloque, 123 Boulevard Port Royal, Paris 75674, France

Catherine S. Peckham, Department of Paediatric Epidemiology, Institute of Child Health, 30 Guilford Street, London WCIN IEH, UK

Herbert B. Peterson, Division of Reproductive Health, National Center for Chronic Disease Prevention and Health Promotion, Centers for Disease Control, Atlanta, GA 30333, USA

R. Hugh Philpott, 26 Kloeflands Road, Kloof, Natal 3610, South Africa

Alan Pinshaw, Beth Israel Hospital/Harvard Medical School, 330 Brookline Avenue, Boston, MA 02215, USA

Philip R. Reilly, E. K. Shriver Genetic Center, 200 Trapelo Road, Waltham, MA 02254, USA

Allan Rosenfield, Columbia School of Public Health, 600 W. 168th Street, 7th Floor, New York, NY 10032, USA

Cristine Russell, Special Health Correspondent for The Washington Post, and Freelance Writer, 43 Huckleberry Lane, Darien, CT 06820, USA

Benjamin P. Sachs, Department of Obstetrics and Gynecology, Beth Israel Hospital, Harvard Medical School, 330 Brookline Ave, Kirstein 317, Boston, MA 02215, USA

Lynne S. Wilcox, Division of Reproductive Health, National Center for Chronic Disease Prevention and Health Promotion, Centers for Disease Control, Atlanta, GA 30333, USA

Paul H. Wise, Harvard Institute for Reproductive and Child Health, Joint Program in Neonatology and Department of Pediatrics, Harvard Medical School/Children's Hospital, Richardson-Fuller Building, 221 Longwood Avenue, Boston, MA 02115, USA

Carl Wood, Monash University and Medical Centre, Department of Obstetrics and Gynaecology, Level 5, 246 Clayton Road, Clayton, Melbourne, Victoria 3168, Australia

Evolving role of women and children in our society

Mary Ellen Avery

Towards the end of the twentieth century, we have reason to celebrate the great advances of child health throughout the industrialized world. Consider the eradication of smallpox world-wide and the eradication of polio in the western hemisphere in 1992. Immunization against diphtheria, tetanus, measles, and now *Haemophilus influenzae* has prevented untold thousands of deaths of infants and children, so that now among the industrialized nations infant mortality rates are at an all-time low level. Central to this remarkable achievement has been a substantial and continuing improvement to the standard of living, which brings with it sanitation, nutritious foods, and the benefits of health education, including family planning.

By contrast, a cause of great concern is the continuing plight of most of the world's children who are nearly half the population of the underdeveloped countries, and are concentrated mostly in Africa and South-East Asia. Their total numbers dwarf the populations in the developed world, with approximately 4.7 million births in India, and nearly 5 million in Indonesia each year. In China alone, there are approximately 23 million births a year. The population of the world was about 3 billion in 1960, but by 1990 it was 5 billion, and the annual net increase is 100 million per year. Where the birth rates are high, so too is infant mortality. In Afghanistan, for example, 1 in 3 infants dies before the first birthday, whereas the numbers for Japan, Sweden, and Finland are approximately seven per 1000 live births.

Striking contrasts exist in the outlook of infants born to impoverished parents in the developing world, compared with that of infants born to parents who want only a few children and plan to nurture and educate them, as is the case in most countries of the industrialized world. Many of these differences are the result of war (as in Somalia, or Iraq, or Afghanistan), or natural disasters (such as recurrent floods in Bangladesh), or in situations where the societal drive is to increase the number of offspring in the face of a high likelihood of an early death. The women of Kenya are either pregnant or breast-feeding for on average 15–20 years of their adult life. Similar figures apply to much of the rest of Africa, and also India and Pakistan. High fertility rates accompany high infant mortality rates. For example, in the USA in the 19th century the fertility rate was eight per woman. Now, with the high probability of infant survival, it is just under two. Even so, the population of the USA has doubled in the last 60 years (partly through immigration).

The outlook for children is inextricably bound to the status of women. When women have the opportunity for education, when they can decide when and how often to become pregnant, and when they have access to good general medical care, as well as advice about reproductive technologies, the number of children will be fewer and their outlook infinitely improved.

The distribution of Depo-Provera to women in more than 90 countries provides suppression of ovulation for a 3 month interval that can be repeated. Use of the contragestion RU486 increasingly permits women to opt for a medically induced interruption of pregnancy within the first 2 months of pregnancy. This drug, invented by the French endocrinologist Baulieu, acts by binding specifically and reversibly to the progesterone receptor. However, barrier contraceptives are the preferred method of prevention of pregnancy, since they also reduce the likelihood of spreading sexually transmitted diseases.

If we do not recognize the dangers to our future from the current logarithmic growth in the world's population, we are destined for increasing environmental contamination of the world, and for the unrest that will inevitably follow the worsening of the disparity between those who have and those who have not.

Certainly, many of our predecessors have worked diligently to create the new knowledge that is the basis of modern obstetrics and pediatrics, and to make it available outside their own environment through participation in global endeavors, such as the World Health Organization and UNICEF. Many nations subscribe to a list of goals enunciated at the World Summit for Children on 30 September 1990. These goals are both feasible and financially affordable, if there is a will to promote them.

It seems self-evident that it should be the right of every infant to be wanted, and the right of every woman to decide when and how often to become pregnant. If these are indeed inalienable human rights, they are clearly in the best interests of the child. Programs that enrich the quality of life of women, and make them available to provide appropriate nurture to their children should be one of our generation's highest priorities.

It is the purpose of this book to bring some of the relevant issues concerning health care for women and babies to a wide audience whose actions on behalf of mothers and babies will be essential to achieving the goals. In words attributed to Abraham Lincoln,

> You may adopt all the policies you choose, but how they are carried out depends on your children. They are going to assume control of your cities, states, and nations. They will take over your churches, schools, universities, and corporations. All your works are going to be judged, praised, or condemned by them. The fate of humanity is in their hands. It is our responsibility to see that those hands are ready to carry forward our very civilization.

Recognizing the responsibility of any civilized society to optimize the health of mothers and children is the first step. Appreciating the fact that we are citizens of a 'global village' in the 1990s sets the agenda for the future.

I Changing Health Risks for Women over their Life-cycle

1 The health risks women face

Cristine Russell

The health gender gap

When it comes to health, women and men are certainly not created equally. From the first breath to the last, women face different health risks than men, not only in how and when they die but in the nagging medical conditions that affect the way they live. Women generally have a strong advantage in terms of life span, but unfortunately they often live less healthy lives than their male counterparts.

Some examples of the health gender gap:

1. An American female born in 1900 could expect to live about 48 years, roughly 2 years longer than men of that time. By 1990, the gap had widened. Average female life expectancy at birth was up to 78.8 years, 7 years longer than men (NCHS 1993*a*). By age 85 there are only about 45 men for every 100 women (Speroff 1992). Women tend to outlive men in most countries around the world. (About Women Inc. 1992, p. 196).

2. Premature deaths under the age of 65 are almost twice as high for males as for females in the USA, with injury deaths from car crashes, homicides, and suicides, as well as lethal heart attacks and AIDS, more common in younger men than women (Desenclos 1992, p. 16). But the incidence of new female HIV infections is now rising more rapidly, and AIDS is the leading cause of death for younger women in some major cities, including New York. According to the World Health Organization, about half of new HIV infections worldwide are in women. (About Women Inc. 1992, pp. 129–130).

3. Women are afflicted by more chronic and debilitating illnesses than men, including osteoporosis, arthritis, and Alzheimer's disease. This increases the likelihood of institutional care in old age, particularly since women often outlive

their spouses. At younger ages, women are more prone to major depression and suicide attempts than men.

4. While heart disease has often been portrayed as a man's disease, it is also the number one killer of women. But women tend to come down with heart disease at least a decade later. The risk rises in the post menopausal years to eventually equal that of men. When heart disease does strike, women often fare worse than men and appear to get different health care treatment (Rosenfeld 1992).

5. Lung cancer has passed breast cancer as the major cancer killer in women. The culprit—cigarettes—continues to attract a new generation of young women who have 'come a long way, baby' toward shortening their life spans with smoking-related illnesses. While there has been a drop in the number of American male smokers over the past 20 years, the number of women smokers in the USA and around the world is on the rise. Lung cancer is now declining in men, while rising in women.

6. American women go to doctors' offices and the hospital more frequently and undergo more surgical procedures than do men. Women visit doctors an average 6.1 times annually, compared to 4.7 for men. In addition to purely female medical diagnoses and procedures involving childbirth and hysterectomy, women are more likely to be treated for back problems, angina, digestive disorders, and mental illness (About Women Inc. 1992, pp. 8–9).

In addition to gender-related health gaps, large differences in relative health risks among women can be related to race, income, and geography. Black and White women in the USA live longer than their male counterparts. White women born today, however, still have a 5-year edge in life expectancy over Black women. Black women have a higher risk of dying from heart disease, cancer, stroke, injuries, and HIV infection and are more than twice as likely to die prematurely before the age of 65 than White women (NCHS 1992*a*, pp. 26–35).

The diseases and disabilities associated with being a woman change throughout the life span. From infancy through childhood, adolescence, young adulthood, middle age, and old age, females face shifting health threats, some well understood, others only now receiving the research scrutiny they deserve.

Recognizing which risks are most important and tackling those that are most preventable in time to make a difference in both quality of life and the risk of death is a challenge not only for the individual woman, but for clinicians, researchers, and public policy makers.

What should women be worrying about? This chapter discusses some of the key diseases and disabilities of particular concern to women throughout their lives, as well as the risk factors and possible interventions of greatest importance.

Age and mortality

One way to answer the question of what women should be worrying about is to focus on what they die from and how this differs from male mortality threats.

But risk information becomes even more meaningful if we look at which killers strike most frequently at what ages. A teenager's mortality risks are far different than those of her grandmother.

Overall, fewer American women die each year at lower rates than men from the leading causes of death. The largest differences occur in the death rates for HIV infection (which is nearly nine times as great for males as females), suicide (four times as high), homicide (3.6 times as high), and unintended injuries (2.6 times as high) (NCHS 1992*b*, p. 7).

For all ages combined, heart disease remains the number one killer for both women and men of all races, in the USA as in other industrialized countries. Cancer is the second leading killer of both sexes. Stroke is the number three killer for American women, while motor vehicle crashes are the third leading killer of men. Altogether, heart disease, cancer and stroke account for two-thirds of all deaths among women annually (NCHS 1992*b*, p. 20).

The remaining top ten mortality threats for American women include pneumonia and influenza, chronic lung diseases, unintended injuries, diabetes, hardening of the arteries, kidney disease, and blood poisoning. The rankings differ somewhat for black women, with diabetes, unintended injuries, newborn conditions, kidney diseases, and homicide greater mortality threats. While HIV infection has moved into the top ten for men, it is not yet in the top 15 causes of death for women in the USA.

Less than 1 per cent of female deaths occur among infants and toddler girls aged 1–4 years. Injury, either in the home or in automobiles, is the top mortality threat for them, followed by birth defects, cancer, homicide, and heart disease. HIV infection moved into seventh place in 1990 (NCHS 1993*b*).

The risk of dying drops by half among girls 5–14 years of age, compared with that of female toddlers. Again, their greatest threat is motor vehicle and other unintended injuries, followed by cancer, birth defects, homicide, and heart disease (NCHS 1993*b*).

As girls move into the young adult years of 15–24, the chance of dying is roughly the same as that when they were toddlers. Motor vehicle and other injuries remain in top place, followed by homicide, cancer, suicide, and heart disease. HIV is in seventh place (NCHS 1993*b*).

For adult women in the 25–44-year-old age group, the risk of dying is more than twice that in the 15–24 age group. But this age group still accounts for less than 5 per cent of all female deaths. For the first time, cancer becomes the number one killer, followed by injuries, heart disease, suicide, and homicide (NCHS 1993*b*).

For women from 45 to 64 years, the risk of dying begins to rise more rapidly, to a rate nearly six times that of the previous age group. Nearly 14 per cent of female deaths are in this middle-aged group. Cancer remains the number one killer, followed by heart disease, stroke, injuries, and chronic liver disease (NCHS 1993*b*).

Women aged 65 years and over account for eight out of ten female deaths each year in the USA, at a rate that is seven times higher than in middle-aged women. Heart disease is by the far the greatest threat, killing at a rate more than twice that for cancer, followed by stroke, chronic lung disease, and pneumonia (NCHS 1993*b*).

Another measure of the substantial differences between young and old in mortality is to look at deaths that strike younger women disportionately and result in premature mortality that could have been prevented. A Centers for Disease Control study of years of potential life lost before age 65 indicates that among American females, motor vehicles are the top premature killer, followed by infectious disease, breast cancer, heart disease, and other unintended injuries. Premature deaths are highest among Blacks, followed by American Indians, Whites, Hispanics, and Asians (Desenclos 1992, pp. 18–19).

While health status in the USA exceeds that of some other Western industrialized countries, it is not universally better. In terms of life expectancy, Japan ranks at the top, with Japanese women expected to live an average of nearly 82 years, 3.6 years longer than US women. The USA also falls slightly behind France, Switzerland, the Netherlands, Canada, Sweden, Italy, Hong Kong, Australia, Spain, Greece, Germany, and England in female life expectancy. In developing countries, however, women fare less well, with those in many African nations facing an average life expectancy of only 54 years (About Women Inc. 1992, p. 196).

Heart disease and stroke

Deaths from cardiovascular disease have dropped dramatically over the past two decades in the USA. But coronary heart disease is still the leading killer, with nearly half of the fatal heart attacks each year suffered by women. More than one-third of all deaths in American women are due to heart disease, with the annual toll—nearly 400 000 deaths each year—more than three times that of deaths from breast and lung cancer combined. The third leading cause of death for US women is stroke, killing another 90 000 women annually (NCHS 1993*b*).

Heart disease tends to strike women about a decade later than men, with middle-aged males about six times more likely to have heart attacks. But the risk gradually rises in women after menopause begins. While about one in nine women between the ages of 45 and 64 have some form of cardiovascular disease, the risk rises to one in three among women 65 years and older (Rosenfeld 1992).

Black women are at greater risk: they are about 60 per cent more likely to die from heart disease than White females and 86 per cent more likely to die from stroke (NCHS 1992*a*, pp. 28–29).

Diet—both the type of food and the amount—is a leading contributor to heart disease. According to recent studies, a diet high in fat may help predispose women to heart disease, breast cancer, and colon-rectal cancer.

Obesity is a leading underlying risk factor for coronary heart disease as is high blood pressure, the leading cause of stroke. Being overweight contributes to about four in ten heart attacks and other cases of heart disease among women.

Among women under the age of 50 who are overweight, the risk of developing coronary heart disease is two and a half times greater than among women of the same age who maintain a desirable weight. The risk of stroke is four times greater in the overweight group. Obesity and hypertension are greater among poor women, as well among minority women, particularly Blacks (Rosenfeld 1992).

Less is known about preventing heart disease in women than in men, in part because research studies in the past have focused on male study populations. Researchers believe, however, that conventional preventive advice applies to women as well as men: stop smoking, exercise more, lose weight, eat less fat, and reduce high blood pressure and cholesterol with diet and sometimes drugs.

The National Institutes of Health are now including women in experimental trials to test cholesterol-lowering drugs. A new study will examine whether taking hormones after the menopause reduces the risk of heart disease in women.

There are also lingering questions about access to medical care. Women who suffer heart attacks are twice as likely as men to die in the first few weeks after a heart attack. They are also more likely to die within the first year.

Cancer

Cancers are the second leading cause of death among American women, accounting for nearly one-quarter of all female deaths (NCHS 1993*b*).

Smoking among women led lung cancer to recently surpass breast cancer as the most deadly female cancer. But breast cancer is perhaps the most feared of female health risks. It remains the most frequent type of cancer among US women and its death rate has also risen, despite medical advances and efforts for early diagnosis.

Some critics are concerned, however, that public information campaigns to alert women to the risks of breast cancer have unnecessarily alarmed them as well, creating a climate in which fear of breast cancer is perhaps as great a threat as the disease itself (Blakeslee 1992).

One of the most oft-quoted statistics from the American Cancer Society is that one in every nine American women will develop breast cancer. More recently, the National Cancer Institute updated that to a one in eight risk when women over age 85 are included. In either case, these are cumulative lifetime risks and tell women very little about their risks at given ages.

In fact, three-quarters of all breast cancer cases strike women over the age of 50. The US National Cancer Institute estimates that the chance of getting breast cancer by age 50 is about one in 50 and the chance that a woman under age 50 will get breast cancer in the next year is about one in 1000.

Many of the known risk factors for breast cancer, including family history, no children or first child born after age 30, early first menstrual period, late menopause, and upper socio-economic status, are not amenable to change.

Instead, the focus has turned to early detection, particularly mammography. Studies have consistently found a reduction in breast cancer deaths in women aged 50 and above on the order of 30 per cent from annual mammograms and breast physical exams. But no significant mortality benefit has been demonstrated in international studies on women under 50 (Russell 1993).

Death rates for other female cancers have been declining, including uterine and cervical cancer, in part because of better early detection through Pap smears. Colon and rectal cancer, the third leading cancer killer in women, still kills more women annually than all reproductive system cancers—ovary, uterus, and cervix—combined.

Racial differences in cancer persist. White women are generally more likely to contract cancer, but Black women are more likely to die from it, perhaps because of later diagnosis and poorer access to treatment. The rate of new breast cancer cases is 17 per cent lower for Black than White women, but 5-year relative survival rates are 24 per cent lower for Black than White females (NCHS 1992*a*, p. 29). One long-term study found that 49 per cent of White women with breast cancer had localized disease at the time of diagnosis, in contrast to 41 per cent of Black women.

The overall US death rate for cancer in women is similiar to that in Canada and many European countries, with mortality slightly higher in Denmark and the United Kingdom and lower in France. Female lung cancer death rates are higher in the USA than most other European, Asian, and South American countries, and breast cancer deaths are higher in England and Wales (Boring *et al.* 1992).

Unintended and intentional injuries

Unintended and intentional injuries take a major toll on the lives of women, with one in five American females sustaining an injury in a given year (Rice and MacKenzie 1989, p. xxii). The largest risk is in the 25–44 year age group and in the elderly over age 75.

While heart disease, cancer, and stroke take more female victims overall, the injury toll among young women is so severe that productivity losses and years of life lost from each death are far higher than those for any of the three top killers (Rice and MacKenzie, p. 66).

Understanding the pattern of injuries is a major new area of public health research, as experts have redefined the field and sought ways of preventing and controlling problems that were once dismissed as inevitable. They have dropped the term accident, which suggests a random action that cannot be foreseen or prevented. Instead, injuries are divided into those that are unintentional—motor vehicle accidents, falls, poisoning, or fire—and those that are intentional, including violence and suicide.

While men suffer more than twice as many injury fatalities, women suffer almost as many non-fatal injuries. Motor vehicle deaths are the leading premature cause of death among women and men (Desenclos 1992, p. 19), with alcohol a factor in roughly half of such deaths (DHHS 1992, p. 19) Falls are the leading cause of non-fatal injury, with elderly females at much higher risk of non-fatal falls than males (Rice and MacKenzie 1989, pp. 9–21). About one-quarter of female injury fatalities are intentional, either homicide or suicide. Alcohol is a factor in about half of all homicides.

For women, deaths from unintended injuries peak in the teenage years. Intentional homicide deaths are highest in the early 20s, with firearms the most common cause and the perpetrators most often family members or acquaintances. The highest suicide rates occur at about age 50, however (Baker *et al.* 1992, p. 19; NCHS 1992*a*, p. 177).

The impact of non-fatal violence is far greater. Nearly one-third of women treated in emergency rooms have suffered some form of physical abuse. One in five women are likely to be raped at some point in their lives, with the majority knowing their assailants (About Women Inc. 1992, p. 213).

White women are at higher risk for motor vehicle deaths than Black women and at twice the risk of suicide. But the rate of homicide among Black females is more than four times higher than that in White females and 1.5 times that of White males (NCHS 1992a, pp. 31–32).

AIDS and other sexually transmitted diseases

Originally recognized as a disease of men, particularly homosexual men, AIDS is now a growing threat to women and their offspring. In 1991, more than 11 per cent of adult and adolescent American AIDS cases were in women and cases among women accounted for the largest annual increases (up about 20 per cent). US projections for the number of AIDS cases diagnosed between 1990 and 1994 suggest that there will be 55 000–75 000 new cases in women compared with roughly 365 000–465 000 cases in men (CDC 1992).

Minority women, particularly those in their early 30s, are hardest hit, with more than half of all female AIDS cases reported in the US by 30 September, 1991, among Black women. The death rate for Black women in the USA is nine times that for White women in 1989 (NCHS 1992*a*, p. 2). In some US cities, including New York, AIDS has become the leading killer of young women (About Women Inc. 1992, p. 130).

Intravenous drug use is the largest risk factor for American women, with half of those with AIDS to date reportedly exposed to the virus by injecting drugs. One-third became infected by heterosexual contact, usually with partners who were IV drug users.

World-wide, about one-third of the adults with AIDS are estimated to be women, with sexual transmission playing a bigger role. About half of new infections, particularly in Africa, are in women (About Women Inc. 1992, p. 129).

AIDS is not the only sexually transmitted disease rising in incidence: syphilis has been increasing among reproductive-age women, putting them and their children at great health risk (NCHS 1992*a*, p. 64).

Reproductive health problems

For women of all childbearing ages, from 15 to 44, birth rates have been on the upswing in the USA, while the overall proportion of women terminating pregnancies by abortion has declined (Horton 1992, pp. 1–12). Women at greatest risk of having health problems from pregnancies, for either themselves or their offspring, include teenagers, unmarried women, and minority women.

Early in this century, about one in every 150 women died from pregnancy-related causes. Today, the risk of giving birth is minimal in industrialized countries: only about eight maternal deaths are reported for every 100 000 live births in the USA (Horton 1992, p. 13). The risk is greatest in Black women, who are more than three times as likely as White women and twice as likely as Hispanic women to die of pregnancy-related problems. Older mothers also face increased health risks (NCHS 1992*a*, p. 53).

The risk to infants is more significant. In 1900, about 10 in every 100 liveborn infants died in the first year of life. The 1991 rate in the USA had dropped to less than one in 100 live births, the lowest ever. But despite the dramatic drop, American infant mortality is still among the highest of Western countries, with US Black infants dying at more than twice the rate of White infants. Most infant deaths are associated with low birth weight.

Nearly one in seven pregnant women has prenatal complications, many of which can cause fetal distress or early labor. Improvements in access to prenatal health care are needed to reduce the risks of poor pregnancy outcome. In 1989, Black and Hispanic women were more than twice as likely to receive little or no prenatal care as White women in the USA (NCHS 1992*a*, p. 37).

Among teenagers, increased sexual activity has been accompanied by rising numbers of unintended births. An estimated eight out of ten teenage pregnancies are unplanned. Birth rates among both Black and White teenagers increased in the late 1980s in the USA, with Black teenagers far more likely to give birth and have a second child than White teenagers (NCHS 1992*a*, p. 27). Unintended births among single American women 15–44 years old also rose dramatically over the last decade. Unintended births among never-married American women also climbed to 55 per cent of births to women below the poverty level in 1988, while those among women of higher incomes stayed steady at less than 30 per cent (NCHS 1992*a*, p. 50).

Chronic physical and mental conditions

Throughout their lives, women are more likely than men to be treated for the most common debilitating physical and mental illnesses, from migraines to varicose veins, sinusitis to cataracts. Among elderly women, it is a mixed blessing: they are more likely to survive, but also more likely to be limited in major activities than men of comparable ages. Particularly debilitating are arthritis and osteoporosis, which are a major threat to the day-to-day comfort and independence of older women (About Women Inc. 1992, p. 145).

Half of women are at risk of developing fractures caused by osteoporosis (About Women Inc. 1992, p. 163). Digestive and bowel disorders are nearly twice as common in women as in men and are most common among elderly women. Fifteen per cent of non-institutionalized women aged 65 years and over reported having hemorrhoids, and 6.4 per cent said they were chronically constipated (LeClere *et al*. 1992, p. 3).

Women are about twice as likely to be in a nursing home as men (NCHS 1992*a*, p. 236).

Major depression is diagnosed twice as frequently in women as in men, with one in four women estimated to suffer from severe depression at some point (About Women, Inc. 1992, p. 221). Depression is more common in teenage girls than boys—one study found nearly one in five girls age 13–15 years have attempted suicide. At older ages, differences in the rates of depression between men and women seem to vanish, in part because depression increases in elderly men. At all ages, men are more likely to be hospitalized in psychiatric institutions than women, however (NCHS 1992*a*, p. 240).

Overall, men are somewhat more likely than women to consider their own health excellent and women are more likely to report their health as fair or poor (NCHS 1992*a*, p. 202). Women go to the doctor more often and are more likely to be hospitalized for short stays, in part because of deliveries and pregnancy-related conditions, and undergo a higher rate of medical procedures in the hospital.

Comparative risk

Assessing female health risks and their relative importance is not merely a matter of numbers. The challenge is to choose the right numbers to answer a given question. While heart disease may be the top killer among all women, cancer is the top killer of childbearing women. The risks to poor minority women are quite different, and often higher, than those to middle or upper income White women. A risk may be low for any given woman, but pose a public health problem if millions of women, or their unborn infants, are at risk.

In a world in which each new health study may be publicized widely, it is important for women and their doctors, as well as public policy makers, to scrutinize just what the numbers mean or do not mean before jumping to conclusions.

Each women should attempt to determine whether she is indeed at risk and, if so, how great the risk is to her health now or in the foreseeable future. More importantly, what if anything can she personally do about it?

Policy makers need to estimate the relative magnitude of a given risk, how many women are potentially at risk, and the costs and benefits of doing something about the risk now or waiting for more data.

There are several questions to consider in assessing a given risk and its practical implications for a given woman (Russell 1990).

1. How certain is the risk? Is it well-known and well-documented or is it a preliminary finding from a single study? A single study should be viewed with skepticism until further evidence is in.

2. What is the absolute versus the relative risk? Too often new medical studies fail to provide meaningful risk data because they focus on the relative risk of a given activity—drug X poses a nine times greater risk of cancer than drug Y—but do not have data on what the actual, or absolute, risk was in the first place. A nine times greater risk of getting a cancer that is originally one in a million is quite different than a nine times greater risk of something that is one in one thousand to start with.

3. Is a given woman really at risk? Often a newly publicized risk, published in a national newspaper or televised on the network news, causes universal panic. Many women may unnecessarily personalize the risk. While a given problem may be of general public concern, most people are not actually at risk unless they were exposed to a toxic substance or took a dangerous drug.

4. If a person was exposed to a risky event, when and how did the exposure take place? Simply being exposed does not always mean a significant level of health risk. The amount of exposure, the timing and the potential health consequence—whether short-term or long-term—will affect the degree of risk. Risk generally increases with more exposure.

5. What are the risk trade-offs? For a menopausal woman considering estrogen therapy, the benefits must be weighed against the risks and the degree of uncertainty about both must be taken into account. A women with severe symptoms may decide that the known short-term and long-term benefits are worth any potential risk. A women with minimal symptoms may make the opposite decision.

6. Can a woman or her doctor really do anything about a given risk? Realistically, a woman is not going to give up driving because she might be involved in a serious car crash. But she can decide to wear a seat belt every time to minimize her risk. A woman who is worried about breast cancer may not be able to do anything about her risk factors—age of first birth or family history—but she can seek careful medical supervision. A woman seeking to minimize her long-term chances of developing heart disease can make life-style changes.

A pound of prevention

Women, by virtue of their sex, carry built-in health dangers. But, fortunately, these are not immutable and many of the most serious health risks are under a woman's own control. A study for the Carter Center in Atlanta, focusing on what can be done with existing knowledge, singled out six major personal health risks: tobacco, alcohol, injuries, high blood pressure, overnutrition (as measured by obesity and high cholesterol), and gaps in primary health care, particularly in prenatal and reproductive health services.

These key risk factors accounted for an estimated two out of three US deaths and one out of three hospitalizations, as well as more than two-thirds of premature deaths before age 65 (Amler and Eddins 1987, pp. 181–7).

By making basic changes in her life-style, a woman can affect several health problems at once. Without question, cigarette smoking is the largest single cause of death and disability. About 23 per cent of American women 25 years old and over still smoked in 1990 (NCHS 1992*a*, p. 24) and young women and women with little education are at greater risk of starting smoking. Stopping smoking or never starting in the first place not only reduces the well-known risks of contracting several forms of cancer, but also reduces risks of heart disease, stroke, lung disease, and harm to unborn children during pregnancy or to young children (DHHS 1991, p. 2).

Diet also crosses disease boundaries. About one-quarter of American women are overweight, with older women and Black women more likely to be overweight. Being overweight is associated with high blood pressure, elevated cholesterol, diabetes, heart disease, stroke, some cancers, gallbladder disease, and some forms of arthritis (NCHS 1992*a*, p. 26).

In addition to helping weight control, eating a diet low in fat and high in fruits and vegetables (five servings a day) is healthy in combating both heart and cancer risks, as well as diabetes. Calcium intake may also need to be boosted with dietary supplements to help prevent osteoporosis.

Elevated blood pressure may require medication to bring it under control, but many women who would benefit from it are not on medication.

Alcohol is a major contributor to injuries, particularly motor vehicle crashes, and plays a major role in other chronic health problems as well, including liver disease, high blood pressure, obesity, and malnutrition. Alcohol use during pregnancy, particularly heavy drinking, poses a risk to the fetus as well. Although women generally drink less than men, alcohol abuse has been increasing among women. Young women and women with little education are more likely to be binge drinkers (M. G. Kovar, unpublished). About one-third of alcoholics are women and alcohol tends to take a greater physical toll in women abusers, particularly liver disease (About Women, pp. 206–7).

Motor vehicle injuries can also be greatly reduced by wearing seat belts, but only about four out of ten American women say they use seat belts all or most of the time. Only about one-quarter of women with less than a high school education used them, compared to just over half of those who were college-educated (M. G. Kovar, unpublished).

Risky sexual behavior, including multiple sexual partners and unprotected intercourse, puts a woman at double risk for unplanned pregnancies and sexually transmitted diseases.

Exercise at all ages appears to contribute to improved health, with potential benefits in controlling weight, strengthening bones, reducing cardiovascular disease and high blood pressure, and improving mental health (DHHS 1988, pp. 36–8). Young women are more likely to report that they exercise regularly.

But a recent Boston study showed that even among 85–100-year-old volunteers, weight-lifting built muscles and helped some participants to move from walking with walkers to walking without assistance (Russell 1992).

Preventive medical care is less common among poor women and older women (M. G. Kovar, unpublished). Many women over 50 who would most benefit from mammograms to detect early cancers are still not getting them. Only 43 per cent of women aged 50–64 and 30 per cent over 65 have had a Pap smear in the previous year (Speroff 1992).

In some cases, controversies abound, the scientific answers are still not in, and healthy choices involve balancing some risks against others before all the information is known. Estrogen replacement therapy in the women experiencing symptoms of menopause, for example, has been on a teeter-totter for three decades as various studies have shifted the benefit–risk equation. Pushed as a boon to women with severe menopausal symptoms in the 1960s, estrogen sales plummeted in the 1970s as alarms sounded about increased uterine cancer risks. In the 1980s, more balance entered the picture as potential benefits, including protection against heart disease and bone loss, were weighed against the possible cancer risks. Women who have not had a hysterectomy take cyclical progesterone with their estrogen to protect against uterine cancer.

The Women's Health Initiative, a massive new $500 million study by the US National Institutes of Health that will carry over into the next century, is designed to provide more definitive answers to many of the health questions facing older women, including hormone therapy and calcium replacement.

Beyond science, the public policy steps for reducing women's health risks are largely issues of cost and access. Increased availability of reproductive health services and pregnancy health care would go a long way toward reducing unplanned pregnancies and improving the outcome of those that do occur, particularly among teenagers and poor women. Careful attention to the health of post-menopausal women, including regular physical examinations and tests such as mammograms, would help detect chronic diseases in their earliest stages.

Conclusion

Better understanding of relative health risks will help women and their advocates focus on what is really worth worrying about in the long run. Women overwhelmed with fear about too many risks may be too paralysed to do anything. Those with a better understanding of true threats and what can be done about them will be more active in preventing health problems, and will be better informed patients when health problems do occur.

References

About Women, Inc. (1992). *About women & health*. About Women, Inc., Boston.

Amler, R. W. and Eddins, D. L. (1987). Cross-sectional analysis: precursors of premature deaths in the United States. In *Closing the gap: the burden of unnecessary illness*, (ed. R. W. Amler and H. B. Dull). Oxford University Press, Oxford.

Baker, S., O'Neill, B., Ginsburg, M., and Li, G. (1992). *The injury fact book*, (2nd edn). Oxford University Press, New York.

Blakeslee, S. (1992). Better odds, faulty math heightens fear of breast cancer. *New York Times*, 15 March, Section 4, p. 1.

Boring, C. C., Squires, T. S., and Tong, T. (1992). Cancer statistics. *Cancer Journal for Clinicians*, **42**, 19–38.

CDC (Centers for Disease Control and Prevention) (1992). Projections of the number of immunosuppressed HIV-infected persons, United States, 1992–94. *Morbidity and Mortality Weekly Report*, **41**, 1–29.

DHHS (Department of Health and Human Services) (1988). *Disease prevention health promotion: the facts*. Office of Disease Prevention and Health Promotion, Washington.

DHHS (1991). *Women's health is a national priority*. Prevention Report, December 1991–January 1992. Office of Disease Prevention and Health Promotion, Washington.

DHHS (1992). *Prevention '91/'92: federal programs and progress*. US Government Printing Office, Washington.

Desenclos, J. C. (1992). Years of potential life lost before age 65, by race, Hispanic origin, and sex—United States, 1986–88. *Morbidity and Mortality Weekly Report*, **41**, 13–23.

Horton, J. A. (ed.) (1992) *The women's health data book: a profile of women's health in the United States*. Jacobs Institute of Women's Health, Washington.

Kovar, M. G. (1987). Women: our health and some risks we take. Unpublished Speech, May 19, 1987.

LeClere, F. B., Moss, A. J., Everhart, J. E., and Roth, H.P. (1992). Prevalence of major digestive disorders and bowel symptoms, 1989. In *Advance data for vital and health statistics*, No. 212, p. 3. National Center for Health Statistics, Hyattsville, MD.

NCHS (National Center for Health Statistics) (1992*a*). *Health, United States, 1991*. Public Health Service, Hyattsville, MD.

NCHS (1992*b*). Advance report of final mortality statistics, 1989. *Monthly Vital Statistics Report*, **40**, 1–52.

NCHS (1993*a*). Advance report of final mortality statistics, 1990. *Monthly Vital Statistics Report*, **41**.

NCHS (1993*b*). *Vital Statistics of the United States*, 1990, Vol. 2, *Mortality*, Part A. (In press.)

Rice, D. P., MacKenzie, E. J., and associates (1989). *Cost of injury in the United States: a report to Congress*. University of California and Johns Hopkins University, San Francisco.

Rosenfeld, L. E. (1992). Women and heart disease. In *Yale University School of Medicine heart book*, (ed. B. Zaret, M. Moser, and L. Cohen), pp. 237–46. Hearst Books, New York.

Russell, C. (1990). What, me worry? *American Health*, June, 45–51.

Russell, C. (1992). The medical search for the fountain of youth, *Washington Post Health Section*, 27 October, 20.

Russell, C. (1993). Do younger women need mammograms? *Washington Post Health Section*, 9 February, 6.

Speroff, L. (1992). Introduction. *Women's Health Issues*, **2**, 57.

2 Reproductive cycles in women: quality of life impact

Bruce Kessel

Each time I have a period—and that has only been three times—I have the feeling that in spite of all the pain, unpleasantness, and nastiness, I have a sweet secret, and that is why, although it is nothing but a nuisance to me, in a way, I always long for the time that I shall feel that secret within me again.

Anne Frank *The Diary of A Young Woman*

Introduction

Through menarche, the reproductive years, and the menopause, both normal and abnormal gynecologic events influence women's health and have an impact on quality of life. The events that most significantly alter psychosocial adjustment include premenstrual syndrome, infertility, childbirth, pelvic pain, abnormal uterine bleeding, and the menopause. Undoubtedly the medical aspects of reproductive health and disease receive far more attention than the psychosocial and cultural aspects. There is only limited knowledge of the impact of reproductive cycles on work, family, and personal sense of well-being. A further limitation to the ability to address health policy issues for women has been the relative disregard for women in much medical research, which is conducted mainly on men, resulting in conclusions that are of little relevance to women. As gynecologic processes are chiefly age related, the effect of reproductive events on quality of life in women may be considered with respect to age-related reproductive milestones.

Adolescents

Although the world's population is getting older, approximately 30 per cent are between the ages of 10 and 24. In addition, most young people live in developing countries; this is expected to be true for as many as 83.5 per cent by the year 2000. The percentage of youths living in urban environments is also increasing. These factors, combined with the improvement in early childhood survival, have caused increased attention to be placed on causes of morbidity and mortality in youth (Blum 1991).

Amenorrhea and dysmenorrhea

Maturation of the hypothalamus and pituitary gland in the brain results in adrenal and ovarian hormone production, leading to pubertal changes and ultimately to menarche, the first menstrual cycle. At this time various adolescent menstrual disorders such as painful menses (dysmenorrhea), absence of menses (amenorrhea), and abnormal bleeding may become apparent. In addition, the teenager is dealing with her attitude to menstruation, body self-image, and psychosocial factors influenced by parents, peers, and schooling. The teenager's response to these pressures and changes in life-style can in themselves induce menstrual dysfunction during this time.

Dysmenorrhea is defined as painful menstrual periods and is often differentiated into primary (no underlying pelvic pathology) or secondary. Primary dysmenorrhea is very common in adolescents, with as many as 72 per cent of adolescent girls reporting pain or discomfort during their periods. In addition to uterine cramps ranging from mild to severe and debilitating, dysmenorrhea can be associated with nausea, vomiting, headaches, and diarrhea. The pathophysiology of primary dysmenorrhea, in the absence of pelvic pathology, is thought to be the release of prostaglandins (substances that cause smooth muscles to spasm) with subsequent increased uterine activity, constriction of blood vessels, and ischemia.

Nonsteroidal anti-inflammatory agents are remarkably effective in primary dysmenorrhea, relieving symptoms in 80 per cent of patients (Dawood 1988). Also highly effective in management of primary dysmenorrhea is the use of the oral contraceptive pill, which relieves symptoms for 80–90 per cent of women. However, even in the adolescent, if dysmenorrhea persists despite medical treatment, laparoscopy may be indicated to find out whether any pelvic pathology is present. In adolescents with chronic pelvic pain and negative laparoscopy, the possibility of psychologic trauma and sexual abuse should be explored.

Both amenorrhea and abnormal uterine bleeding may exist in the adolescent. Amenorrhea may be defined as the absence of menses by the age of 14 in the absence of secondary sexual characteristics, or by the age of 16 in all women, and, in menstruating women, the absence of menses for either a time equivalent to three normal cycles or 6 months. The causes of primary amenorrhea include abnormalities of the genital tract (imperforate hymen, müllerian anomalies), ovarian failure (either premature ovarian failure or secondary to chromosomal abnormalities), pituitary tumors (especially hyperprolactinomas), other endocrinopathies (thyroid or adrenal disease, polycystic ovarian disease), or functional hypothalamic amenorrhea. The commonest cause is physiologically delayed menstruation which will resolve spontaneously. The evaluation of amenorrhea includes a careful history including life-style variables, examination, and selected laboratory tests (thyroid-stimulating hormone, follicle-stimulating hormone, prolactin). Therapy is directed at the cause, including counseling for life-style changes in hypothalamic amenorrhea.

In adolescents the incidence of significant abnormal bleeding is low, although in the first year after menarche many episodes of bleeding are anovulatory. In teenagers with heavy bleeding, an investigation for possible causes, particularly coagulation disorders (found in up to 19 per cent of teenagers hospitalized with heavy bleeding) should be performed (Claessens and Cowell 1981).

Impact on quality of life

Medical and social attitudes toward menstrual symptoms have been clouded until recently with folklore and psychosomatic implications. Such feelings may be particularly unresolved in adolescents. There are socio-cultural beliefs that menstruation is 'unclean', and some adolescents continue to accept any number of myths related to menstruation (for examples avoidance of exercise or swimming). In addition, adolescents may have limited medical knowledge of the menstrual cycle. More than half the teenagers in one study were unaware of when ovulation occurred or when pregnancy was likely. Other young women, however, have accurate knowledge of menstruation and accept their menstrual periods without negative feelings (Cumming *et al.* 1991).

Psychological and social pressures and life-style habits can have a profound effect on menstrual cyclicity in the adolescent. Functional hypothalamic amenorrhea is defined as the absence of menses when no identifiable anatomic abnormalities of the hypothalamic–pituitary–ovarian–endometrial axis can be found. This type of amenorrhea is commonly caused by factors which predominate in the adolescent population, including excessive exercise, psychogenic stress, weight loss, and eating disorders (Liu 1990). Involvement in athletics by women in the USA is steadily increasing as a result of changes in school district policies, and a 'wellness' attitude, or health consciousness, that is often associated with concerns about weight. Although amenorrhea is common in certain athletes, there is a wide range in incidence and the mechanisms are unclear. Psychogenic stress alone can cause some episodes of amenorrhea. Weight loss is another cause in the adolescent population, and is the product of eating disorders associated with dissatisfaction with body self-image. In a national school-based survey, 43.6 per cent of female students were trying to lose weight, including 27.4 per cent of those who said they considered themselves to be at the right weight. These students reported exercising, missing meals, taking diet pills, and inducing vomiting (Morbidity and Mortality Weekly Report 1991).

Important to the adolescent population is absenteeism from school. In one study of 182 adolescents, 72.7 per cent reported pain or discomfort during their menses, 58.9 per cent had associated decreased activity, and 45 per cent reported school or work absenteeism. Despite this, only 15 per cent had used a prescription medication and 14 per cent could not name any non-steroidal anti-inflammatory agent except aspirin (Johnson 1988).

There is a marked disparity between health problems that are medically recognized as important and those accepted by the adolescent population. Health policy concerns center around reproductive health morbidity and mortality (for example, contraceptive behavior, sexually transmitted disease, maternal mortality), as well as non-reproductive problems (for example, substance abuse, suicide, accidents, and homicide). Adolescents tend to regard these as outside their sphere of experience, and concentrate more on acne, weight, dental problems, and emotional concerns such as school stress, peer and parent relationships, and loneliness (Blum 1991).

In addition, availability of health care does not ensure that the adolescent will access this care. In one study, although youths had sought medical assistance for stomach pains, headaches, and coughing, nearly half had not sought help for other health problems. These included concerns regarding weight, birth control, and emotional upset. Although 24 per cent reported being sexually active, only 4 per cent sought medical advice, 20 per cent used illicit drugs, but only 1 per cent requested help, and 38 per cent felt they had a weight problem, but only 10 per cent had seen a physician (Marks *et al.* 1983).

Both health and life-style patterns established in adolescence have far-reaching implications for later morbidity and mortality. Examples include: the effect of safe sex on future infertility and death from AIDS; the effects of obesity and diet on cardiovascular disease; and the effects of calcium intake, eating disorders, and amenorrhea on peak bone mass and therefore later risk for osteoporotic fracture. This emphasizes a need among adolescents for alternative education programs and for studies on access to health care in this population.

Women of reproductive age

Premenstrual syndrome

The underlying pathophysiology of premenstrual syndrome (PMS) is poorly understood, and research in this area is in its infancy. This lack of knowledge, together with the inconsistent use of strict diagnostic criteria and the preponderance of poorly controlled studies, has frustrated both clinicians and patients who seek satisfactory care for this syndrome.

Premenstrual syndrome may be defined as 'the cyclic recurrence, in the luteal phase of the menstrual cycle, of a combination of distressing physical, psychologic, and/or behavioral changes of sufficient severity to result in deterioration of interpersonal relationships and/or interference with normal activities' (Reid 1985). Although more than 150 symptoms have been ascribed to PMS, none is particularly specific. In almost all patients, there is repeated irritability or depression and fatigue during the luteal phase, accompained by a bloated sensation, breast tenderness, and/or headache. The diagnosis of PMS is dependent on the prospective recording of symptoms. It can then be diagnosed if:

(1) repetitive physical and behavioral symptoms occur in the luteal phase of the cycle, and are followed by a symptom-free interval in the follicular phase of the cycle;

(2) other pathologies have been ruled out;

(3) symptoms result in a level of impairment (Mortola *et al.* 1990).

Other conditions that may give rise to similar symptoms are drug ingestion, alcohol abuse, perimenopausal state, use of hormonal agents, thyroid dysfunction, and a concurrent psychiatric disorder. Estimation of the prevalence of PMS has been greatly hampered in the past by the lack of consistent diagnostic criteria. When strict criteria are used to diagnose premenstrual syndrome, the prevalence is quite low and in the range of 2.5–10 per cent. Certainly most of the estimated 70–80 per cent of women who notice premenstrual symptoms ('molimina') are not considered to have PMS.

The etiology of PMS is unknown; however, research efforts have made some progress over the past decade. Mounting evidence supports the hypothesis that alterations in central neurotransmitters (opioids, nor epinephrine, serotonin, and GABA) are involved. As an example, central serotonin uptake and receptor levels are regulated by progesterone or state of cycle in animals. In women, altered serotonin uptake by platelets has been reported in the premenstrual phase of the cycle and correlated with severity of PMS symptoms. Furthermore, serotonin reuptake inhibitors, which prevent neuronal uptake of serotonin and thereby increase serotonin concentrations in the synapse, are effective in treating PMS patients (Wood *et al.* 1992).

The approach to PMS can include treatments designed to address a single symptom, to eliminate menstrual cyclicity, or to influence a proposed etiological basis for PMS. Controlled studies have demonstrated the value of suppression of ovarian activity by gonadotropin-releasing hormone analogues, benzodiazepines (which reduce anxiety), and serotonin reuptake inhibitors. Education, emotional support, and exercise also help to reduce the severity of the condition.

Impact on quality of life

By definition, a diagnosis of PMS implies some impairment to the quality of life. Some investigators feel that the level of impairment must be an identifiable disruption in socio-economic performance as ascertained by marital or relationship discord, difficulties in parenting, poor work or school performance, increased social isolation, legal difficulties, or seeking medical attention for somatic symptoms (Mortola 1992).

Despite the difficulty in study design and in quantifying the effect of PMS on family life and work, the few published reports suggest that PMS does have adverse effects. They suggest that it increases marital discord as well as tending to produce harsher disciplining of children. Husbands develop strategies during these times which include spiritual coping, passivity (the problem will go away), becoming more supportive, and expressing anger. One survey examining prevalence of PMS reported that 10 per cent of women missed more than 1 day of work during the premenstrual week in the preceding 6 months. The cost of loss of productivity secondary to PMS has been estimated at $5 billion annually in the USA. The family and social impacts of PMS remain unclear. Better understanding awaits larger epidemiologic studies in which strict diagnostic criteria are used and methodology is sound.

Infertility

In some countries there has been a steady increase in involuntary infertility. The problem affects nearly one in six couples attempting pregnancy in the USA. The demand for infertility services has increased rapidly and in the USA in the 1980s there were over 2 million visits per year to infertility specialists. The precise reasons are not known; however, a prominent factor is likely to be the trend toward delaying childbearing. The age at first child has steadily increased because of increasing emphasis on completing higher education programs and establishing careers prior to beginning a family. During this delay factors related to fertility may come into play. These include the effect of age itself on fecundity, the increased incidence with age of gynecologic pathology associated with infertility, such as endometriosis, and the potential for increased exposure to sexually transmitted disease.

Approximately 40 per cent of infertility in the USA is thought to be due to a male factor. Depending on the patient population, infertility is due to ovulatory disturbance in about 40 per cent of infertile women and tubal pathology in 30–50 per cent.

The investigation of an infertile couple follows from these etiologies. A semen analysis is performed, assessing sperm count, and motility and morphology of the sperm, as well as ejaculate volume, viscosity, and pH. Evaluation of the infertile female involves documentation of ovulation and, in anovulatory women, hormonal testing to determine the cause of anovulation. Pelvic and tubal pathology may be assessed by ultrasound scan, hysterosalpingography, laparoscopy, and hysteroscopy to identify endometriosis, pelvic adhesions, and other pelvic pathology, and to determine whether or not the fallopian tubes are patent. Treatment is based on either correcting the underlying abnormality or attempting to increase fecundity rates. The rapid development of assisted reproductive technologies including *in vitro* fertilization and gamete intrafallopian transfer have improved the outlook for some infertile couples.

Impact on quality of life

The simple decision of a couple to seek medical advice for infertility is an emotional decision. Several phases then ensue. Initially, the couple may react with shock, disbelief, or denial. They may examine present or past behavior to formulate a theory to explain the infertility, and may become preoccupied with fault-finding or determining what is wrong. The second phase in unsuccessful initial treatments involves mourning the loss of the children the couple will never bear and an examination of what parenthood means to them. The couple may experience a modified grief reaction. This is followed by a period of coming to terms with the outcome and proceeding with plans for adoption, trying assisted reproductive technologies, or living without children (Mahlstead 1985; Golombok 1992).

The decision to try assisted reproductive technologies then brings an additional emotional stress ('the last chance') and possibly a tremendous financial burden, and may bring out feelings of ambivalence depending on the couple's ethical and religious views of the technology being recommended (Herz 1989). These issues are dealt with in greater depth in Chapter 11.

Postpartum health and children

Little attention has been placed on the evaluation of health in the postpartum period or the impact on women of caring for children in a work-oriented society. With regard to postpartum health, it is clear that, despite the return to normal of reproductive organs by 6 weeks after birth, many symptoms persist long after this. Fatigue, emotional lability, and sexual dysfunction are reported up to 4–6 months postpartum by 25 per cent of women. Two studies found a majority of women had dyspareunia (painful intercourse) at 3 and 4 months postpartum. In a comparison of first-time mothers, adoptive mothers, and controls (married women with no children) at 6 weeks after birth, first-time mothers had more breast complaints, urogenital symptoms, and fatigue (Gjerdingen and Froberg 1991). A recent study examined 436 first-time mothers during the first 12 months postpartum. Physical problems at 1 month included expected symptoms such as breast symptoms, hemorrhoids, fatigue, and vaginal discomfort. Of interest was an increase in many other medical problems between 3 and 12 months postpartum, including hair loss peaking at 6 months and a greater than 40 per cent incidence of respiratory symptoms especially in women who returned to work (Gjerdingen *et al.* 1993).

The clinical manifestations of postpartum depression encompass a wide range of symptom severity. A period of dysphoric mood following childbirth occurs in as many as 40–60 per cent of new mothers, with such a high prevalence suggesting that this is not due to chance. As with PMS, the pathophysiology is poorly understood. Possible mechanisms include hormonal changes such as in thyroid function, or an effect on central neurotransmitters secondary to the abrupt fall in sex steroids on expulsion of the placenta. Alternatively, difficulty in adjusting to increased responsibility and interference with life-style by the demands of a new baby have been proposed as a cause for postpartum blues. In most cases the symptoms are mild and self-limited, but they may interfere with a mother's pleasure in caring for her baby. Relatively rarely, postpartum depression is either a severe impairment of psychological functioning or not self-limited; in these cases, consultation and consideration of counseling and pharmacologic therapies are useful (Hamilton 1989).

Women are increasingly working outside the home and this, combined with an increase in mothers who are not supported by the father, has lead to increased concern about child care. In addition, although employment has become common, equal opportunities and pay for women have lagged, adding to personal and financial pressures. The effects of the significant life stressor of a new baby on the increasing percentage of working women (the 'superwoman syndrome') have received little study. The timing of marriage, family, and career have diverged. There are increased parenting demands, with less societal consensus on parenting. Further research is needed on the effect of out-of-home care on newborn development, issues related to availability of child care, maternity benefits, and parental leave, and workplace adaptations allowing parents to be with young children (Hopper and Zigler 1988; Presser 1989).

There has been a steady increase in the percentage of working women, in postponement in timing of first birth, in single-mother households, and in single mother households as a proportion of poor families. In the USA women account for 44 per cent of the work force, and 48 per cent of working women with children under the age of 3 are the sole provider for the family.

Chronic pelvic pain

Pelvic pain occurs commonly in women of reproductive age. Most women regard pelvic discomfort such as dysmenorrhea and mid-cycle ovulatory pain as a normal part of their reproductive life. Severe and acute pelvic pain is often secondary to identifiable pathology such as an ectopic pregnancy, acute pelvic infection, or rupture of an ovarian cyst. In contrast chronic debilitating pelvic pain that interferes with normal life is the cause of great suffering in women and poorly understood or managed by physicians.

In the USA chronic pelvic pain is estimated to cause about 600 million lost working hours, and cost $2 billion annually (Dawood 1988). Chronic pelvic pain for which no cause can be found is estimated to affect at least 350 000 young women in Britain (Davis *et al.* 1992). Approximately 10 per cent of all referrals to a gynecology clinic in the USA are for pain and about 40 per cent of diagnostic laparoscopies are performed for pelvic pain. Chronic pelvic pain is the principal preoperative indication for about 10 per cent of hysterectomies, and approximately 20 per cent of hysterectomies are performed for endometriosis (Carlson *et al.* 1993).

Pain occurring with the onset of menstrual flow is very common in women. Although this pattern of pain is not often associated with any detectable underlying pathology it occasionally seriously disrupts the lives of young women (see p. 19). It is thought to be due to the release of prostaglandins, and is often alleviated by antiprostaglandins or by the use of the oral contraceptive pill. Pain occurring cyclically before the onset of the menstrual flow is more often associated with detectable underlying pathology. This pain can also be initially treated with a trial of the contraceptive pill or antiprostaglandins.

Pelvic pain that has been present for more than 6 months is regarded as being chronic. It is a very common reason for women to present to their gynecologist (Reiter 1990). Numerous causes have been suggested for this condition, but even today little is known about it and in consequence it is poorly managed. Presumed etiologies related to pelvic pathology include endometriosis and pelvic scar tissue (adhesions). Endometriosis is a condition in which tissue similar to the endometrial lining of the uterus is implanted elsewhere in sites such as the ovary, abdominal cavity, and muscle of the uterus. Endometriosis grows under the influence of estrogen and can be treated by suppressing ovulation and by medications that create a temporary 'menopause'. In addition, conservative surgery (cautery or laser treatment) may alleviate symptoms. When all medical and conservative therapies have failed, removal of the ovaries may be indicated. Although pelvic infection which recurs and leads to the formation of adhesions is also said to be a cause of chronic pelvic pain, there is little evidence to support this, unless the adhesions are extensive and, in particular, involve the ovaries or bowel.

In about 60 per cent of women who complain of chronic pelvic pain, no obvious cause can be found when a laparoscope is used to look inside the abdominal cavity. Endometriosis and adhesions are present in no more than 15–20 per cent of the remaining women. The unclear role of pelvic pathology in chronic pelvic pain is emphasized by a blinded prospective study which found that the prevalence of endometriosis or pelvic adhesions as documented at laparoscopy was similar in chronic pelvic pain patients and pain-free controls (reviewed in Reiter and Milburn 1993).

Recently a group of researchers in the UK (Beard *et al.* 1988) have described a condition, the pelvic pain syndrome, which they consider is caused by congestion. The pain is aching, and is present most of the time, but occasionally is so severe as to require admission to the hospital (Beard *et al.* 1988). It is made worse by standing and exercise and commonly occurs after rather than during sexual intercourse. It may be so severe as to cause many women to cease intercourse altogether. Beard and colleagues have demonstrated pelvic varicosities in this group of patients by using X-ray techniques and ultrasound. Further support for their theory is the finding that administration of an agent that causes veins to constrict provided relief when given to patients during an acute attack of pain (Reginald *et al.* 1987). They have also demonstrated that suppression of ovarian function with high doses of a progestin (medroxyprogesterone acetate) was effective in relieving pain, particularly when combined with psychotherapy (Farquhar *et al.* 1989). Beard and colleagues hypothesize that in women with pelvic congestion there is a delay in the drainage of blood out of the pelvis, which in turn leads to the release of pain-producing substances.

To what extent a history of physical and sexual abuse should be considered in the evaluation of women with chronic pelvic pain is still undetermined. It is certainly true that adult victims of childhood physical and sexual abuse are found to have increased risk of depression and of problems with somatization, self-esteem, and sexual dysfunction, among others. Reiter *et al.* (1991) evaluated 99 women with chronic pelvic pain lasting longer than 6 months, who had a negative laparoscopy for any organic disease of the pelvis. These patients were further divided into those with a probable somatic cause of pain (such as myofascial pain, or gastroenterologic disease), and those without a somatic abnormality. The women without a somatic abnormality had a higher prevalence of sexual abuse before age 20. A study comparing idiopathic chronic pelvic pain patients with pain-free control patients had similar results. There was a history of childhood sexual abuse in 40–60 per cent of chronic pelvic pain patients. However, these findings have not been substantiated in a large survey of women with pelvic congestion (Fry 1993).

Women with chronic pelvic pain are also apt to have concurrent medical conditions such as irritable bowel syndrome, abdominal cutaneous nerve pain, and urologic disease. Furthermore, as many as 70 per cent of such patients have concurrent psychologic conditions. This highlights the complexity of the approach needed for these patients in assessing pelvic pathology, medical pathology, and the psychologic overlay to the presenting problem (Reiter and Milburn 1993). In light of these complexities, researchers in the USA and UK are now advocating multidisciplinary management of these patients with emphasis on counseling and assistance with underlying emotional disturbance. This type of management aims for 'optimization of symptom control, education, maximization of function, modification of maladaptive beliefs and behaviors, and cognitive pain therapies' (Reiter and Milburn 1993). Evidence for such an approach demonstrated that pain management, optimization of adaptive and coping skills, and help with restoring function was significantly more effective in these patients than traditional medical approaches (Peters *et al.* 1991).

Quality of life impact

The reception and interpretation of a painful stimulus plays a major part in the effect pain may have on daily life. It is well known that pain is better tolerated by individuals who are in a relaxed and well-balanced mood than by those who are anxious. There is also good evidence that people subject to repeated attacks of pain become sensitized and fearful of it (Fry *et al.* 1993). Fear of the unknown when the cause is undiagnosed also heightens the response to pain. These are important factors that must be taken into account when managing a woman who presents with any form of pain but particularly when it is chronic. A careful history that elicits details of the emotional as well as physical problems will often provide insight into the reason why the sufferer has sought help. The physician responsible for care of the patient should never forget that while the short-term objective of treatment is amelioration of pain, the ultimate objective is to return her to normal life.

With this in mind it is essential that the expectations of the patient concerning the results of treatment are modified. It may not be possible to achieve immediate and complete relief of pain, particularly if it has been present for many years. Initially amelioration of the pain, allowing the woman to return to a normal daily life-style, is a more realistic outcome. Unless patients' views are modified from the outset, there is a real possibility that they will be disillusioned if the pain does not disappear completely, or shortly after treatment has begun. Research and initial trials of a multidisciplinary approach taking account of the psychosocial profile of these patients have shown promising therapeutic results (Peters *et al.* 1991).

Abnormal menstrual bleeding

Abnormal uterine bleeding may be manifest by excessive bleeding at the time of expected menses (hypermenorrhea or menorrhagia), or too frequent or irregular bleeding episodes (polymenorrhea or metrorrhagia). The etiologies of abnormal uterine bleeding can be broadly divided into two groups: those involving an abnormality of the pelvic organs; and those which are the result of ovarian dysfunction (anovulation), which are termed dysfunctional uterine bleeding.

Dysfunctional uterine bleeding is increased at either extreme of reproductive age group (perimenarchal and perimenopausal) as a result of the increased incidence of anovulation, and is also associated with specific gynecologic disorders such as polycystic ovary syndrome. Organic causes include complications resulting from pregnancy (miscarriage, ectopic pregnancy), benign and malignant tumors of the uterus, infection, and more generalized diseases (coagulation disorders, severe liver disease). Pelvic causes of abnormal bleeding include uterine fibroids, polyps in the uterus, endometrial hyperplasia, and cancer of the cervix or uterus. Diagnosis involves a careful history and physical examination followed by laboratory tests and consideration of ultrasound of the pelvis. Laboratory tests include a complete blood count, pregnancy test, Pap smear, and cervical cultures. Sampling of the endometrium may also be necessary, depending on the clinical presentation and the patient's age. In the adolescent with significant bleeding, coagulation studies should be performed.

Dysfunctional uterine bleeding responds well to the oral contraceptive pill or progestins. Non-steroidal anti-inflammatory drugs decrease mean blood loss, and antifibrinolytic agents are also effective in dysfunctional uterine bleeding. Abnormal uterine bleeding secondary to fibroids may be treated with gonadotropin-releasing hormone analogs for limited periods. Dilatation and curettage is not curative for abnormal uterine bleeding, and newer techniques of endometrial ablation await the results of long-term follow-up.

Quality of life

When menstrual blood loss repeatedly exceeds 80 ml per cycle, iron deficiency anemia will ensue. Progressive anemia may be associated with lethargy and decreased productivity at work and at home as well as absenteeism. Patients who experience abrupt and heavy bleeding episodes may also avoid work or social activities because of the risk of unexpected break-through bleeding. Abnormal uterine bleeding is common and may account for as many as 15 per cent of out-patient visits and 25 per cent of gynecologic operations. The impact of two causes of abnormal uterine bleeding—dysfunctional uterine bleeding and uterine fibroids—as preoperative indications for hysterectomy is profound.

Hysterectomy is the second most common major operation performed in the USA after cesarean section, with approximately 590 000 hysterectomies performed per year, at a cost exceeding $5 billion (Carlson *et al.* 1993). There is substantial variation in hysterectomy rates according to country (high in the USA, low in Norway, Sweden, and England), within regions of a country, and related to patient and physician factors. It appears that professional uncertainty about appropriate indications is a primary reason for these differences. Common indications for hysterectomy include uterine leiomyomas (30 per cent), dysfunctional uterine bleeding (20 per cent), genital prolapse (15 per cent), endometriosis or adenomyosis (20 per cent), and chronic pelvic pain (10 per cent). Of interest is a study in which a criteria-based quality assurance process for hysterectomy was instituted. The overall frequency of hysterectomy decreased by 24 per cent, and significant reductions were seen for the indications of chronic pelvic pain (77 per cent), recurrent uterine bleeding (46 per cent), preinvasive disease of the uterus (55 per cent), and severe infection (70 per cent). Clearly indications for hysterectomy as a treatment for benign gynecologic conditions are not established and require further evaluation.

Women at the menopause

The menopause, defined as a woman's last menstruation, usually occurs between the ages of 48 and 55 years. This has been consistent for at least a century. Prior to the last menses, there is a perimenopausal period in which there may be a change in menstrual patterns and fluctuations in ovarian hormone production. Following menopause, ovulation ceases and the production of estrogen and progesterone falls. The menopause is heralded by an increase in the pituitary hormone FSH (follicle-stimulating hormone) and a fall in the ovarian hormone estradiol.

The postmenopausal years are influenced by the effects of low estrogen, the process of aging, and socio-cultural factors. Estrogen decline may abruptly result in flushing and sweats, with bladder and vaginal symptoms appearing later, and osteoporosis (loss of bone density), stroke, and coronary artery disease lagging by many years. Late consequences of menopause and aging, specifically osteoporosis and cardiovascular disease, are receiving increasing attention as women's longevity increases. Whereas the age of menopause does not appear to have changed over the centuries, there has been an increase in life expectancy, so that a 60-year-old woman may expect to reach the age of 80. Many women now spend more than one-third of their lives after the menopause.

Consequences of the menopause

The possible medical effects of hypoestrogenism and aging can be divided into four groups: vasomotor symptoms, changes in urogenital estrogen target tissues, osteoporosis, and atherosclerotic heart disease. To what extent hypoestrogenism results in behavioral changes is debated. The degree to which a menopausal woman is at risk for any of these effects depends on numerous factors such as race, genetic predisposition, diet, exercise, concurrent risk factors (smoking), and concurrent medical disease (such as diabetes mellitus or hypertension).

Vasomotor instability, often referred to as hot flushes, affects 70–80 per cent of perimenopausal women. For 30 per cent, the symptoms are serious and they seek medical help; 25 per cent still have hot flushes 5 years after menopause. A flush is usually felt as heat arising in the torso or neck and spreading upward over the head, giving rise to sweating and reddening of the face which may cause embarrassment at work or during social activities. Night flushes may cause debilitating sleep disturbance. There are changes in skin temperature, core temperature, cutaneous electrical resistance, and heart rate (Ravnikar 1990). In addition, a pulsatile release of luteinizing hormone coincides with the hot flush.

The vagina and urethra have a common embryological origin. Estrogen deficiency may result in tissue changes related to both vaginal and bladder symptoms. There are well documented changes in the vaginal wall, including changes in epithelial cytology, electrical conductance, and amount of vaginal secretion. Such changes can lead to a more alkaline pH and vaginitis. Thinning of the vaginal mucosa and decreased vaginal secretions may result in painful intercourse. Urologic symptoms include urinary frequency and urgency.

Osteoporosis is a reduction in bone density to the point that fractures may occur. About one in four northern European women has vertebral fractures by the age of 65 and about half have them by the age of 75. In the USA, about 15 per cent of women have a hip fracture by the age of 80 and 25 per cent by the age of 90 (Stevenson, 1990). Determinants of the development of osteoporosis include both the maximal bone mass achieved and the subsequent rate of bone loss. Bone is constantly being remodeled, with osteoblasts forming new bone and osteoclasts resorbing bone. After attaining peak bone mass during their 30s, men and women progressively lose bone as they age. In women, the hypoestrogenism that follows menopause is associated with acceleration of bone loss. Other risk factors for osteoporosis include Caucasian or Asian race, family history, leanness, inactivity, low calcium intake, smoking, and therapy with glucocorticoids.

Cardiovascular disease is the leading cause of death in postmenopausal women in the USA and is more than 12 times more common as a cause of death than breast and uterine cancer. Approximately 500 000 deaths per year result from cardiovascular disease, including stroke and atherosclerotic heart disease. Despite the common public perception that cardiovascular disease primarily affects men, in the USA it kills roughly as many women as men, and accounts for more than half of all deaths in women older than 50 (Bush 1990; Gunby 1992). Factors associated with coronary artery disease are divided into non-modifiable risk factors including age, family history, and prior atherosclerotic heart disease, and modifiable factors including cigarette smoking, hypertension, hypercholesterolemia, obesity, diabetes mellitus, and estrogen use.

Management

The sequelae of hypoestrogenism are managed by a number of approaches, including life-style and risk factor modification, and use of estrogens. A variety of types of estrogens (natural and synthetic) and routes of administration (oral, transdermal, vaginal) are available. Progestins are given with estrogen to women with an intact uterus, to prevent endometrial hyperplasia and carcinoma. Nonhormonal management is directed at specific complaints (vaginal moisturizers and lubricants for vaginal dryness, clonidine for hot flushes), at life-style changes that would alter a specific risk (calcium and weight-bearing exercise for maintenance of bone mass), or at life-style change that affects not only aging-related processes but also other causes of morbidity and mortality (cessation of smoking). In all menopausal patients an empathic carer who can provide validation of experiences, education, and psychosocial support is of clear benefit (Hamburger and Anderson 1990).

Vasomotor symptoms are successfully treated by estrogens. In addition, both progestins and the antihypertensive agent clonidine reduce hot flushes. Over time after the menopause, many women will experience a decline in frequency of hot flushes. Vaginal dryness and urinary urgency are also highly amenable to estrogen therapy. In addition, sexual activity itself has beneficial effects on the vaginal wall and acidity. Alternatives to estrogen include lubricants and vaginal moisturizers for dyspareunia, and anticholinergics for urgency symptoms.

Administration of estrogens to postmenopausal women also decreases the rate of bone loss and incidence of fracture (Ettinger *et al.* 1985; Kiel *et al.* 1987). A retrospective analysis indicated a possible 50 per cent reduction in hip fracture with estrogen use, and a prospective study revealed as much as a 90 per cent reduction in vertebral fracture. The addition of progestins does not attenuate the estrogen effect and may in fact enhance it. Calcium supplementation and weight-bearing exercise are important adjuncts to preserving bone mass; however, neither is as potent as estrogen administration. Calcium supplementation may need to be higher in postmenopausal women than the current recommendation of 800 mg per day. Postmenopausal women not on estrogen may require 1500 mg per day, and women on estrogen therapy 1000 mg per day. Weight-bearing exercise for as little as 30 min three times a week is beneficial. Research is active on two other promising approaches to osteoporosis, which might be alternatives to estrogens. The first is the use of calcitonin, a hormone that inhibits osteoclast function and thereby diminishes bone resorption. The second is the use of bisphosphonates, which also interfere with osteoclast function.

Further work is needed on preventative health measures for osteoporosis and identification of women at risk. Preventative health measures may include education about diet, exercise, and calcium and vitamin D intake in young women (adolescents) as this may alter peak bone mass and therefore change the timing of postmenopausal development of osteoporosis. Technological advancements in bone density measurements have made it easier to identify women at risk. Dual energy X-ray absorptiometry makes it possible to assess the spine and hip with greater precision than earlier methods and may help identify those women who are losing bone more rapidly. Bone density is not the sole factor in fracture risk; bone quality and the woman's propensity to fall are also important.

The role of estrogen therapy in modifying risk for atherosclerotic heart disease in women is of great public health import. The 22 available studies in combination (and by meta-analyses) lead to the conclusion that in postmenopausal women estrogen administration reduces the risk of heart disease by about half (Lobo 1990; Lobo 1991; Barrett-Connor and Bush 1991). The effect of concurrent administration of progestins is not known. The mechanism by which estrogen is cardioprotective was initially felt to be predominantly alteration of circulating lipoproteins, including an increase in HDL-cholesterol. This is now believed to account for only about one-third of the effect. Other cardioprotective mechanisms of estrogens are not known but may involve direct actions on vascular wall, antioxidant properties, or other unexplored mechanisms.

Controversies in menopause management

There is a lack of data and a lack of a consensus regarding the appropriate management of menopause. Biomedical conflicts surround the effects of hormone replacement therapy on cardiovascular disease and breast cancer, and the appropriate use of progestins. Specifically, the protective effect of estrogens with regard to cardiovascular disease, although based on large epidemiologic studies, has never been tested in a large, randomized, placebo-controlled trial. If estrogen treatment results in a 50 per cent reduction in cardiovascular disease, this could be used as an argument for estrogens as a preventative health measure in otherwise asymptomatic women (Grady *et al.* 1992). Increasing data on the effects of estrogen on the cardiovascular system will become available over the next two decades, from large controlled epidemiologic trials in both the USA and Europe.

The important issue of postmenopausal hormone replacement and breast cancer remains unresolved; conflicting reports suggest that hormone replacement reduces, does not change, or slightly increases breast cancer risk. Recent meta-analyses are also not clear, and suggest that the breast cancer risk may be related to the type of estrogen, the duration of use, and the presence or absence of progestin therapy. Progestin therapy also remains under examination, as the ideal type of progestin, dose, and necessary length of duration to prevent unwanted endometrial changes are not established. Furthermore, the adverse lipid changes seen with some progestins, and the lack of epidemiologic data on this issue, raise the hypothetical concern that progestins may partially negate the beneficial effect of estrogen on cardiovascular disease.

Further controversies relate to the 'medicalization' of menopause, and conflicts between biomedical and psychosocial models (Flint and Samil 1990; Voda 1992). Some hold that menopause is a normal biologic event, that there is a lack of proof of causality between hormone changes and symptoms, and that women often experience menopause with a minimum of difficulty. From this stance, as menopause is a normal process with no risk to health, the use of hormones in healthy women is condemned. The opposing view is that the reason for re-evaluating hormone replacement is not menopause *per se*, but the recent dramatic changes in life expectancy, allowing the late sequelae of osteoporosis and heart disease, which may be ameliorated by estrogen therapy. The appropriateness of short-term hormone replacement for symptomatic patients versus long-term preventative health use of hormones in women who have no symptoms, to reduce risks of osteoporosis and cardiovascular disease, remains controversial.

Clearly, the question as to who should receive postmenopausal hormone replacement has not been answered. Presently, decisions must be made only after a full discussion of the effects of hypoestrogenism and aging with the woman and a risk–benefit analysis of hormone replacement therapy individualized to the woman's medical history and family history. Such a discussion cannot occur in a brief 'gyn visit'. Women with symptoms will address the impact of these symptoms on quality of life.

Future research on estrogen replacement in menopause will focus on a number of factors, including the results of large controlled clinical studies evaluating the effect of estrogen on atherosclerotic heart disease and breast cancer, the increasing ability to identify and treat women at risk for osteoporosis, and new methods to protect against estrogen-induced endometrial hyperplasia. In addition, cost analysis and health policy decisions on the use of estrogen as preventative health care for osteoporosis and heart disease in asymptomatic postmenopausal women will be critically examined.

Impact on quality of life

The change from the reproductive years to menopause is an important physiological and social milestone for women in the middle years. The impact on quality of life is variable and to some degree culturally determined. The menopause signified the end of reproductive capacity and childbearing, until donor egg *in vitro* fertilization became possible. It is often considered to be a negative life event and the beginning of an aging process in Western culture. In contrast, in some cultures menopause is viewed positively, freeing women for leadership in the extended family and community.

While there is general agreement that hot flushes and urogenital symptoms are associated with estrogen deficiency, there is no evidence that the low estrogen level of menopause results in psychological symptoms. A review of gynecologic and psychiatric publications from the mid-nineteenth century to the present revealed that recent epidemiological and clinical studies not only fail to demonstrate a specific entity of menopausal depression but, in fact, show a decline in depression among women in this age group (Youngs 1990). In addition, changes in mood felt to be related to the menopause can often be explained as secondary effects—for example, irritability may result from sleep loss due to repetitive hot flushes, or other factors may be involved such as negative cultural stereotypes, and concurrent socio-economic and psychosocial factors. Although irritability, anxiety, increased tension, and depressed mood have been associated with the menopause, a direct cause and effect has not been established. It is difficult to determine whether they are related to changes in the central nervous system because of decreased estrogen levels, or have a different etiology. Contemporary research has produced conflicting data on minor psychological and somatic complaints, with some studies reporting an increase in symptoms, and others no change. Rubinow and Schmidt (1991), in their review of menopause-related affective disorders agree that recent research has not been able to confirm disturbance of mood or behavior related to the menopausal years but suggests that it is premature to conclude that a relationship does not exist.

Specific changes that effect sexual life do occur during the climacteric period. A later effect of decreased estrogen levels is genital atrophy, of which the most evident symptom is vaginal dryness giving rise to painful intercourse. Kinsey's data show a decrease in frequency of intercourse in women 50–60 years old. However, studies by Masters and Johnson indicate that among women who were sexually active at the age of 60, overall sexual activity did not decrease until the age of 75. Coital frequency is not the most accurate indicator of sexual satisfaction. Current studies do not demonstrate a consistent or predictable decline in sexual activity or interest and in fact suggest that 'the presence of a suitable male partner appears to play a more important role than age *per se*' (Youngs 1990). As physiologic sexual responses are maintained in the menopause, sexual activity appears related more to availability of a partner and the prior pattern and enjoyment of sexual activity. Traditional and widely held beliefs and assumptions about the relationship between menopause and psychologic symptoms or a decline in sexual activity and interest are controversial and not well supported by more contemporary studies.

Aging women

Medical problems of the aging woman include the processes that begin in the early postmenopausal years (osteoporosis and atherosclerotic heart disease) as well as other physiologic changes and medical conditions associated with aging. Physiologic changes associated with aging include:

(1) cardiovascular changes, including a decrease in cardiac output and responsiveness to sympathetic stimulation, and increased valvular calcification;

(2) pulmonary function changes, such as reductions in vital capacity, forced expiratory volume, and chest wall compliance;

(3) renal function changes, including a decline in glomerular filtration rate;

(4) endocrine changes—in addition to hypoestrogenism, these include a decline in carbohydrate metabolism and thyroid function;

(5) a relative impairment in immune function.

Medical problems associated with aging include:

(1) an increase in the incidence of stroke, diabetes mellitus, and degenerative arthritis;

(2) urinary incontinence becoming a larger problem, with a prevalence of 5–15 per cent in the community at large and more than 30 per cent in institutionalized women (Resnick and Subbarao 1985);

(3) complications associated with osteoporosis increasing progressively with age—the incidence of hip fractures doubles every 5 years after the age of 60;

(4) accidents, especially falls, resulting in a high degree of disability in the elderly population (many factors account for this, including changes in gait and stability,

postural hypotension, visual or neurological problems, environmental factors, and medications);

(5) an increase in atherosclerotic heart disease, the cause of 50 per cent of all deaths in women over the age of 50;

(6) a progressive increase in breast cancer risk with age.

In addition, geriatric women are at risk of depression and dementia. The depression associated with aging appears to involve depressive symptoms more often than the onset of major depressive illness. These feelings of dysphoria may not be directly related to menopause or aging but rather to grief associated with loss of partner, and social, economic, and physical problems encountered by geriatric women. Cognitive and functional impairment affects 20 per cent of those over the age of 80, and in a large percentage this dementia is caused by Alzheimer's disease or infarction and is not currently reversible. Attention is being focused on tools for assessment of functional capacity, depression, and cognitive measures.

Impact on quality of life

It is estimated that there will be 31 million people aged 65 and older in the USA by the year 2000. Of these, almost 70 per cent will be women. Women over the age of 65 are currently the fastest growing segment of the USA population. As women live longer than men, the disparity in ratio of women to men increases with increasing age, and in the 85 plus age group there are about 224 women for every 100 men. World-wide, there are approximately 342 million people over the age of 65 comprising 6.2 per cent of the population. Current demographic trends indicate that by the year 2050 there may be 2.5 billion people over the age of 65, accounting for one-fifth of world population (Olshansky *et al.* 1993).

Complications related to aging leave more than 4 million people more than 65 years old in the USA severely limited in activity, as a result of physical or mental disability. The morbidity and mortality from hip fractures is enormous. The disability may result in a patient being institutionalized and the mortality rates following hip fracture may be as high as 15–20 per cent in the first 3 months owing to complications of surgery, postoperative thromboembolic events, and postoperative cardiopulmonary complications. One study showed that only half of hip fracture victims survived 1 year (Beals 1972).

In addition to medical complications, stressors also commonly include losses as a consequence of longevity, affecting home, work, and social life. In addition, people may have fears of dependency, physical disability, and cognitive impairment. More older women live alone than men, and about two-thirds of women over the age of 65 are widowed, compared with 13 per cent of men. Family support is also jeopardized, with about 25 per cent of older women having no surviving children. In addition, the percentage of older women at below poverty incomes is greater than men of the same age. Increasing emphasis is being placed on the elderly population as the percentage of elderly women steadily increases.

The impact of the aging population is felt in terms of families and health care expenditures (Rice and LaPlante 1992). Osteoporosis-related pathology is estimated at $10 billion annually in the USA. The cost of cardiovascular diseases is even higher, with a US estimate of $108.9 billion for 1992. In addition, a significant proportion of the frail elderly are taken care of by family members, and these are commonly daughters and wives.

The well woman and health maintenance strategies

Preventative health measures, the role of periodic health examinations in asymptomatic patients, and health policies specific to women are critical issues that continue to be refined. Groups addressing these issues and publishing guidelines include the Canadian Task Force on the Periodic Health Examination, the American Medical Association Council on Scientific Affairs, the Medical Practice Committee of the American College of Physicians, and the US Preventive Services Task Force (Rosen 1990).

Discussions of screening for risk factors and disease must consider that the ability to reduce risk factors by life-style alterations (smoking cessation, diet, exercise, safe sexual practices, drug and alcohol abuse) would probably have a greater impact on health than a screening program for specific disease. In addition, selecting screening tests that are sensitive enough and incorporating appropriate testing related to the individual risk factors is necessary. Also, a complete data base that includes a woman's life-style, health practices, and medical and family history is critical. Lastly, these general health maintenance strategies then need to be specifically modified to women's health risks and needs.

Health policy must be modified if it is to address women's health issues in an appropriate manner, but efforts at modification have been hampered by the lack of research on women in areas not related to gynecologic pathology. Major studies of risk factors for atherosclerotic heart disease, death following myocardial infarction, and the use of aspirin to prevent heart attacks, were all predominantly or initially performed in men. It is impossible to generalize from these studies to make recommendations or polices for women (Wallis and Klass 1989; Snowe 1990).

Furthermore, the assessment of women's health cannot rely solely on a medical model. A bio-psychosocial model that evaluates wellness and function in the context of psychological and socio-economic factors is required (Flint and Samil 1990). This leads to a multidisciplinary team approach in many circumstances. In addition, the complexities of women's life experiences today include an overlap and interplay of the biologic–reproductive circle with the family–marital circle, and the educational–vocational circle. The impact of reproductive processes on quality of life must be constantly modified and re-examined in the context of the evolving role of women in society. Women contribute increasingly to the national workforce, yet are expected to continue to care for the children and elderly in their families. Clearly, investment in research, socio-economic reform, and health policy to ensure good health throughout life for women should be an international priority.

References

Beard, R. W., Reginald, P. W., and Wadsworth, J. (1988). Clinical features of women with chronic lower abdominal pain and pelvic congestion. *British Journal of Obstetrics and Gynaecology*, **95**, 153.

Barrett-Connor, E., and Bush, T. L. (1991). Estrogen and coronary heart disease in women. *Journal of American Medical Association*, **265**, 1861–7.

Beals, R. K. (1972). Survival following hip fracture: long term follow-up of 607 patients. *Journal of Chronic Disease*, **25**, 235.

Blum, R. (1991). Global trends in adolescent health. *Journal of American Medical Association*, **265**, 2711–9.

Bush, T. L. (1990). The epidemiology of cardiovascular disease in postmenopausal women. *Annals of the New York Academy of Sciences*, **592**, 263.

Carlson, K. J., Nichols, D. H., and Schiff, I. (1993). Indications for hysterectomy. *New England Journal of Medicine*, **328**, 856–60.

Claessens, E. A. and Cowell, C. A. (1981). Acute adolescent menorrhagia. *American Journal of Obstetrics and Gynecology*, **139**, 277–80.

Cumming, D., Cumming, C., and Kieren, D. (1991). Menstrual mythology and sources of information about menstruation. *American Journal of Obstetrics and Gynecology*, **164**, 172–6.

Davies, L., Ganger, K. F., Drummond, M., Saunders, D., and Beard, R. W. (1992). The economic burden of intractable gynaecological pain. *Journal of Obstetrics and Gynaecology*, **12(2)**, 854–6.

Dawood, M. Y. (1988). Nonsteroidal anti-inflammatory drugs and changing attitudes toward dysmenorrhea. *American Journal of Medicine*, **84(5A)**, 23–9.

Ettinger, B., Genant, H. K., and Cann, C. E. (1985). Long-term estrogen replacement therapy prevents bone loss and fractures. *Annals of Internal Medicine*, **102**, 319.

Farquhar, C. M., Rogers, V., Franks, S., Pearce, S., Wadsworth, J., and Beard R. W. (1989). A randomized controlled trial of medroxyprogesterone acetate and psychotherapy for the treatment of pelvic congestion. *British Journal of Obstetrics and Gynaecology*, **96**, 1153.

Flint, M. and Samil, R. (1990). Cultural and subcultural meanings of the menopause. *Annals of the New York Academy of Sciences*, **592**, 1.

Fry, R. P., Crisp, A. H., Beard, R. W., and McGuiyan, S. (1993). Psychosocial aspects of chronic pelvic pain, with special reference to sexual abuse. A study of 164 women. *Postgraduate Medical Journal*, **69 (813)**, 566–74.

Gjerdingen, D. K., Froberg, D. G., Chaloner, K. M., and McGovern, P. M. (1993). Changes in women's physical health during the first postpartum year. *Archives of Family Medicine*, **2**, 277–83.

Gjerdingen, D. K. and Froberg, D. G. (1991). The fourth stage of labor: the health of birth mothers and adoptive mothers at six weeks postpartum. *Family Medicine*, **23**, 29–35.

Golombok, S. (1992). Psychological functioning in infertility patients. *Human Reproduction*, **7**, 208.

Grady, D., Rubin, S., Petitti, D., Fox, C., Black, D., Ettinger, B., *et al.* (1992). Hormone therapy to prevent disease and prolong life in postmenopausal women. *Annals of Internal Medicine*, **117**, 1016–37.

Gunby, P. (1992). Cardiovascular diseases remain nation's leading cause of death. *Journal of American Medical Association*, **267**, 335–6.

Hamburger, S., and Anderson, E. (1990). The value of education and social–psychological support in a menopause clinic. *Annals New York Academy of Sciences*, **592**, 1.

Hamilton, J. A. (1989). Postpartum psychiatric syndromes. *Psychiatric Clinics of North America*, **12**, 89.

Herz, E. K. (1989). Infertility and bioethical issues of the new reproductive technologies. *Psychiatric Clinics of North America*, **12**, 117.

Hopper, P. and Zigler, E. (1988). The medical and social science basis for a national infant care leave policy. *American Journal of Orthopsychiatry*, **58**, 324–38.

Johnson, J. (1988). Level of knowledge among adolescent girls regarding effective treatment for dysmenorrhea. *Journal of Adolescent Health Care*, **9**, 398–402.

Kiel, D. P., Felson, D. T., Anderson, J. J., Wilson, P. W. F., and Moskowitz, M. A. (1987). Hip fracture and the use of estrogens in postmenopausal women: the Framingham study. *New England Journal of Medicine*, **317**, 1169.

Liu, J. H. (1990). Hypothalamic amneorrhea: clinical perspectives, pathophysiology, and managment. *American Journal of Obstetrics and Gynecology*, **163**, 1732–6.

Lobo, R. A. (1990). Cardiovascular implications of estrogen replacement therapy. *Obstetrics and Gynecology*, **75**, 18S.

Lobo, R. (1991). Effects of hormonal replacement on lipid and lipoproteins in postmenopausal women. *Journal of Clinical Endocrinology and Metabolism*, **73**, 925.

Mahlstead, P. P. (1985). The psychological component of fertility. *Fertility and Sterility*, **43**, 335–46.

Marks, J., Malizio, J., Hoch, J., Brody, R., and Fisher, M. (1983). Assessment of health needs and willingness to utilize health care resources of adolescents in a suburban population. *Journal of Pediatrics*, **102**, 456–60.

Morbidity and Mortality Weekly Report (1991). Body-weight perceptions and selected weight-management goals and practices of high school students—United States, 1990. *Journal of American Medical Association*, **266** (20), 2811–12.

Mortola, J. F., Girton, L., Beck, L., and Yen, S. S. C. (1990). Diagnosis of premenstrual syndrome by a simple prospective, and reliable instrument: the calendar of premenstrual experiences. *Obstetrics and Gynecology*, **76**, 302–7.

Mortola, J. F. (1992). Assessment and management of premenstrual syndrome. *Current Opinions in Obstetrics and Gynecology*, **3**, 877–85.

Olshansky, S., Carnes, B., and Cassel, C. (1993). The aging of the human species. *Scientific American*, April, 46–52.

Peters, A. A. W., van Dorst, E., Jellis, B., van Zuuren, E., Hermans, J., and Trimbol, J. Z. (1991). A randomized clinical trial to compare two different approaches in women with chronic pelvic pain. *Obstetrics and Gynecology*, **77**, 740.

Presser, H. (1989). Can we make time for children? The economy, work schedules, and child care. *Demography*, **26**(4), 523–43.

Ravnikar, V. (1990). Physiology and treatment of hot flushes. *Obstetrics and Gynecology*, **73**, (Supplement), 3–7.

Reginald, P. W., Beard, R. W., Kooner, J. S., Mathias, C. J., Samarage, S. U., Sutherland, I. A., *et al.* (1987). Intravenous dihydroergotamine to relieve pelvic congestion with pain in young women. *Lancet*, **ii**, 351–3.

Reid, R. L. (1985). Premenstrual syndrome. *Current Problems in Obstetrics and Gynecology*, **8**, 1.

Reiter, R. C. (1990). A profile of women with chronic pelvic pain. *Clinical Obstetrics and Gynaecology*, **33**, 130.

Reiter, R. C., and Milburn, A. (1993). Chronic pelvic pain. In *Gynecology and obstetrics: a longitudinal approach*, (ed. T. R. Moore, R. C. Reiter, R. W. Rebar, and V. V. Baker), pp. 857–67. Churchill Livingstone, Edinburgh.

Reiter, R. C., Shakerin, L. R., Gambone, J. C., and Milburn, A. K. (1991). Correlation between sexual abuse and somatization in women with somatic and nonsomatic chronic pelvic pain. *American Journal of Obstetrics and Gynecology*, **165**, 104–9.

Resnick, N., and Subbarao, V. Y. (1985). Management of urinary incontinence in the elderly. *New England Journal of Medicine*, **313**, 800.

Rice, D. and LaPlante, M. (1992). Medical expenditures for disability and disabling comorbidity. *American Journal of Public Health*, **82(5)**, 739–41.

Rosen, M. (1990). Health maintenance strategies for women of different ages. *Obstetrics and Gynecology Clinics of North America*, **17**, 673–94.

Rubinow, D. R. and Schmidt, P. J. (1991). Menopause-related affective disorders: a justification for further study. *American Journal of Psychiatry*, **148**, 844–52.

Snowe, O. (1990). Women's health: a focus for the 1990s. *Academic Medicine*, **65**, 684–5.

Stevenson, J. C. (1990). Pathogenesis, prevention, and treatment of osteoporosis. *Obstetrics and Gynecology*, **75**, (Supplement), 36–41.

Voda, A. M. (1992). Menopause: a normal view. *Clinical Obstetrics and Gynecology*, **35**, 923–33.

Wallis, L., and Klass, P. (1989). Toward improving women's health care. *Journal of American Medical Women's Association*, **45**, 219–21.

Wood, S. H., Mortola, J. F., Chan, Y.-F., Moossazadeh, F., and Yen, S. C. (1992). Treatment of premenstrual syndrome with fluoxetine: a double-blind, placebo-controlled, crossover study. *Obstetrics and Gynecology*, **80**, 339–44.

Youngs, D. D. (1990). Some misconceptions concerning the menopause. *Obstetrics and Gynecology*, **75**, 881–3.

3 Female adolescent health care: international perspective

Roxane Gardner

Attention has long been directed towards improving the health status of infants and children. The time has come to focus a greater portion of this attention towards improving the health of adolescents, especially female adolescents. This chapter is a discussion of demographics and socio-economic issues which affect the health of teenagers throughout the world, and a review of specific reproductive health issues. It has been said that children are our future. With adolescents, this statement becomes more cogent and immediate because adolescents are our tomorrow.

General comments

The period of adolescence embodies the passage from childhood to adulthood. This transition is often turbulent with emotion, risk-taking behaviours, and physical growth as the child becomes increasingly independent and autonomous. Although there are societies in the world which define the period of adolescence as extending to the age of 24 years, most describe adolescence as the ages of 10–19 years. The World Health Organization (WHO) is in agreement with this definition of adolescence (WHO 1989). World statistics, however, generally collect and group data on adolescents between the ages of 15 and 19 years, thereby omitting the 10–14 year age group.

The global young adolescent population, of ages 10–14 years, is rapidly increasing (Blum 1991). Physical changes of puberty often begin around the age of 10. Developmental issues related to sexuality and self-identity can be complex and confusing to the early adolescent as the myriad of physical changes evolve through puberty. With breast development beginning as early as the age of eight years, and testicular enlargement as early as nine, data collection should be broadened to include this younger age group in statistics normally compiled on the adolescent period.

Despite societal variations in socio-economic status, level of education, and cultural beliefs that exist within each country, the task of adolescents is the same, that is, to become functioning and competent adults. The cognitive ability to think abstractly is usually achieved by the age of 15–16 years. Full psycho social development—the way an individual relates to self and society—necessitates effective separation from parents and family, attainment of a mature level of sexuality, a realistic vocational goal, and, most importantly, a realistic and positive self-image (Strasberger and Brown 1991). How successfully the adolescent achieves adulthood is directly affected by local and regional socio-economic factors and cultural practices that exist within each society. Adolescents may reach the age defined as adulthood, but these cognitive ability and/or psychosocial development may be deficient or delayed. However, it is important to remember that most adolescents traverse this period successfully. Adolescence is not just a time of trouble.

Demography

Adolescents, comprise at least 30 per cent of the world's population (United Nations 1989). Accurate data for the size of the world's 10–19 year age group is not available. In some countries the 15–19 year old age group has been reported to be 45–50 per cent of the total population. The Population Reference Bureau estimates that 60 per cent of the population in developing countries is under 25 years old and 40 per cent under 15 years old (UNESCO 1991).

Within the USA, the US Bureau of Census (1990) estimates that adolescents between 10 and 19 years old represent approximately 14 per cent of the total population. The trend in the USA in the 1990s has been towards a slight decline in total numbers from the peak in the mid-1970s; however, the percentage is expected to remain constant to the year 2000. The early adolescent age group is expected to form an increasing percentage of the adolescent population, though (US Bureau of Census 1984). The US adolescent population is currently experiencing a shift in ethnic composition and geographic concentration. By the year 2000 it is estimated that Whites will comprise 69 per cent and non-Whites 31 per cent. Within the non-White subgroups, African-Americans will predominate; however, the Hispanic population will continue to grow. The majority of the various non-White subgroups will reside in urban communities in the northeast, West Coast, and southwest. Forty-nine per cent of the US adolescent population are female, consistent with other industrialized countries.

Most of the world's adolescents—83 per cent—reside in developing countries (WHO 1986*a*). They largely dwell in urban centers, where the population exceeds 50 000. In almost every developing country there is heavy migration from rural communities to large cities, with young females migrating at rates greater than young men (Singh and Wulf 1991). In 1985, there were approximately 245 million women aged 15–19 years, 82 per cent of whom were living in developing countries, and 75 per cent residing in Asia. By the year 2000 there will be 75 million more adolescent women residing in developing countries. Half of the adolescent population in developing countries is female (UNESCO 1991).

Mortality and morbidity

The general health of adolescents is good and, therefore, often taken for granted. An individual who survives to adolescence has successfully traversed two periods of life where mortality is high—namely infancy (birth to 1 year) and early childhood 1–5 years). Before examining the factors affecting the health of female adolescents, it is instructive to review the causes of death and major morbidity for adolescents in general, and then for females in particular.

Mortality

In most countries, accidental injury is the leading cause of death, accounting for at least 50 per cent of all deaths of adolescents (Taket 1986). Males are at much greater risk for unintentional injury, but the risk for females is growing. Most unintentional injuries are due to motor vehicle and traffic accidents, reflecting the growing shift in the population from rural to urban areas. Other causes are drowning, poisoning, burns, falls, and firearms. Intentional injury is the second leading cause of death for adolescents, and includes suicide, homicide, and war. Intentional and unintentional injuries account for 80 per cent of deaths in this age group. Mortality due to suicide, homicide, and motor vehicle accidents in the USA has increased by 300–400 per cent over the past two decades (Fingerhut and Kleinman 1989). Increases in mortality have been even greater in Mexico, and Central and South America. Japan, Australia, and many European countries have experienced a slight reduction in deaths from unintentional injury (Taket 1986).

Suicides are the second most common single cause of death for adolescents in developed and developing countries. Suicide attempts are more common among adolescent females; however, males are more successful at completing their attempts. Death by suicide occurs more frequently in industrialized countries such as the USA, Canada, Norway, Switzerland, Sweden, Japan, and Germany (Diekstra 1989). Blum (1991) states that social stress due to high unemployment rates, divorce rates, the percentage of women in the workplace, the increase in alcohol abuse, access to drugs and weapons, social disruption, and urban crowding contribute to high suicide rates. Less obvious contributory factors include poor self-esteem, dissolution of a relationship, and poor school performance. Suicide in developing countries may also be associated with objection to arranged marriage or dissatisfaction within a marriage.

Intentional injury—is the third most frequent cause of death for adolescents, affecting primarily adolescent males. In the USA, homicide is the leading cause of death for young adolescent Black males, with a death rate that is 50 per cent greater than the rate for young White males. The USA, in fact, has the fifth highest homicide rate in the world (Fingerhut and Kleinman 1990). The relative ease with which teenagers can access firearms contributes in a major way to this statistic. The mortality associated with war is greatest in developing countries. Absolute numbers are difficult to obtain because of poor reporting procedures. However, many countries in Central and South America, the Middle-East, Africa, and many former Soviet republics have high adolescent mortality rates attributable to the conflicts of war and civil unrest.

Adolescent maternal mortality

The leading cause of death for adolescent females in most developing countries is directly related to pregnancy and childbearing. There are at least 13 million births per year world-wide from the adolescent female population. Maternal mortality rates for adolescent females in industrialized countries are lower where there is good access to legal abortion, so that deaths related to childbirth exceed those related to abortion (Jones *et al.* 1986). Death secondary to abortion-related complications such as hemorrhage and sepsis can account for up to 50–60 per cent of pregnancy-related deaths, especially in developing countries where abortions are illegal and/or not medically supervised.

The WHO estimates that half a million women die per year from pregnancy-related complications (WHO 1986*b*). Ninety-nine per cent of these deaths occur in developing countries. Maternal death rates as high as 1270 per 100 000 births have been reported in some rural African communities (WHO 1986*b*). Compare this with industrialized countries where maternal death rates as low as 10 per 100 000 births have been reported. Seventy-five per cent of these pregnancy-related deaths take place in India, Pakistan, Bangladesh, Indonesia, and Malaysia. Death from childbirth complications, such as hemorrhage, infection, hypertension–toxemia, and obstructed labor, is often a result of poor access to prenatal and obstetrical delivery services. Starrs (1987) has stated that women in developing countries have a greater risk of death with each pregnancy and become pregnant more often. WHO (1987) asserts that in some developing countries most maternal deaths go unregistered. Not only are these women more likely to die from pregnancy or childbirth, their death is less likely to be reported by national statistics.

The group most vulnerable to complication from pregnancy and childbirth is the early adolescent, aged 10–14 years. This age group is more likely to deny being pregnant, and therefore less likely to seek medical attention when pregnancy is suspected. Confirmation of pregnancy may not happen until an advanced gestational age, thereby delaying initiation of prenatal services. Termination of pregnancy may be unobtainable, unaffordable, performed at more advanced gestational ages than for adults, or performed illegally. It has been estimated that this early adolescent age group has a maternal mortality rate twice or three times that of the older adolescent, and four to five times that of the young adult (Chen *et al.* 1974; Rochat 1981; Harrison 1985; Royston and Armstrong 1989, p. 38) Obstructed labors are more common because of immature skeletal development and smaller pelvic diameters (Moerman 1982).

Royston and Armstrong (1989, p. 79) acknowledge that poor nutrition and low socio-economic status may be responsible for immature skeletal development and obstructed labor, as opposed to young maternal age *per se*.

Lee and Corpuz (1988) and Friede *et al.* (1987) each have shown that young adolescent females are at greater risk for giving birth to low and very low birth weight infants. Friede *et al.* (1987) demonstrated a strong association between young maternal age and higher neonatal and infant mortality rates. Extensive study by Hardy and Zabin (1991) implicates a stronger association between socio-economic status, excess low birth weight rates, and high neonatal and infant mortality rates. Complicating matters further, young adolescents are less likely to use contraception, especially those who live in developing countries such as Africa, Asia, and Latin America where access to family planning services is limited or services are absent (United Nations 1987*a*, *b*). It may also be culturally and morally unacceptable for these younger females to seek contraceptive services.

Morbidity

As with mortality data, intentional and unintentional injuries contribute in large part to overall adolescent morbidity. In the USA, it is estimated that for every injury resulting in death of an adolescent, there are approximately 1500 injuries requiring hospitalization or emergency medical treatment. These injuries occur primarily because of the risk-taking behaviors characteristic of adolescence (Neinstein 1991). These include: substance abuse such as alcohol, tobacco, and licit and illicit drug use; unprotected sexual activity resulting in unwanted pregnancy and sexually transmitted diseases; and dare-devil activities to validate their worth or strength, often resulting in motor vehicle accidents, non-fatal stabbing or gunshot wounds, falls, drownings, or poisonings. Nutrition and dietary practices, poverty, and chronic medical illness contribute to adolescent morbidity and are less obvious causes of intentional and unintentional injury.

Factors affecting female adolescent health

Poverty

Poverty is and continues to be the most common factor resulting in adverse adolescent health outcomes throughout the world, in developing and developed countries alike. The socio-economic level of an adolescent female profoundly affects access to medical care and nutritional status, increasing the risk of maternal mortality and morbidity. The lower the socio-economic status, the higher the maternal death rate (Royston and Armstrong 1989, p. 45).

Poverty is closely associated with early initiation of sexual activity, failure to use adequate contraception, and, therefore, unintended pregnancy and sexually transmitted disease. This association has been repeatedly substantiated in studies in the USA. The US Panel on Adolescent Pregnancy and Childbearing (Hayes 1987) reported that 18 per cent of people between 14 and 21 years old lived in families with incomes well below the poverty level. Fifty-four per cent of families headed by single mothers lived at or below the poverty level. Sixty-six per cent of Black and Hispanic children under the age of 18 living in single parent families had incomes below the poverty level. The rise in the number of single female head-of-household families translates into the 'feminization and juvenilization' of poverty. More recently the Children's Defense Fund (1992) Report on *the health of children in America* states that the situation for poor women and children has worsened during the 1980s. In 1988, children under 18 represented nearly 40 per cent of the population living at or below the poverty line. Global figures for children aged 10–19 living at or below poverty are not available. Developing countries have reported that as many as 80 per cent of their adolescent females live in poverty.

Poverty is a significant factor contributing to poor educational achievement. In the USA, it is a more significant predictor of school drop-out than race or ethnicity. Failure to complete high school is associated with decreased economic opportunity and success, resulting in lower income and poorer health. Burstin *et al.* (1992) confirmed that the inability to pay for medical care significantly increases the likelihood of receiving substandard medical care due to physician negligence. The cycle of poverty is vicious and unrelenting.

Women living in poverty may resort to prostitution for their own survival and/or to support their families. They are less likely to use barrier method contraceptives, and more likely to contract sexually transmitted diseases (Padian 1988). Unintended pregnancies are common by-products of the failure to use contraception. Prostitution is prevalent where there is poverty, social upheaval, and where there is a double standard of sexual behavior, so that men are allowed greater sexual liberty than women (Day 1988). When a relatively small number of women are having sex with a large number of men, prostitution significantly contributes to the transmission of sexually transmitted diseases, including HIV infection. The urban poor of industrialized countries may become enmeshed in drug abuse, and therefore resort to prostitution to support their habit. Abuse of crack cocaine is strongly correlated with sexual behavior involving multiple sexual partners whether or not prostitution is used to support the habit (Schonberg 1992).

The relationship between poverty and poor nutritional status is well known. Growth retardation, chronic anemia, and higher lead levels have been more prevalent in low-income children (Royston and Armstrong 1989, p. 62). Poor nutritional status and chronic malnutrition contribute directly and indirectly to higher rates of maternal mortality and morbidity. Poor children are more likely to experience a more severe course of illness not only because of poor nutritional status, but also because of poor access to medical assistance, and delayed acquisition of medical care. A country entrenched in famine easily illustrates the relationship between poverty, nutritional status, and poor health. The plight of the inner-city poor, compared to the victims of famine in developing countries, is easy to ignore. The inner-city poor of developed countries, however, are just as vulnerable to poor nutrition and its consequences.

Education

Young women in developing countries have even less of an opportunity to pursue an education, therefore, even less of a chance to advance their economic standing. The value of a woman may be judged by the ability to have children, thereby advancing social status, if not economic standing. Teenage marriages are more common in developing countries, and result in higher fertility and adolescent pregnancy rates. Teenage marriages are most common in rural communities, especially within the countries of Asia, India, Africa, Bangladesh, and Latin America. Literacy and education are strongly correlated with delayed childbearing and lower maternal mortality rates (Royston and Armstrong 1989, p. 56). Approximately 70 per cent of women in developing countries are illiterate.

Industrialized countries, by comparison, have high levels of literacy and educational success, and lower fertility rates. Adolescents residing in these industrialized countries have experienced earlier onset of puberty, earlier initiation of intercourse, greater access to information on contraception and family planning, and delay in the age of marriage. The exception to this is the USA where, despite higher literacy rates and overall economic and educational success, the teenage pregnancy rate is 96 per 1000 females aged 15–19, compared with 14 per 1000 in the Netherlands. The pregnancy rate of adolescent American teenagers is twice that of Great Britain, France, and Canada, and three times that of Sweden (Jones *et al.* 1986).

Of the underestimated 13 million births per year to adolescents world-wide, the US adolescent population aged 15–19 accounts for approximately 1 million pregnancies per year. US adolescents have consistently contributed an average of 1 million pregnancies per year for the past 12 years. Adolescent pregnancies comprise 13 per cent of all births and 33 per cent of abortions performed in the USA. While the rate is higher than other industrialized countries, it is hardly an 'epidemic'. However, it is important to remember that while the majority of American teenagers do not become pregnant, 30 per cent of sexually active, never married teenagers are not using any contraception. An estimated three-quarters of pregnancies to unmarried American teenagers are unintended. Much has been written in an attempt to understand and diminish the occurrence of teenage pregnancy, yet accurate data on teenage sexual behavior is not available in the USA. Even as recently as 1991, the Secretary for Health and Human Services refused to sponsor a comprehensive survey of adolescent sexual behavior (Marshall 1991; Roberts 1991). Most of the available data on adolescent sexuality has been obtained by surveys of high school seniors, which necessarily excludes high-risk adolescents who are truant, who have already dropped out of school, or who are homeless or incarcerated.

Industrialized countries promote safe sex through liberal, accessible, and affordable education, coupled with widespread provision of affordable contraceptive services. The predominant attitude in these countries, excluding the

USA, is that all unintended pregnancies, including adolescent pregnancies, can be resolved through practical means, unencumbered by moralism. Sex education typically begins as early as the age of 10 years in many of these industrialized countries. The primary principle guiding US policy has been to decrease the incidence of teenage pregnancy by insisting teenagers refrain from sexual intercourse. The Guttmacher Institute (Singh and Wulf 1990) asserts that the reasons for high adolescent pregnancy rates in the USA are a consequence of government policy and cultural attitudes. Since the incidence of teenage pregnancy has not decreased dramatically over the last 12 years, this principle must be re-evaluated. The provision of sex education and family planning services has been shown to delay first sexual intercourse and to increase the likelihood that a contraceptive method will be employed during intercourse (Hardy and Zabin 1991). Similarly, it has been shown that government welfare assistance programs do not encourage adolescents to have children (Jones *et al.* 1986).

Abuse

An under-reported cause of intentional and unintentional injury for the adolescent female is physical, emotional, and sexual abuse. A 1988 study in the USA on child abuse and neglect reports that 25 per cent of all child abuse victims were between the ages of 12 and 17 years old. Finkelhor *et al.* (1990) found that 20–30 per cent of adult women and 16 per cent of adult men report having been sexually abused as children. Fifteen per cent of adolescent females have been sexually abused before the age of 16 years. All of these numbers are low estimates because of poor reporting by the victims and because, in many societies, these events are poorly documented. Finkelhor and Korbin (1988) assert that undoubtedly millions of cases of child abuse occur in areas where reporting is not institutionalized. Females account for up to 80 per cent of all sexual abuse victims. The mean age for females at time of the abusive episode is 10 years. Further examination reveals that the two peak ages when most abuse occurs are: 5–6 and 14–15 years.

It is difficult to obtain accurate numbers that reflect the world-wide prevalence of female battery. In the USA, a conservative estimate of 2 million women are beaten each year by a spouse or boyfriend. Newberger *et al.* (1992) estimates that 7–17 per cent of pregnant women are abused. The adolescent female is particularly vulnerable to sexual and physical abuse because of the developmental changes of puberty, growing sexual awareness, and tendency towards engaging in risk-taking behavior. Older males, such as relatives or acquaintances, are most often the perpetrators of the abuse. Half of all female rape victims are under the age of 18 years. Boyer and Fine (1992) suggested that sexual victimization and abuse have been overlooked as a potential key factor in promoting or provoking initiation of adolescent risk-taking sexual behavior, early initiation of intercourse, adolescent pregnancy, and repeat pregnancy. These investigators found that 62 per cent of adolescents who became pregnant reported a history of sexual abuse prior to their first pregnancy. The mean age of this study population was 17.6 years.

Genital mutilation

The traditional practices of female circumcision and gishri deserve special comment since both contribute to female adolescent morbidity and mortality (Royston and Armstrong 1989, p. 149). They directly and indirectly affect reproductive health, including pregnancy outcome and birth, acquisition of infectious diseases, such as human immunodeficiency virus (HIV) infection and acquired immune deficiency syndrome (AIDS), tetanus, and urinary tract infections. They can lead to long-term sequelae such as anal incontinence, recto-vaginal fistula formation, disfiguring keloid scar formation, depression, psychosis, and even suicide. Linke (1986) noted the association of HIV infection and AIDS with regions of Africa practising female circumcision. This practice is common in Africa; particularly southern Egypt, the Sudan, Somalia, Senegal, Mali, northern Kenya, and northern Nigeria, and has been documented in more than 26 African countries. Hosken (1983) states that, millions of continental African women have undergone the procedure. The practice continues to be widespread in these areas. Additional areas where the practice occurs include the southern Arab Peninsula and Persian Gulf, certain Moslem groups in Yemen, Bahrain, Oman, Pakistan, Jordan, Syria, Malaysia, Indonesia, and the Philippines. The practice has also been reported in Brazil, El Salvador, Peru, eastern Mexico, Australia, and in some sects in Russia. Women in Western Societies, including the USA have undergone female circumcision primarily as treatment for nymphomania, depression, or hysteria. France, Sweden, and Norway have taken strong measures to ban the practice altogether (Koso-Thomas 1986).

Female circumcision encompasses both simple clitoridectomy and excision of all or part of the labia minora, or majora, or both. The extreme form—infibulation—includes radical excision of the clitoris and vulva. The cut edges are then sutured with thorns, cat gut or sticky paste so that a small opening is left to allow passage of urine and menstrual blood. The woman's legs are then bound together for weeks until the wound has healed. However the genital mutilation is performed, it is usually considered a rite of passage for young girls aged between 10 and 14 years. The procedure may be performed on children as young as 4–8 years old, or even on infants a few days old. The procedure is usually performed without anesthesia, often with dull instruments or primitive objects such as broken glass. Intense pain and shock, hemorrhage, infection (tetanus, sepsis), and death are common immediate sequelae of the procedure. Broken bones may result when the girl struggles against her attendants. Poor cosmetic results may occur from incomplete wound healing or keloid scar formation. Adhesions, dyspareunia, obstructed birth fistula formation, hematocolpos, infertility, and anal or urinary incontinence are later sequelae. HIV infection may result from the use of unsanitized, instruments in sequentially performed procedures. Obliteration of the vaginal orifice promotes the practice of anal intercourse which further increases the risk of heterosexual transmission of HIV (Padian *et al.* 1987; European Study Group 1989).

Gishri involves incising the vaginal vault and/or orifice to widen the birth canal during childbirth. These incisions are also commonly performed with primitive tools, knives, or razor blades. Anesthesia is not usually employed during this procedure. This practice is largely confined to northern Nigeria (Trevitt 1973).

Female circumcision procedures flourish in areas where patriarchal societies seek to control the sexual behavior of females, especially where females are regarded as the property of males. Furthermore, where virginity is cherished, sex talk taboo, and illiteracy among females is high, economic incentives encourage families to have their young daughters undergo the procedure. These women have no power to voice their opinion or to resist or refuse the procedure. If they resist, they are ostracized from the community.

Recommendations to improve their health of female adolescents

There have been many interventions both world-wide and in individual countries which have directly and indirectly served to improve the health status of female adolescents. It is clear that no one intervention or management plan will serve all communities throughout the world in the effort to improve conditions for female adolescents. The following recommendations stress the importance of women's rights as the means by which to improve the health status world-wide.

Women's rights

A document entitled *World plan of action* was assembled during the Women's International Conference which convened in 1975 and was sponsored by the United Nations. This document highlighted the important role women serve as homemaker, parent, and spouse, and thereby affirmed the need to improve the status of women on a global basis. The *World plan of action* designated the decade 1975–1985 as the 'international decade of women.' Efforts were made by participants in the UN's call to action to increase global awareness about the effects of sex discrimination on the health and economic status of women, and the health of families. The importance of advancing the educational status of women was also stressed. Guidelines to assist governments to these ends were delineated. The international decade of women led to the development of another document entitled, *Forward looking strategies for the advancement of women to the year 2000*. This document further promoted the importance of women's economic contribution to society, encouraged governments to provide adequate childcare to working parents, especially for the urban poor, and to provide adequate support, in both time and money, of maternity leave. The UN later held a separate convention calling for the elimination of all forms of discrimination against women, especially in the areas of employment, wages, benefits, and social security. Guidelines were established to help countries eliminate job discrimination for women.

If there were any one identifiable intervention that would improve the health status of adolescent females, it would be to genuinely implement the principles that were put forth in these documents.

Germain and Ordway (1989) of the International Women's Health Coalition emphasize that placing women at the center of reproductive health would strengthen family planning and health programs, and in the process help women attain dignity, health, and basic human rights. Advancing the health status of women necessarily involves human rights, not simply because women are childbearers and child rearers, but also because women are the equal of men. Women are not property to be traded, discarded, or abused. Barzelatto (1990) strongly supports dialog between feminist groups and health professionals in order to improve the reproductive health of all women. The Ford Foundation (1991) has strongly supported this approach in their 1990 program stategy on reproductive health.

Children's rights

Promoting global respect and support of women's rights in an effort to improve the health status of adolescent females is the most straightforward method by which to achieve this goal. Attention must also be given towards improving the circumstances in which children live. Promoting the rights of children on a global basis is strongly supported by the United Nations and WHO. The Children's Defense Fund in the USA serves as a strong advocate for children's rights. A children's bill of rights has long been supported by this and other organizations in the USA, such as the American Academy of Pediatrics, the National Education Association, and the Parent Teacher Association. Building coalitions such as these can force a change in public policy. There is currently no national policy on adolescent health despite the three-volume report by the US Congress Office of Technology Assistance on adolescent health issued in 1991. Such a policy would need to ensure access to and provision of medical care, adequate nutrition and housing, and quality education, including sex education. It would also have to provide for protection from abuse and violence.

Education

Interventions must be multidimensional. Increasing access to, and support of, general educational pursuits and job-training skills for female children advances the social status and self-image of women. Quality education must be legally protected and guaranteed. Job-training programs should not be limited to instruction in domestic or manual labor. While there is no overnight solution for the abolition of poverty, education provides the means by which female children and adolescents can become familiar with life-style options, become familiar with the basic biology of their own bodies, make their own decisions, and voice their own opinions. In some societies, however, a female child with an independent mind is not valued. Socio-cultural obstacles contribute to systems whereby female children fail to receive equal education. As developing countries become more like industrialized countries, these obstacles will be surmounted. In the meantime, consistent effort must be made to support equal education and employment opportunities for adolescent females throughout the world.

Sex education, family planning, and contraceptive services

Preventing unintended pregnancy should be a primary goal. Sex education and the provision of affordable contraceptive services allow women to control their own reproductive potential and prevent or diminish the acquisition of sexually transmitted diseases. Provision of contraceptive information and services delays the age of first coitus, delays the age of first marriage, and promotes the use of contraceptives when there is coitus. Hardy and Zabin (1991) make a strong argument to these ends in their treatise on adolescent pregnancy in the urban environment. Kirby (1985) and Marsiglio and Mott (1986) illustrate how integrated and comprehensive school- and community-based sex education leads to lower rates of adolescent pregnancy by delaying the start of sexual activity and promoting consistent use of contraception.

In many developing countries there are programs which promote family planning education through the efforts of native community outreach workers and health educators at local family planning or community health centers. The grassroots of health promotion is education, whether by individual community outreach worker, health educator, or by consistent attendance at primary and secondary schools. While education is universally recognized as important in improving the health status of females, it is not universally provided. Roemer and Paxman (1985) concluded that 'the process of education go forward for health reasons, if for no other.'

Uniform definition of terms and enhanced data collection

The current failure to collect data on the young adolescent age group often results in poorly designed health policy and programs that do not adequately target the problems that these adolescents encounter. Expanding data collection to include the early adolescent in the usual statistics compiled for the adolescent period will enhance the ability of health policy and program development to adjust to the demands of the future. Data collection should include accurate information on reproductive behavior of 10–19 year olds, broken down into 10–12, 14–16, and 17–19 age groups. An accurate picture of adolescent sexual behavior will result in programs which address the true needs of this population. Ennew and Milne (1990) assert that 10–12 year olds are least visible in current statistics and are the group least known in any country. They emphasize that combining statistics on 10–12 year olds with the 15 year and older age groups ignores physical, sexual, social, and emotional differences between these age groups. Accurate information about adolescents categorized by age groups will enhance efforts to change behaviors and improve outcomes. This may obviate the temptation to yield to moralistic approaches, especially when the goal is to decrease the occurrence of adolescent pregnancy and reduce the prevalence of sexually transmitted disease.

Equally important is the need to report accurately female adolescent deaths. Direct and indirect causes of death related to pregnancy and childbirth should be accurately recorded on death certificates. Accurately registering a death implies regard for that individual as a worthwhile human being; acknowledging a woman's death and clarifiying the cause of that death validates her birth and intrinsic worth to society. Clarifying these causes of death will help direct program intervention to minimize their occurrence.

Defining an adolescent mortality rate, similar to the infant mortality rate, will help to focus international attention on this age group and provide objective evidence on whether improvements in health status have been accomplished. Furthermore, the adolescent mortality rate should be subdivided into the different age groups of early, middle, and late adolescents, and uniformly categorized by cause of death. This will facilitate identification of age-related global trends in specific causes of death, and thereby direct program strategy and policy interventions to better target the health needs of this population.

Medico-legal interventions

Adequate medical services must be made accessible and affordable, whether the pregnancy is continued or terminated. This implies that basic reproductive medical services be provided in a network of primary care clinics located within a reasonable distance from home. Strengthening the existing network may be the important task in some communities, whereas helping to establish a network of primary care services would be the primary goal in other communities. Wherever primary care services are strengthened or established, they should be provided with an attitude of respect and genuine concern for the adolescent females who attend these facilities. In addition, greater use of trained traditional birth attendants and certified nurse–midwives will augment obstetric services currently provided in isolated rural communities as well as in inner-city poor neighborhoods.

World-wide legalization of abortion and widespread provision of accessible, affordable abortion services would result in lower maternal mortality rates for all women, not just adolescent females. These services may best be provided at more regional or secondary care facilities, where strict adherence to proper medical procedure and sanitation is assured. The role of RU-486 in primary care facilities has yet to be explored and defined.

In addition to providing accessible and adequate contraceptive, abortion, and obstetrical services, global attention must be paid to efforts to diminish violence and injury. It is impossible to condone or permit female battery. The USA has several projects under way to diminish domestic violence, as well as to reduce adolescent deaths from interpersonal violence and unintentional injury (Prothrow-Stith 1986; Prothrow-Stith *et al.* 1987).

Raising the legal age of teenage marriage would diminish the occurrence of childbearing at a young age. Progress has been made to this end; however, there still exist developing countries where teenage marriages involve females as young as age 12. Given the varied cultural traditions world-wide, it would be futile to attempt to abolish completely teenage marriage.

Finally, establishing and implementing strong international regulations to outlaw female circumcision and gishri would significantly diminish morbidity and mortality for young females. The UN and WHO in separate conferences held in 1979, condoned efforts to eradicate female genital mutilations via legislation and coordinated health education and health care programs. The need to eradicate these procedures was again highlighted in 1988, during an international seminar held in Mogadishu, Somalia. Participants formulated a plan that would involve religious leaders and organize local health educators in the campaign against female genital mutilation. They also stressed the importance of international solidarity and financial support to ensure the success of their campaign. International solidarity and financial support of these efforts in conjunction with active participation of women directly affected by these practices could eradicate genital mutilation within the next decade.

Promoting male responsibility for family planning and childcare

The responsibility for contraception, pregnancy, and childrearing cannot rest solely on women. Comprehensive sex education and family planning services must actively reach out and be made available to all men, not just adolescent males since the majority of fathers of teen pregnancy are older than age 20 (Hardy and Zabin 1991, p. 102). Greater responsibility by the fathers of teen pregnancy to provide financial and emotional support for mother and child should be emphasized world-wide. Several programs in the USA are currently addressing these issues (Hardy and Zabin, p. 359; Hayes 1987). Some include classes on parenting and child rearing, especially for fathers of teen pregnancy.

Conclusion

The task of adolescence is uniform throughout the world; the ability to avoid major morbidity and mortality and enter adulthood in good health is the challenge. Female adolescents, regardless of their country of residence, experience greater difficulty meeting this challenge because of sexual discrimination, socioeconomic status, and their reproductive capabilities. The challenge is formidable but it is possible to effect major changes and ease the difficulties female adolescents confront in their daily lives. Statistics should incorporate the adolescent mortality rate, subdivided by early, middle, and late age groups, in quality assurance and outcomes analysis of female adolescent service programs. The recommendations suggested here also address issues of rights, namely the rights of women and the rights of children, the importance of education, and the needs to emphasize and strengthen family planning and contraception services, and to improve access to medical care. The responsibility men have towards this end cannot be overstated. The health status of female adolescents can be improved the world over if these socio-economic interventions are genuinely implemented, and coupled with a global change in attitude and priorities.

References

Barzelatto, J. (1990). Comments. In *Special challenges in Third World women's health*, pp. 29–33, presented at the 117th meeting of the American Public health Association, Chicago, IL October 1989. International Women's Health Coalition, New York.

Blum, R. (1991). Global trends in adolescent health. *Journal of the American Medical Association*, **265**, 2711–9.

Boyer, D. and Fine, D. (1992). Sexual abuse as a factor in adolescent pregnancy and child maltreatment. *Family Planning Perspectives*, **24**, 4–11.

Burstin, H., Lipsitz, S., and Brennan, T. (1992). Socioeconomic status and risk for substandard medical Care. *Journal of the American Medical Association*, **268**, 2383–7.

Chen, L. C., Gesche, M. C., Ahmed, S., Chowdhury, A. I., and Moseley, W. H. (1974). Maternal mortality in rural Bangladesh. *Studies in Family Planning*, **5**, 334–41.

Children's Defense Fund (1992). *The Health of America's Children: 1992*. Washington DC.

Day, S. (1988). Prostitute women and AIDS: anthropology. *AIDS*, **2**, 421–8.

Diekstra, R. (1989). Suicidal behavior in adolescence and young adults: the international picture. *Crisis*, **10**, 16–35.

Ennew, J. and Milne, B. (1990). *The next generation: lives of third world children*. New Society Publishers, Philadelphia, PA.

European Study Group (1989). Risk factors for male to female transmission of HIV. *British Medical Journal*, **298**, 411–5.

Fingerhut, L. A. and Kleinman, J. C. (1989). Trends and current status in childhood mortality, United States 1900–1985. *Vital and Health Statistics*, Series 3, No. 26. DHHS Publication No. (PHS) 89–1410. National Center for Health Statistics, US Government Printing Office, Washington DC.

Fingerhut, L. A. and Kleinman, J. C. (1990). International and interstate comparison of homicide among young males. *Journal of the American Medical Association*, **236**, 3292–5.

Finkelhor, D., Hotaling, G., Lewis, I. A., and Smith, C. (1990). Sexual abuse in a national survey of adult men and women: prevalence, characteristics, and risk factors. *Child Abuse and Neglect*, **14**, 19–28.

Finkelhor, D. and Korbin, J. (1988). Child abuse as an international issue. *Child Abuse and Neglect*, **12**, 3–23.

Ford Foundation (1991). *Reproductive health: a strategy for the 1990s*. Ford Foundation, New York.

Friede, A., Baldwin, W., Rhodes, P., Buehles, J., Strauss, L., Smith, J., and Hogue, C. (1987). Young maternal age and infant mortality: the role of low birth weight. *Public Health Reports*, **102**, 192–9.

Germain, A. and Ordway. K. (1989). *Population control and women's health: balancing the scales*. International Women's Health Coalition, New York.

Hardy, J. and Zabin, L. (1991). *Adolescent pregnancy in urban environment: issues, programs and evaluation*. Urban and Schwarzenberg, Baltimore.

Harrison, K. A. (1985). Childbearing health and social priorities. A survey of 22774 consecutive births in Zaira, northern Nigeria. *British Journal of Obstetrics and Gynecology*, **92**, (Suppl. 5), pp. 1–119.

Hayes, C. (ed.) (1987). *Risking the future: adolescent sexuality, pregnancy, and childbearing*, Vol. 2. National Academy Press, Washington DC.

Hosken, F. (1983). *Hosken report: genital and sexual mutilation of females* (3rd edn). WIN News, Lexington, MA.

Jones, E. F., Forrest, J. D., Goldman, N., Henshaw, S., Lincoln, R., Rosoff, J. I., *et al.* (1986). *Teenage pregnancy in industrialized countries*, pp. 64–65, 239–240. Yale University Press, New Haven, CT.

Kirby, D. (1985). Sexuality education: a more realistic view of its effects. *Journal of School Health*, **55**, 421–4.

Koso-Thomas, O. (1986). *The circumcision of women: a strategy for eradication*. Zed Press, London, UK.

Lee, K., and Corpuz, M. (1988). Teenage pregnancy: trend and impact on rates of low birth weight and fetal, maternal and neonatal mortality in the United States. *Clinics in Perinatology*, **15**, 929–42.

Linke, U. (1986). AIDS in Africa (Letter). *Science*, **231**, 203.

Marshall, E. (1991). Sullivan overrules NIH on sex survey (news). *Science*, **253**, 502.

Marsiglio, W. and Mott, F. L. (1986). The impact of education on sexual activity, contraceptive use, and premarital pregnancy among American teenagers. *Family Planning Perspectives*, **18**, 151–62.

Moerman, M. L. (1982). Growth of the birth canal in adolescent girls. *American Journal of Obstetrics and Gynecology*, **143**, 528–32.

Neinstein, L. S. (1991). *Adolescent health care: a practical guide*, (2nd edn). Urban and Schwarzenberg, Baltimore.

Newberger, E. H., Barken, S. E., Lieberman, E. S., McCormick, M. C., Yllo, K., Gary, L. T., *et al.* (1992). Abuse of pregnant women and adverse birth outcome: current knowledge and implication for practice. *Journal of the American Medical Association*, **267**, 2370–2.

Padian, N., Marquis, L., Francis, D. P., Anderson, R. E., Rutherford, G. W., O'Malley, P. M., *et al.* (1987). Male to female transmission of Human Immunodeficiency Virus. *Journal of the American Medical Association*, **258**, 788–90.

Padian, N. S. (1988). Prostitute women and AIDS: epidemiology. *AIDS*, **2**, 413–9.

Prothrow-Stith, D. (1986). Interdisciplinary interventions applicable to prevention of interpersonal violence and homicide in black youth. In *Surgeon General's Workshop in Violence and Public Health*, pp. 35–43. US Department of Health and Human Services, Publication HRS-D-MC86-1, Washington DC.

Prothrow-Stith, D., Spivak, H., and Hauman, A. J. (1987). The violence prevention project: a public health approach. *Science Technology and Human Values*, **12**, 67–9.

Roberts, J. (1991). American sex survey cancelled. *British Medical Journal*, **303**, 263.

Rochat, R. W. (1981). Maternal mortality in the United States of America. *World Health Statistics Quarterly*, **34**, 2–13.

Roemer, R. and Paxman, J. (1985). Sex education laws and policies. *Studies in Family Planning*, **16**, 219–30.

Royston, E. and Armstrong, S. (ed.) (1989). *Preventing maternal deaths*, pp. 30–74, 79–82, 149–50, 187, 200–2. World Health Organization, Geneva.

Schonberg, S. K. (1992). Substance use and abuse. In *Textbook of Adolescent Medicine*, (ed. E. McAnarney, R. Kreipe, D. Orr, and G. Comerci), pp. 1063–77. W. B. Saunders, Philadelphia.

Singh, S. and Wulf, D. (1990). *Today's adolescents, tomorrow's parents: a portrait of the Americas*. Alan Guttmacher Institute, New York.

Starrs, A. (1987). *Preventing the tragedy of maternal deaths: a report on the international safe motherhood conference*, pp. 4–55. World Bank Publications, Washington, DC.

Strasberger, V. and Brown, R. (ed.) (1991). *Adolescent health. A practical guide*, pp. 1–10. Little Brown, Boston.

Taket, A. (1986). Accidental mortality in children, adolescents and young adults. *WHO Statistics Quarterly*, **39**, 232–56.

Trevitt, L. (1973). Attitudes and customs among the Hausa in Zaire City, *Savanna*, **2**, 223–6.

United Nations (1975). *World Plan of Action*. United Nations World Conference of the International Women's Year, adopted at Mexico City July, 1975.

United Nations (1985). *Forward looking strategies to the year 2000*. Adopted at Nairobi, Kenya, July 1985 (Paragraphs 59 and 73).

United Nations (1987*a*). *World contraceptive use. 1987 data sheet*. Department of International Economic and Social Affairs, Population Division, New York.

United Nations (1987*b*). *Fertility behavior in the context of development: evidence from the World Fertility Survey*. Department of Economic and Social Affairs, New York.

United Nations (1989). *Demographic Yearbook 1987*. United Nations, New York.

UNESCO (1991). *Adolescence education*. UNESCO, Bangkok.

US Bureau of Census (1984). *Projections of the population of the United States by age, sex and race: 1983–2080*. Current Population Reports, series P-25, No. 952. US Government Printing Office, Washington DC.

US Bureau of Census (1989). *Money, income and poverty status in the United States: 1988*. Current Population Reports, series P-60, No. 66. US Printing Office, Washington DC.

US Bureau of Census (1990). *United States population estimates by age, sex, race and Hispanic origin: 1989*. Current Population Reports, series P-25, No. 1057. US Printing Office, Washington DC.

WHO (1986*a*). *Young people's health: A challenge for society. Technical Report 731*. World Health Organization, Geneva.

WHO (1986*b*). *Maternal mortality rates: a tabulation of available information*, pp. 1–3, (2nd ed). World Health Organization, Geneva.

WHO (1987). *Evaluation of the strategy for health for all by the year 2000*. Seventh report on the world health situation. Vol. 1: *Global Overview*, pp. 41, 74–75. World Health Organization, Geneva.

WHO (1989). *The health of youth*. World Health Organization, Geneva.

4 Sexually transmitted diseases

Willard Cates, Jr

Introduction

Just as syphilis predominated in the beginning of the twentieth century, sexually transmitted diseases (STDs) remain a major international public health priority in its last decade (Holmes *et al.* 1990). Trends in STDs are important indicators of both high-risk sexual behavior and the adequacy of control programs in both developed and developing countries. Variations in STD prevalence serve to monitor the effectiveness of our public policies, especially strategies aimed at the human immunodeficiency virus (HIV). This chapter will emphasize the epidemiologic patterns of STDs, their historic perspective, their impact on the health of women and children, the role of diagnosis and treatment in prevention, and current ethical problems in controlling STDs.

Epidemiology

Data on STDs

Estimates of the incidence and prevalence of STDs vary according to the source of data (Rothenberg 1990). Sources generally include diseases reportable to official health agencies (such as gonorrhea and syphilis in most industrialized countries), visits to office-based practices (for example, The National Drug and Therapeutic Index in the USA), national surveys of representative populations (NHANES in the USA), and data on patients attending specialized health facilities (such as STD clinics, family planning clinics).

Unfortunately, each of these sources has limitations. Data on reported diseases are affected by the completeness of reporting, and differences exist between public and private health care sources. Therefore, the data are susceptible

Table 4.1 Estimated levels of sexually transmitted diseases, USA, 1993

STD	Estimated annual incidence	Estimated cumulative prevalence
Syphilis	30 000 (P/S) 113 000 (all stages)	1.5 million
Gonorrhea	800 000	–
Chlamydia	4 million	–
Genital herpes (first visits)	300 000	31 million (HSV)
Genital warts (first visits)	800 000	45 million (HPV)
Hepatitis B (sexually transmitted)	53 000	–
Human immunodeficiency virus	70 000	1 million

Abbreviations: P/S, primary and secondary; HSV, herpes simplex virus; HPV, human papillomavirus
Source: updated from Cates (1990), Division of STD/HIV Prevention (1994)

to biases caused by characteristics of people who tend to use public clinics. Likewise, data from private physicians' practices are generally affected by the absence of laboratory diagnostic validation. National surveys are limited by their sporadic nature and the superficial nature of the analytic variables. Finally, data from specific health facilities suffer from the problem of patient selection bias, as well as geographic differences. Therefore, interpretations of trends need to be undertaken cautiously (Quinn and Cates 1992).

In developing countries, data sources have even more limitations (WHO 1989; Wasserheit 1989; Meheus *et al.* 1990). Few developing nations have rudimentary national surveillance systems. Therefore, STD incidence is derived from attendance at health care facilities, and prevalence is extrapolated from studies performed on selected populations. Although these data provide useful estimates, they must be viewed with even more caution than reports from the developed world.

Data on specific STDs also vary by the type of infection (Division of STD/HIV Prevention 1994), depending on whether the measure is current or previous infections. On the basis of estimates from the USA (Table 4.1), syphilis has a much lower incidence—and even cumulative prevalence—than other bacterial STDs, probably because STD control programs have targeted this infection. Symptomatic viral infections (measured by physician visits) occur less frequently than serologic or cytologic indicators of the cumulative number of infected persons. Thus, care must also be used in making comparisons among the different measures.

Epidemiology of STDs in developed countries

In North America and Europe, the incidence of genital chlamydial infections and viral STDs steadily increased during the 1970s and 1980s, while the incidence of gonorrhea generally declined during the same interval (Cates 1990). Depending on the individual country, levels of syphilis have varied among different population subgroups.

Syphilis is the STD about which we have the most consistent information and which is most amenable to traditional control measures (Cates *et al.* in press). In developed countries, syphilis incidence rose during the Second World War, but began to decline thereafter, coinciding with the introduction of penicillin. The lowest levels were observed at the end of the 1950s, but from the 1960s on, syphilis trends increased. The rapidly rising male : female ratio characterized the spread of syphilis among homosexuals throughout the 1970s.

However, in the 1980s, syphilis rates among gay men declined precipitously probably indicating safer sexual behaviors stimulated by HIV prevention messages. Simultaneously, in the USA and other developed countries with heterogeneous populations, syphilis rates climbed during the mid-1980s among heterosexuals of minority races. These trends in subpopulations were initially obscured by crude data. When the data were stratified by gender and race, the increases in heterosexual syphilis among Black men and women in the USA had actually begun in 1986, even though they were not recognized by public health authorities until a full year later.

Gonorrhea trends have been consistent among the developed countries. Gonorrhea generally increased in the 1960s, and then declined at different times in different countries during the 1970s. In the USA most of the decline occurred among older, white populations, with gonorrhea rates remaining high among minority races and adolescents. The male : female ratio was lower than with syphilis, indicating that a larger proportion of gonorrhea was being transmitted among heterosexuals. In addition, among all gender and race categories, gonorrhea patients have a younger mean age than do syphilis patients.

Chlamydia infections became recognized as the most prevalent bacterial STD in the developed world in the 1970s, at the time that gonorrhea trends began declining. Chlamydia is not a universally reported infection, so syndromes have been used as proxies to monitor trends. In the UK and the USA, diagnoses of non-gonococcal urethritis exceeded those of gonorrhea in the early 1970s, with the gap widening in recent years (Division of STD/HIV Prevention 1994). In one rural Candian province, active surveillance showed rates of chlamydia nearly three times higher than gonorrhea (Alary *et al.* 1989). In all industrialized countries, chlamydial infections among women exceed those among men. Moreover, chlamydial prevalence is strongly correlated with younger age and heterosexual orientation.

Sexually transmitted viral infections are widespread within the developed countries. In the UK and the USA, the numbers of symptomatic cases of genital herpes and genital warts increased 5–15-fold during the 1970s and 1980s (WHO 1989; Division of STD/HIV Prevention 1994). In the developed world, symptomatic genital herpes causes over ten times more cases of genital ulcer than does syphilis. Moreover, recent investigations have shown that symptomatic herpes simplex virus (HSV) infections are only the tip of the iceberg (Johnson

Table 4.2 STD control in selected countries

	Australia	Poland	UK	USA
Estimated percentage GNP for health expenditures %	7	2	7	11
Crude estimate percentage GNP for STD control %	0.003	0.002	?	0.003
Reported rates (per 100 000)				
Gonorrhea	48	20	142	400
Early syphilis	16	3.2	1.8	12

Abbreviation: GNP, gross national product
Source: Hart *et al.* (1990)

et al. 1989; Koutsky *et al.* 1992). An estimated 31 million Americans have been infected with HSV-2, even though less than one-quarter preceive themselves ever to have had genital herpes.

Likewise, the diagnosis of both symptomatic and asymptomatic genital warts caused by the human papillomavirus (HPV) has been skyrocketing in the developed world during the last two decades (WHO 1989; Division of STD/HIV Prevention 1994). HPV infections of the cervix have emerged as the most common STD among sexually active adolescents. Since no serologic test is available to determine previous infections, and HPV cannot be recovered through tissue culture, determining the full extent of these infections is difficult. However, polymerase chain reaction testing demonstrates that up to half of sexually active young women have evidence of HPV infection (Bauer *et al.* 1991).

Comparative estimates of the scale of the STD problem have been presented for four developed countries (Hart *et al.* 1990): Australia, Poland, the UK, and the USA (Table 4.2). Despite consistent percentages of health resources being devoted to STD control, the reported rates of gonorrhea and early syphilis were remarkably different. In these countries, the discrepancies between expenditures and rates of STD were apparently due to differences in the composition of the populations, the sexual behaviors of these populations, the system of delivering health care, and the effectiveness of STD interventions.

Epidemiology of STDs in developing countries

The epidemiology of STDs in developing countries differs greatly from the situation in industrialized nations (WHO 1989; Cates 1990). First, STDs overall are a more frequent health problem in developing countries. For example, they are among the top five causes of consultation at health services in Cameroon, which is representative of many African countries; among adults, an STD is the leading

Table 4.3 Prevalence of sexually transmitted diseases among pregnant women in developing countries in the 1980s

	Percentage positive		
Country	Syphilis (TPHA/FTA/Abs)*	Gonorrhea (culture)	Chlamydia (culture)
Cameroon	–	14.5	–
Central Africa Republic	9.5	9.5	–
Ethiopia	16.9	–	–
Kenya	–	6.6	29.0
Gambia	11.0	6.7	6.9
Gabon	–	5.5	9.9
Ghana	–	3.1	–
Malaysia	2.0	0.5	–
Malawi	13.7	–	–
Mozambique	6.3	–	–
Nigeria	2.1	5.2	6.5
Saudi Arabia	0.9	–	–
Somalia	3.0	–	–
South Africa	20.8	11.7	12.5
Swaziland	33.3	3.9	–
Tanzania	16.4	6.0	–
Zambia	12.5	11.3	–
Zaire	2.0	–	–
Zimbabwe	–	7.0	9.9

*Specific syphilis serologic tests
Sources: WHO (1989) and Wasserheit (1989)

diagnosis (Meheus *et al.* 1990). Second, cases of STDs among homosexuals are less common in the developing world. Third, among the STDs, bacterial genital ulcer disease occurs at higher relative frequency. Syphilis and chancroid are the major causes of genital ulcers in tropical countries, with genital herpes accounting for a smaller proportion.

Syphilis in developing countries remains at levels seen half a century ago. The interpretation of serological tests for syphilis is difficult since seropositivity could be due to this sexually transmitted infection, or to a previous infection with non-venereal treponematoses. When these limitations are taken into account, rates of past syphilis infections among pregnant women in the developing countries have ranged from 1 per cent in Saudi Arabia to 33 per cent in Swaziland (Table 4.3). In one population of rural Somalia, nearly one-quarter of men and women in the general population had evidence of past syphilis (WHO

1989). Thus, syphilis is highly prevalent in many developing countries, and the risk of congenital syphilis is high in many areas.

Gonorrhea, like syphilis, is more prevalent in the developing world than in industrialized countries. Estimates for large cities in Africa suggest an annual rate of gonorrhea from 3000 to 10 000 cases per 100 000 inhabitants. These frequencies have been extrapolated mainly from attendance at general health care centers or from special surveys of prevalence in selected populations. Surveys of gonorrhea in pregnant women have ranged from less than 1 per cent in Malaysia to 40 per cent in Uganda (Table 4.3). Among women attending family planning clinics, rates have ranged from 2 per cent in Swaziland to 17 per cent in Kenya.

Genital chlamydial infections are highly prevalent in both the developing and developed worlds. Among pregnant women, chlamydial infections are more frequent than gonococcal, with rates ranging from 6 per cent in Nigeria to 29 per cent in Kenya (Table 4.3). Among men with symptoms of urethritis, rates of non-gonococcal infection appear to be lower than in the developed world. However, because chlamydia causes less severe infections, both women and men may not seek treatment in areas where health care is difficult to obtain.

Chancroid is highly endemic in many tropical countries, in particular Southeast Asia and eastern and southern Africa. The global incidence of chancroid is probably equivalent to that of syphilis, and interest in this STD has heightened because of the recent availability of a selective media for isolation of *Haemophilus ducreyi*, its etiologic agent. As in the developed world, prostitues play a crucial role in the spread of chancroid in developing countries.

Interpretation

In most industrialized countries, the incidence of classical STDs such as gonorrhea and syphilis declined rapidly during the 1980s among the middle and upper classes; in North America, however, the incidence of the same diseases increased within low-income, minority populations, which are the most difficult to reach with traditional community health education messages. In the developing world, the absence of any national commitment to reducing levels of STDs, even in the face of the HIV epidemic, has allowed high levels of all such diseases to continue in these populations.

History

Social attitudes

Throughout history, STDs have caused society to wrestle with its moral feelings about this public health problem. In recent years, the human tragedies suffered by people with STDs have led to more effective social and political responses designed to interrupt transmission and reduce complications, rather than to stigmatize those with disease.

Before 1900, physicians were known to withhold treatment for STDs, fatalistically regarding infection as evidence of (and even punishment for) 'promiscuous' behavior (Brandt 1985). Prior to the First World War, the increasing professionalization of medicine coincided with the rise of venereology as an established specialty. Syphilis became the disease upon which the skills of twentieth-century physicians were judged. Knowledge in this field rapidly progressed from acceptance of the germ theory, to fascination with serologic tests, to use of toxic cures. The foundations were laid for a medical, rather than a moralistic, approach to STD control.

In USA during the New Deal era, Surgeon General Thomas Parran seized an opportunity to dramatize the plight of those with STDs. With the availability of penicillin and the national imperative of winning a war, the image of these diseases shed a portion of its stigmatic cloak during the 1940s. Sexually transmitted infections could be diagnosed and treated on an out-patient basis, thus allowing a more convenient approach toward finding and treating both patients and partners.

Finally, during recent decades, the changing social roles of women and minorities and the greater acceptance of homosexuality have been accompanied by a slow shift in the developed world's attitude toward human sexuality. The population at risk of STDs increased, creating a growing constituency that demands personal and public health solutions. Feminists, realizing that women and children bear the brunt of the sexually related complications, became increasingly active in politics. Homosexual organizations, spurred by the availability of a hepatitis B vaccine and the tragedy of HIV and acquired immunodeficiency syndrome (AIDS), lobbied for a greater share of resources being directed to their health concerns. Finally, those interested in minority health are increasingly acknowledging STDs and HIV as priorities for their constituency. Thus, society has apparently become more concerned about STDs as the scope of the problem has increased and public health interventions have become more available.

STD control programs

Current public health approaches to STDs and HIV greatly resemble those used for syphilis in the preantibiotic era. In the USA, national programs to control STDs were established during the early days of the First World War (Brandt 1985). For the next half century, the focus was almost exclusively on the control of syphilis and its complications. Diagnosis was complex, and treatments were dangerous; these factors stimulated the continued development of the specialty of venereology. Federal grants to support venereal disease control initiatives were begun in 1939. Treatment centers for syphilis and gonorrhea were eventually established to cure the large number of people with these infections identified during the Second World War screening programs.

After World War II, the widespread availability of penicillin led to a dismantling of the treatment centers and a decline of the clinical specialty of venereology. However, particularly during the 1960s, federal assistance continued to support of tracing sex partner, serologic testing for syphilis, and health education of patients. The STD 'epidemiologist', who focused on locating and treating people exposed to syphilis, emerged as a central figure in syphilis control efforts.

By the late 1960s, officials became concerned with the rapidly escalating number of gonorrhea cases. The gonorrhea epidemic, together with the development of selective culture media for isolating the gonococcus, stimulated the implementation of a national strategy to control gonorrhea. Beginning in 1968, pilot projects had been initiated to evaluate case-finding of infected women, both by using culture diagnosis and by identifying sex partners of infected men. During the 1970s, gonorrhea control gradually received a larger portion of the STD federal grant, at the expense of syphilis control. By 1980, expenditures for gonorrhea control accounted for almost three-quarters of federal STD grants.

Simultaneously, the growing variety and recognition of other syndromes causing patients to seek care produced a need for major improvements in clinical skills, clinic services, and physical facilities (Holmes *et al.* 1990). This upgrading was necessary both to encourage infected people to obtain treatment and to provide additional capability to diagnose the broad array of STDs. Once again, technological change required hard choices. In the 1980s, increased availability of laboratory diagnostic testing for chlamydial infection created opportunities for chlamydia control, requiring further trade-offs among resources primarily directed to gonorrhea and syphilis control. By the late 1980s, the need to provide testing and counseling for people with HIV infection had placed additional demands on STD personnel and facilities and contributed to a delay in implementing chlamydia control programs.

In addition, the role of the so-called STD core group in sustaining high levels of these infections within communities is better understood (Brunham 1991). Mathematical models have demonstrated that endemicity of various STDs can be sustained by a relatively small subgroup of the population engaging in high-risk sexual practices with a large number of partners. This concept has been supported by considerable empiric evidence showing the entrenchment of particular gonococcal strains in demographically and behaviorally identifiable subgroups within cities such as Rochester, New York; Miami, Florida; Colorado Springs, Colorado; Seattle, Washington; and Baltimore, Maryland. Similar patterns for syphilis have been demonstrated in New York State and Oregon (Cates *et al.* in press). Recent investigations have highlighted the role of illicit drugs—especially the exchange of sex for crack cocaine—as a factor both enlarging the core population and facilitating high-risk sexual behaviors (Turner *et al.* 1989).

Effect on women

Recent trends in STDs have serious implications for reproductive health. To begin with, chlamydia and gonorrhea influence the chances of becoming pregnant. Moreover, virtually every organism that is sexually transmitted can be passed to the fetus or infant—often with tragic consequences.

Pelvic inflammatory disease

The term pelvic inflammatory disease (PID) has come to represent clinically suspected endometritis, salpingitis, or both, that has not been objectively confirmed pathologically or visually (Kahn *et al.* 1991). This diagnosis is usually made in sexually active women who complain of lower abdominal pain and are found to have cervical motion and uterine or adnexal tenderness or both. Laparoscopy has helped clarify the relationship between clinical PID and upper genital tract infection. Approximately two-thirds of women with a clinical diagnosis of PID have laparoscopically evident salpingitis.

Investigations over the past decade have emphasized the polymicrobial nature of PID. In general, three major groups of microorganisms play an etiologic role: *Neisseria gonorrhoeae, Chlamydia trachomatis*, and a wide variety of anaerobic and aerobic bacteria. A leading hypothesis is that *N. gonorrhoeae* and *C. trachomatis* initiate tubal infection and that anaerobic and aerobic bacteria from the cervix and vagina are secondary invaders (Cates and Wasserheit 1991). Recent studies have identified bacterial vaginosis as a risk factor for PID (Eschenbach *et al.* 1988). The organisms involved in bacterial vaginosis are similar to the non-gonococcal, non-chlamydial bacteria frequently isolated from the upper genital tract in women with acute PID.

The rate at which gonococcal and chlamydial organisms have been recovered in patients with symptomatic PID varies widely, probably because of differences among the populations studied, differences in the time during which the investigations took place, and variations in the severity of infection. *N. gonorrhoeae* has a particularly wide range of recovery rates among women with PID. In some European locations, the organism is cultured from less than 10 per cent of these women, whereas in some urban southern American populations with PID *N. gonorrhoeae* has been cultured in up to 80 per cent.

Studies in which risk factors have been examined have usually failed to distinguish the intervening influence of lower genital tract infections. Because cervicovaginal STDs are frequently in the pathogenic cycle of PID, any of the risk factors and risk markers correlated with these infections would be expected to show a similar association with PID. Thus, such factors as age, race, marital status, number of sexual partners, type of contraception, or even douching, which have been associated with PID in some studies, must be carefully examined to see whether lower genital tract STD is the intervening variable.

Teenagers have a particularly high rate of PID, especially when the data are corrected for level of sexual activity (Shafer and Sweet 1989). Sexually active 15–19 year old females have a one in eight estimated risk of suffering PID. If current trends continue, half of young women who were 15 years old in 1970 will have experienced at least one episode of PID by the turn of the century. Both biological and behavioral factors raise the risks of STDs and PID in teenagers, so creative interventions will have to be developed to reach this high-risk age group.

Vaginal douching is another behavior that has been associated with PID (Forrest *et al.* 1989). The temporal pattern of onset of PID symptoms may be linked to douching and menses. The nature of the douche solution and the douching technique may also be important variables. Mechanisms by which douching could facilitate PID include altering the vaginal environment toward more pathogenic organisms, and flushing vaginal and cervical pathogens into the uterus and fallopian tubes.

Contraceptive choice also influences the occurrence of PID. The intrauterine device (IUD) is associated with an increased risk, primarily in the first several months after insertion (Farley *et al.* 1992).

Although laparoscopy is useful in diagnosing salpingitis in women with clinical symptoms of PID, other approaches to detecting upper genital tract infection have been more objectively defined in the past several years. The diagnosis of endometritis has been based on a pathologic finding of plasma cells within the endometrium, which has been highly correlated with *C. trachomatis* and to a lesser degree with *N. gonorrhoeae*. Chronic, subacute, or latent endomaterial and tubal infection may be present in a large number of women, but a consensus definition of these clinically subtle infections is lacking. Diagnosing endometritis through objective histologic measures may complement laparoscopy as a tool to increase the sensitivity of PID diagnosis.

The role of silent (asymptomatic) PID in causing adverse reproductive sequelae is becoming increasingly appreciated (Cates *et al.* 1990). Silent salpingitis accounts for a sizable proportion, probably the majority, of tubal infertility. A variety of investigations has found that more than half of women with documented tubal occlusion reported no history of previous PID, despite serologic evidence of past chlamydia or gonococcal infection (Osser *et al.* 1989; Cates and Wasserheit 1991). Moreover, morphologic and physical analysis of tubal epithelium from women with distal tubal obstruction found extensive ultrastructural damage, even among women who had no knowledge of previous PID (Patton *et al.* 1989). Women with silent salpingitis had levels of tubal abnormalities similar to those with overt salpingitis. Moreover, no demographic or clinical risk factors or markers were able to differentiate those with silent salpingitis from those with symptomatic PID. Thus, clinical evidence of symptomatic PID is not a necessary precursor for the eventual development of tubal dysfunction or obstruction.

Further experience with atypical symptoms (such as oligomenorrhea) or biochemical markers may help identify subclinical PID before it progresses to tubal occlusion. Recent investigations have evaluated the role of tumor-associated trypsin inhibitor, C-reactive protein, and protein CA-125 as markers for subclinical tubal inflammation (Paavonen *et al.* 1989*a*,*b*). Unfortunately, these markers have had relatively low sensitivity among patients with symptomatic PID, being found in less than one-third of such patients. Specific microorganisms were not associated with these serum markers.

Despite a multitude of studies evaluating some of the newer antibiotic regimens in treating acute PID, no single agent or combination of therapies has emerged as superior to others. At the time the decision is made to initiate therapy, clinicians will not have results on the microbiologic etiology—if indeed they ever know. Therefore, treatments chosen for PID should be broad spectrum, based in part on the typical spectrum of organisms found in acute PID in their locations. Current recommendations for treating ambulatory patients involve a combination of cefoxitin and doxycycline for the broadest coverage. Alternatively, ofloxacin, clindamycin, and metronidazole can be used.

Infertility

Infertility as a consequence of STD occurs primarily through the damage caused by PID, which in turn leads to tubal dysfunction and occlusion. Usually this damage involves antecedent lower genital tract infections with either *N. gonorrhoeae* or *C. trachomatis*.

An estimated 2 million American women are infertile (Mosher 1985); approximately 20 per cent of this infertility can be related to STDs (Moore and Cates 1990). Women with a self-reported history of PID are more likely to be infertile than those without. A World Health Organization (WHO) multicenter study of infertile couples defined the proportion of infectious causes of infertility in different parts of the world; in Africa, nearly four-fifths of couples had an infectious etiology compared with about two-fifths of infertile couples in other developing countries and one-fifth in the developed world (Cates *et al.* 1985).

The etiologic role of previous chlamydial infection in tubal infertility has been exhaustively studied. Multiple retrospective investigations have examined the relationship between serologic evidence of past chlamydial infection and tubal infertility. Despite wide variations in study design, results uniformly document that tubal infertility is significantly associated with previous chlamydial infections (Brunham *et al.* 1985; Cates and Wasserheit 1991). The majority of women with tubal infertility have no prior history of clinical PID; thus the role of subclinical (chronic) tubal inflammation in the pathogenesis of tubal infertility is important.

Contraceptive use also affects STD-related infertility. The Dalkon Shield was implicated as the IUD that contributed most to tubal infertility, while barrier methods provided the expected protection (Cramer *et al.* 1987; Cates and Stone 1992). Prior IUD use and chlamydia antibody appeared to be independently associated with a threefold increased risk of tubal disease among infertile women.

Effect on pregnancy

Ectopic pregnancy

After conception, post-STD tubal occlusion still influences pregnancy outcome by increasing the risk of ectopic implantation. The public health impact of ectopic pregnancy has been well defined, both in its increasing incidence and its decreasing death-to-case rate (Centers for Disease Control 1992). In the USA, the annual rate of ectopic pregnancy has tripled over the last decade, while the number of cases diagnosed in hospitals increased from 19 000 in 1971 to nearly 90 000 in 1992. Several factors have contributed to these trends, but the most powerful etiologic correlate is PID (Chow *et al.* 1987). Moreover, many of the other conditions frequently associated with ectopic pregnancy—lower genital tract infection, past IUD use, post-abortion infection, tubal infertility, and pelvic surgery—have a primary link with PID, which in turn affects ectopic pregnancy.

However, few studies have examined the pathogenesis of ectopic pregnancy. The roles of such possible co-factors as douching, diethylstilbesterol exposure, previous abdominal or pelvic surgery, history of induced abortion, and cigarette smoking require clarification. Finally, as with tubal infertility, the preventive impact of both antibiotic treatment of PID and oral contraceptives remains to be established.

Perinatal sexually transmitted diseases

Perinatal transmission of nearly all STDs can influence pregnancy outcome—for both the mother and the neonate (Table 4.4).

Gonorrhea

Among pregnant women, the incidence of gonorrhea has ranged from less than 1 per cent to 7.5 per cent (Beck-Sague and Alexander 1987). As at other times, the majority of women with gonococcal infection during pregnancy are asymptomatic. Preterm delivery, premature rupture of membranes, and histologic evidence of chorioamnionitis are more frequent in mothers with gonorrhea than in comparison groups. Clinical symptoms of sepsis in the newborn, as well as maternal puerperal fever, are associated with positive *N. gonorrhoeae* cultures of the orogastric contents of newborns.

Prevention of neonatal gonococcal ophthalmia relies on ocular prophylaxis with silver nitrate or antibiotics. However, prenatal screening with an endocervical culture at the first prenatal visit would allow primary prevention. Moreover, follow-up cultures should be performed in previously infected women in the third trimester or at delivery, because the rate of reinfection during pregnancy has been reported to be as high as 30 per cent.

Chlamydia

The prevalence of cervical infection with *C. trachomatis* may range from 2 to 25 per cent, but in most samples is 8–12 per cent (Alexander and Harrison 1983). The consequences for the infant of maternal infection include conjunctivitis and pneumonia. Inclusion conjunctivitis of the newborn characteristically occurs at 7–15 days and is clinically indistinguishable from gonococcal conjunctivitis, which typically occurs in the first week. The laboratory diagnosis can be made by recovery of the organism in cell culture, but cytologic scraping of the conjunctiva, followed by staining with either Geimsa or fluoroscein-conjugated *C. trachomatis* antibody, is nearly as sensitive as culture. (This is not true for infection at other sites.)

Ideally, prevention of chlamydial disease among infants relies on detecting and treating maternal infection during pregnancy. However, because prenatal screening for chlamydia is still not widely applied, maternal treatment is

Table 4.4 Neonatal risks of sexually transmitted organisms

Organism	Maternal infection rate (%)	Effects in infant	Transmission risk from infected mother	Prevention	Treatment of neonate
Neisseria gonorrhoeae	1–30	Conjunctivitis, sepsis, meningitis	Approximately 30%	Screening by maternal culture; ocular prophylaxis	Penicillin; ceftriaxone
Chlamydia trachomatis	2–25	Conjunctivitis, pneumonia, bronchiolitis, otitis media	25–50% conjunctivitis 5–15% pneumonia	Screening by maternal culture; ocular prophylaxis	Erythromycin
Treponema pallidum	.01–15	Congenital syphilis, neonatal death	50%	Serologic screening in early and late pregnancy	Penicillin
Herpes simplex virus	1–30	Disseminated central nervous system, localized lesions	3% recurrent at delivery, 30% primary at delivery	Cesarean delivery if lesions present at delivery	Vidarabine, acyclovir
Human papillomavirus	10–35	Laryngeal papillomatosis	Rare	None	Surgical
Human immunodeficiency virus	0.01–20	Pediatric AIDS	22–39% (if no Zidovudine) 7% (if Zidovudine)	Pregnancy prevention, Zidovudine	Zidovudine

Source: adapted from Cates and Alexander (1988)

uncommon. A tertiary prevention strategy is neonatal ocular prophylaxis with erythromycin ophthalmic ointment. No similar strategy exists for preventing chlamydial pneumonia among newborns.

Syphilis

Syphilis can be transmitted transplacentally at any stage of untreated maternal disease, from incubation to tertiary syphilis. The early stages, when spirochetemia is highest, pose the highest risk to the fetus. Untreated syphilis in pregnant women results in adverse pregnancy outcome, including prematurity, stillbirth, or neonatal death in about half of exposed fetuses and congenital syphilis in the other half (Centers for Disease Control 1988). The risk of infection to the fetus falls to about 80 per cent in early latency and gradually to less than 50 per cent after more than 1 year since maternal infection. Fetal infection after 4–6 months of gestation often results in either abortion of the fetus or congenital syphilis.

Prevention depends on prenatal diagnosis and treatment. Effective treatment of the mother, even late in pregnancy, generally results in cure of the fetus. Despite maternal treatment being at least 95 per cent effective, prenatal penicillin and other antibiotics may fail to arrest fetal disease. Most congenital syphilis occurs because the current health care system fails either to detect maternal infection or to treat it adequately. Current prevention recommendations emphasize extending prenatal care throughout society.

Herpes

The prevalence of symptomatic genital herpes infection among pregnant women is less than 1 per cent at the time of delivery. Intermittent asymptomatic shedding occurs from either the cervix or vulva, and the majority of neonatal herpes is transmitted from asymptomatic mothers. The incidence of neonatal herpes is approximately one in 7500 live births (ACOG Technical Bulletin 1988).

The rate of transmission of virus from mother to infant varies with the stage of maternal illness. Primary HSV infection during the third trimester carries the highest risk of transmission. Because of cost and accuracy considerations, routine herpes cultures during the third trimester are no longer recommended. Cesarean delivery is necessary only if active herpetic lesions are present at the time of labor, with emphasis shifting to vigorous monitoring of the neonate for early symptoms that can be treated.

As with other viral sexually transmitted infections, the best prevention is primary, although because of the extent of asymptomatic carriage, this must be on non-specific grounds. The role of helpes simplex screening in pregnancy is being evaluated. Acyclovir may have a role in treatment of primary infection among pregnant women or in prophylaxis of infants born to mothers who demonstrate cervical infection at delivery.

Human papillomavirus

Human papillomavirus (HPV) infection is transmitted from mother to newborn during delivery by direct contact with infected cervical and vaginal tissue. Little is known about what factors may predispose the infant to symptomatic infection.

No effect of maternal HPV infection on infant birth weight or gestational age has been reported (Rando 1988); however, vaginal delivery is sometimes complicated by large warts. Although infants delivered to women with genital HPV infection occasionally have oral and anogential warts, the most important complication for the infant is laryngeal papillomatosis—luckily a rare outcome of a highly prevalent infection.

Human immunodeficiency virus

Human immunodeficiency virus may (HIV) may be transmitted from infected women to their offspring during pregnancy or soon after. Perinatal transmission rates vary from 22 to 39 per cent (Scott *et al.* 1989). However, prophylactic Zidovudine administered during pregnancy can markedly decrease perinatal HIV transmission (Centers for Disease Control 1994) Acquired immunodeficiency syndrome has been diagnosed in infants who had no contact with their mothers after birth, including some delivered by cesarean section, suggesting probable transmission during pregnancy, labor, or delivery (see chapter 5). Breastfeeding can transmit infection to an infant whose mother was infected before or after delivery. Clinical symptoms of HIV infection among children infected perinatally occur earlier in the course of illness than among adults. Moreover, the overall mortality rate after diagnosis of HIV infection is relatively high for those infected perinatally; half die before they reach 36 months of age.

Strategies for treatment and prevention

Treatment based on presumptive diagnosis should be inexpensive, simple, safe, and effective. Early and adequate treatment of patients and their sex partners is an effective means of preventing the community spread of STDs. National treatment recommendations are an essential part of the STD control strategy in any country (Centers for Disease Control 1993). Initially, in the USA these recommendations covered only syphilis and gonorrhea, but they were expanded in the 1980s to include 18 other sexually transmitted organisms and syndromes. Current regimens for treating common STDs have been derived from clinical consensus among a group of experts (Table 4.5).

Selective prophylactic (preventive or epidemiologic) treatment also has a major role in STD control strategies (Hart 1980). In certain clinical instances, as with many other infectious diseases, treatment should be offered on the basis of presumptive diagnosis or exposure, before the specific diagnosis is confirmed. In addition, based on epidemiologic indications, antibiotics can be administered to people at high risk when infection is considered likely, in the interest of public health. This approach interrupts the chain of transmission and prevents complications that might occur between the time of testing and treatment, insures treatment for infected people with false-negative laboratory tests, and guarantees treatment for those who might not return when notified of positive tests.

Most recently, this approach of selective preventive treatment has helped to limit outbreaks of syphilis, resistant gonorrhea, and chancroid in metropolitan

Table 4.5 Current regimens for treating common sexually transmitted diseases

Neisseria gonorrhoeae	Ceftriaxone 125 mg IM once, or cefixime 400 mg orally once, or ciprofloxacin 500 mg orally once, or ofloxacin 400 mg orally once, plus doxycycline 100 mg orally twice a day for 7 days
Chlamydia trachomatis	Doxycycline 100 mg orally twice a day for 7 days, or azithromycin 1 gm orally once
Treponema pallidum	Primary, secondary, or early syphilis of less than one year's duration: benzathine penicillin G, 2.4 million units IM. Syphilis of indeterminate length or of more than 1 year's duration: benzathine pencillin G, 7.2 million units total, administered as 2.4 million units IM given 1 week apart for 3 consecutive weeks. Neurosyphilis (inpatient therapy recommended; see STD treatment guidelines for out-patient regimen): aqueous crystalline pencillin G, 12–24 million units total, administered as 2–4 million units every 4 h IV, for 10–14 days
Herpes simplex virus	No known cure. Systemic acyclovir treatment may reduce symptoms and signs of herpes episodes and may accelerate healing but does not eradicate the infection or effect subsequent recurrence. **First clinical episode of genital herpes**: acyclovir 200 mg orally five times daily for 7–10 days or until clinical resolution occurs; **Recurrent episodes**: acyclovir 200 mg orally five times daily for 5 days initiated within 2 days of onset, or acyclovir 800 mg orally two times a day for 5 days. **Suppression of recurrent genital herpes infection**: continous treatment reduces the frequency of active disease by at least 75% among patients with frequent (at least six per year) recurrences. Dosage must be individualized for each patient. Acyclovir 400 mg orally twice daily or acyclovir 200 mg orally two to five times daily
Human papillomavirus	Cryotherapy with liquid nitrogen (or cryoprobe for external genital/perianal warts). **Alternative treatments for external genital, perianal, or vaginal warts**: podophyllin, 10–25% in compound tincture of benzoin; trichloroacetic acid 80–90%. Note: for women with cervical warts, dysplasia must be excluded before treatment is begun.

Source: Centers for Disease Control (1993)

areas. In addition, within certain closed communities with high prevalence of infection, selective mass penicillin treatment has been useful. The same philosophy underlies the recommendation for giving tetracycline concurrently with penicillin to patients with confirmed gonococcal infection, since a relatively high proportion are likely to be harboring co-existent *C. trachomatis* (Stamm *et al*. 1984).

Screening in pregnancy

Early detection of infection is crucial to STD intervention strategies. In pregnant women, screening improves both primary prevention (by decreasing the duration of infectiousness) and secondary prevention (by leading to treatment before pregnancy complications can occur). Case-finding methods include presumptive clinical diagnosis based on symptoms and signs, confirmatory laboratory testing in women with suggestive symptoms or signs, targeted screening among women at high risk for infection, broader screening without regard to likelihood of STD (such as general prenatal testing), and locating pregnant sex partners of men with an STD.

Whether for making specific diagnoses in those with symptoms or for screening persons without symptoms, tests for STDs should ideally be inexpensive, rapid, simple, and accurate. Our current methods for diagnosing the common STDs incorporate these principles (Table 4.6). However, for many developing countries, constraints on expense, rapidity, and simplicity are so great that few of these tests can be used, except in specialized central laboratories. For example, because cultures are not available for detecting gonorrhea among women, the control of gonorrhea is problematic. In developed countries, constraints on expense have delayed introduction of some diagnostic test—for example, *C. trachomatis*—even in setting in which such tests are considered cost effective.

The usual parameters for assessing diagnostic techniques—sensitivity, specificity, and predictive value—have certain unique implications for STD control. STD treatment is generally shorter and safer than therapy for many chronic conditions. Moreover, as discussed earlier, curing an STD in one person frequently prevents infection in others. Consequently, achieving high sensitivity by reducing false negatives becomes a priority. Achieving high specificity by reducing false positives is less important from the public health perspective when treatment is safe, simple, and inexpensive. However, when false-positive tests trigger partner notification, additional expenses must be considered. Furthermore, from the individual's perspective, the human and emotional costs of erroneously stigmatizing someone as having an STD mean specificity is also crucial.

Deficiencies in sensitivity cause particular problems among populations with a high prevalence of a disease with serious morbidity. For example, a new test for gonorrhea with a sensitivity of 80 per cent in women would fail to identify 20 per cent of infected women. If the prevalence of gonorrhea in women at a prenatal clinic is 30 per cent, then six women out of 100 tested would not be identified and would be at risk for spreading the infection to their offspring and partners.

Table 4.6 Current methods for diagnosing common sexually transmitted diseases

Organism	Presumptive Diagnosis	Definitive Diagnosis
Neisseria gonorrhoeae	Microscopic identification of typical Gram-negative intracellular diplococci on smear of urethral exudate (men) or endocervical material (women); or growth on selective medium demonstrating typical colonial morphology, positive oxidase reaction, and typical Gram-stain morphology	Growth on selective medium demonstrating typical colonial morphology, positive oxidase reaction, and typical Gram-stain morphology, and confirmed by sugar utilization, coagglutination or antigonococcal fluorescent antibody (FA) testing. A definitive diagnosis is required if specimen is extragenital, from a child, or medico-legally significant.
Chlamydia trachomatis		
Mucopurulent cervicitis	The presence of yellow mucopurulent endocervical exudate or the finding of this exudate on a white cotton-tipped swab of endocervical secretions. In women without visible mucopus, the presence of > 10 polymorphonuclear (PMN) leukocytes per $\times$ 1000 field on a Gram-stained specimen of endocervical mucus (without contamination by vaginal cells) also allows a presumptive diagnosis	Definitive diagnosis is made by growth on cycloheximide-treated McCoy cells. Flourescent monoclonal antibody stains or enzyme immunoassay tests are also widely available. DNA amplification tests may soon have wider clinical application. If confirmatory tests are not available, empirical therapy can be given on clinical grounds
Non-gonococcal urethritis (NGU)	Symptomatic men are presumed to have NGU when their gonorrhea tests are negative and they have either white blood cells on Gram stain of urethral discharge or sexual exposure to an agent known to cause NGU. Asymptomatic men with negative gonorrhea tests are also presumed to have NGU if they have >4 PMN leukocytes per $\times$ 1000 field on an intraurethral smear.	Same as above

Table 4.6 (*cont.*)

Organism	Presumptive Diagnosis	Definitive Diagnosis
Treponema pallidum	*Primary*: patients have typical lesion(s) and either a newly positive serologic test for syphilis (STS), or their present STS titer is at least fourfold greater than the last, or there has been syphilis exposure within 90 days of lesion onset. *Secondary*: patients have the typical clinical presentation and a strongly reactive STS. *Latent*: patients have serologic evidence of untreated syphilis without clinical signs	Primary and secondary syphilis are definitively diagnosed by demonstrating *T. pallidum* with dark-field microscopy or FA techniques in material from a chancre, regional lymph node, or other lesion. A definitive diagnosis of latent syphilis cannot be made under usual circumstances
Herpes simplex virus (HSV)	When typical genital lesions are present or a pattern of recurrence has developed, herpes infection is likely. A presumptive diagnosis is further supported by: direct identification of multinucleated giant cells with intranuclear inclusions in a clinical specimen prepared by Papanicolaou or other serological techniques. Morphology by electron microscopy; or detection of HSV antigens by monoclonal or polyclonal antibody detection systems	An HSV virus tissue culture demonstrates the characteristic cytopathogenic effect (CPE) following inoculation of a specimen from the cervix, the urethra or the base of a genital lesion. The isolates can be identified as type 1 or type 2 by FA, neutralization, or other histochemical stain; or typical HSV
Human papillomavirus	A diagnosis may be made on the basis of the typical clinical presentation. Colposcopy may also aid in the diagnosis of certain cervical lesions. Exclude the possibility of condylomata by obtaining a darkfield and/or serologic test for syphilis	A biopsy, although usually unnecessary, is required to make a definitive diagnosis. Very atypical lesions, where neoplasia is a consideration, should be biopsied before initiating therapy. A Pap smear of cervical lesions shows typical cytologic changes

Table 4.6 (*cont.*)

Organism	Presumptive Diagnosis	Definitive Diagnosis
Human immunodeficiency virus	Usually based on clinical evidence	A diagnosis of asymptomatic HIV infection usually is made on the basis of a repeatedly reactive EIA (enzyme immunoassay) test followed by a reactive supplemental test (e.g. western blot or immunofluorescent assay). Polymerase chain reaction (PCR) is a gene amplification technique which has been used as a research tool to detect infection before detectable levels of antibody are found by EIA or western blot techniques. Although isolation of the virus from body fluids is the most highly specific means to make a definitive diagnosis of HIV infection, such testing is not widely available

Source: Cates and Holmes (1991)

Deficiencies in specificity can also cause difficulties, especially among populations with a low prevalence of infection. For example, a new test for *N. gonorrhoeae* with a specificity of 90 per cent and sensitivity of 100 per cent, when used in a low-prevalence population (1 per cent), would produce almost ten times as many false-positive tests as true-positive tests. Referring and evaluating 11 people and their sex partners to identify a single infected person and that person's exposed partner(s) would tax clinical personnel and cause unnecessary anxiety. In public health terms, testing 20 000 000 women using the new test would increase the follow-up burden from approximately 200 000 with culture diagnoses to 2 200 000 individuals from the new test. Such an increase could overwhelm clinical resources.

Even with highly specific tests (specificity more than 99 per cent), screening for an STD of very low prevalence (less than 0.1 per cent) creates many false positives. Thus, tests such as the FTA-ABS or TPHA test for syphilis, although highly specific and having high positive predictive value in patients with positive reagin tests for syphilis, are not recommended for screening the general population for syphilis. In the USA, the prevalence of syphilis has become so low in many areas that the cost-effectiveness of serologic screening with the less expensive and less specific reagin tests (for example, in premarital examinations, blood banking services, and new admissions to hospitals) is even being debated.

To make most effective use of resources, targeted screening has been recommended among high-prevalence groups such as commercial sex workers, homosexual men, and illicit drug users, in facilities such as jails and emergency rooms where high levels of STDs might be expected, and in pregnant women for whom an STD could cause adverse pregnancy outcomes. In the USA, testing prostitutes for syphilis, chancroid, and gonorrhea has proved particularly useful for stemming specific outbreaks in Los Angeles and New York City. Recent experience using mobile vans to provide STD screening to those visiting crack houses in Philadelphia has also been encouraging.

Ethical questions

Partner notification

Because screening is inconsistently applied and clinical diagnosis is inefficient, rapid investigation of sex partners is essential for bringing people with STD to treatment before they can spread the infection within the community. For women, partner notification and treatment help insure reinfection will not occur, and an STD in the lower genital tract will not ascend. However, some have criticized the concept of partner notification because it intrudes on patient privacy and requires labor-intensive use of human resources.

Traditionally, STD control programs in the developed countries have emphasized active intervention by health providers to interview patients, identify sex partners, and assure that partners are evaluated and treated (Rothenberg and

Potterat 1990). The privacy of patients and partners is rigorously protected. Whether applied in isolated rural communities, selected urban neighborhoods, or prison, rapid sex partner identification, location, and treatment has been shown to be effective in reducing the occurrence of STDs.

However, during the past two decades, the growing number of cases limited the personnel available for notifying sex partners. During the 1970s in the USA, in large part due to the expanded spectrum of infections, the process of partner notification was modified in many settings to encourage the patient to assume responsibility for locating and referring his or her sexual partners (Parra *et al.* 1985). Thus, for purposes of efficiency, partner notification was categorized into referral by the patient and referral by the provider. The patient referral approach actively involves the patient in the STD control effort, is relatively inexpensive, is acceptable to many patients, and reserves scarce staff time for targeted provider referral. Potential shortcomings of patients referral methods, however, include its limited effectiveness with non-compliant patients, and difficulty in evaluating its outcomes. Active provider referral (contact tracing by the public health staff) is more labor intensive, time-consuming, and expensive; therefore, this effort, especially in recent years, is concentrated on high-risk core environments. Despite the initial cost, provider referral can be cost beneficial because of its greater yield of infected persons and because these persons tend to transmit syphilis at high rates.

The provider referral process involves a series of interrelated activities: interviewing the infected patients to obtain a complete list of their sex partners, finding these people in the community, and getting them treated promptly. In the USA, interviewing techniques have been developed to encourage patient cooperation in full disclosure of their partners. However, during the 1960s and 1970s, the contact index—a measure of the yield of the STD interview—steadily declined. Possible reasons for this trend include a true decrease in the number of sex partners per infected person; changing environments for sexual relations so that a greater percentage of partners are anonymous (for example, gay bathhouses, crack houses); an increasing atmosphere of distrust of all governmental organizations, including those delivering public health services; deteriorating interviewing techniques; and increasing competition of other STDs.

Locating patients may also have become more difficult in recent years. Distrust of government agencies may have worsened in the Black community after revelations of the Tuskegee syphilis study (Brandt 1985). Moreover, the association of high-risk sexual behavior with environments where illicit drug use and violence are common has made the safety of the STD outreach worker an issue.

Using specific populations, rather than infected individuals, as the units for STD intervention is a means for overcoming problems with naming and locating sex partners. In the past, this community-oriented approach was a type of cluster interviewing. STD patients and their known sex partners were queried about other persons to whom—and social settings in which—syphilis transmission may have occurred. Although this cluster approach produced a lower yield of infected, previously untreated patients than following up those specifically named as sex partners, it still identified a relatively high percentage of person who might not have been reached in any other way. In fact, depending on how the socially related group was defined, as many as one in five people examined had untreated syphilis (Kaufman *et al.* 1974).

In recent years, similar population-based approaches have been used to identify particular communities at high risk of STD. Examples of situations in which this community intervention was successful in stemming syphilis outbreaks include a Native American tribe whose members were reluctant to name any partners to outside officials (Gerber *et al.* 1989) and a Philadelphia neighborhood where crack cocaine use led to unsafe sexual behaviors and high levels of syphilis (Mellinger *et al.* 1991).

Finally, apart from health workers specifically trained in STD interviewing techniques, other health providers are often unwilling to question their patients about sexual activity. For example, private physicians may find it especially difficult to notify the sex partner(s) of their longstanding patients. Not only do such issues as infidelity, homosexuality, or child abuse generate human anxieties, but also the potential need for marital counseling may require skills and time that the clinician does not have. In one study, more than half of primary care physicians questioned said that, to avoid dealing with this situation, they would lie to a patient's spouse about the implications of a sexually transmitted infection if requested by their infected patient (Novack *et al.* 1989). Clearly, additional medical training in this delicate area is necessary to provide skills in partner notification for private clinicians.

Resource priorities

State and local resources mainly support laboratory, diagnostic, and treatment services for STDs. After the data are adjusted for inflation, these non-federal resources have remained relatively stable during the past 40 years. However, federal appropriations for STD control (not including HIV), which support surveillance and outreach activities, have been more variable (Fig. 4.1). From the high of over $17 million in 1949, resources decreased quickly to $13 million a year later, to $700 000 in 1955, when the availability of penicillin permitted the closing of the rapid treatment centers and when sharp declines in early syphilis incidence suggested that the STD problem had been solved (Brandt 1985).

During the 1960s, resources for STD control were further eroded by the expanding spectrum of infections recognized as being sexually transmitted. Although additional funds were appropriated for gonorrhea control in the 1970s and chlamydia control in the 1980s, these new resources were never enough to support all the necessary STD control activities. Policy makers were forced to choose alternatives among secondary prevention approaches for the different organisms. For example, because of the greater burden of disease caused by gonorrhea, chlamydia, and viral STDs, syphilis was relegated to a smaller share of the STD resources available during the 1970s and 1980s.

After the data are adjusted for inflation, total federal STD resources in 1990 were less than in 1950 (Fig. 4.1), despite the expanding spectrum of infections. For syphilis alone, the inflation-adjusted level of investment (in 1990 dollars)

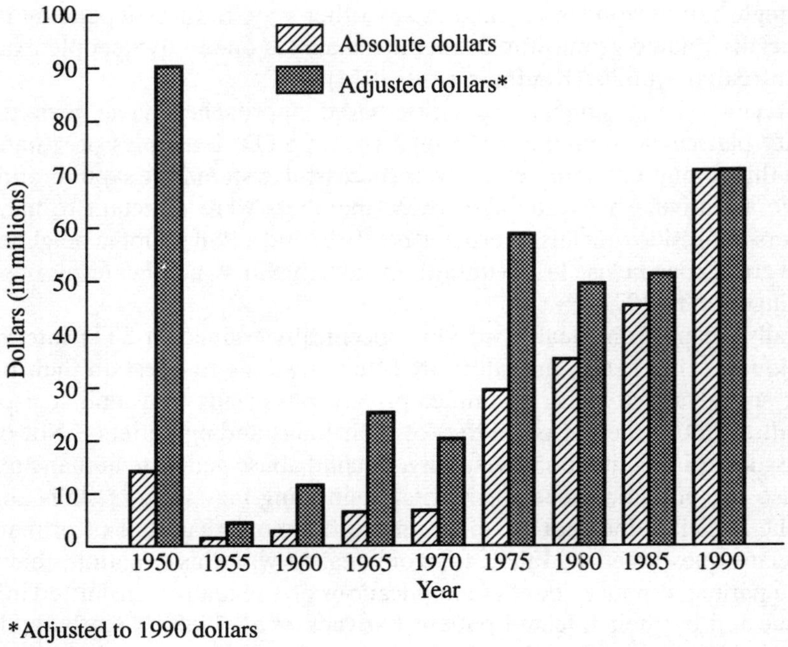

Fig. 4.1 Resources for STD control, fiscal years 1950–1990.

declined from over $100 million in 1949 to just over $20 million in 1990. Since the reported number of primary and secondary syphilis cases was similar in both years, the effect has been to drain the per case investment in syphilis control to one-fifth that of 40 years earlier. To some extent, the dilution of funds has been offset by investments in HIV primary prevention. None the less, the funding level for STD control has ebbed considerably during the past half century.

Recommendations

What does the future hold for sexually transmitted diseases and reproductive health? In the research arena, we must define the etiologic interrelationships between a number of different sexually transmitted infections and their reproductive sequelae. For example, what is the interaction between chlamydia and bacterial vaginosis, if any? How important is trichomoniasis as a cause of reproductive sequelae? Can we identify a specific potentiating organism that, if eradicated, will lead to markedly lower levels of adverse reproductive outcomes?

Better knowledge in STD diagnosis and treatment is vital. Regarding new diagnostic approaches, can we develop an effective method to detect subclinical PID? Regarding new therapies, will the 1993 CDC recommendations for PID treatment—using antibiotics effective against gonorrhea, chlamydia, and anaerobic organisms—reduce the postinflammatory occlusive sequelae? Will research into new treatments for HIV lead to spin-off benefits in antiviral therapy for other viral STDs?

Future efforts must also increase both public and private attention to preventing STDs, as well as making the most cost-effective use of our limited resources. Building on the common approaches to preventing HIV infection and the other STDs can pay mutual dividends. The increased public awareness that has accompanied concern for incurable STDs may stimulate further commitment to reducing the effects of STDs on reproductive health. Prevention programs aimed at reducing perinatal HIV transmission can be extended to involve other sexually transmitted organisms. Finally, outreach efforts to identify high-risk women of reproductive age can also build broad STD screening into their formats.

Within the history of STD control, our quest for rapid, simple magic bullet solutions has tended to ignore the complexities of human sexual behavior. Now that the STD spectrum includes organisms that are also spread by intravenous drug use, the level of complexity is further amplified. History has shown that our quest for a single absolutist solution to complex problems usually falls short. Rather, a myriad of different good approaches are necessary to build on one another to achieve a cumulative solution (Cates and Hinman 1992).

In conclusion, we face a continuing challenge to reduce the major public health impact of STDs on reproductive health. As technology advances and as public interest grows, we will have a greater opportunity to diagnose and treat both the bacterial and viral agents which are related to difficulties in conceiving, problems in carrying pregnancies to term, and complications in the neonate.

References

ACOG Technical Bulletin (1988). *Perinatal herpes simplex virus infections*, number 122, November. Washington DC.

Alary, M., Joly, J. R., and Poulin, C. (1989). Incidence of four sexually transmitted diseases in a rural community: a prospective study. *American Journal of Epidemiology*, **130**, 547–56.

Alexander, E. R. and Harrison, H. R. (1983). Role of *Chlamydia trachomatis* in perinatal infection. *Reviews of Infectious Diseases*, **5**, 713–21.

Bauer, H. M., Ting, Y., Greer, C. E., Chambers, J. C., Tashiro, C. J., Chimera, J., *et al.* (1991). Genital human papillomavirus infection in female university students as determined by a PCR-based method. *Journal of the American Medical Association*, **265**, 472–7.

Beck-Sague, C. and Alexander, E. R. (1987). Sexually transmitted diseases in children and adolescents. *Infectious Disease Clinics of North America*, **1**, 277–304.

Brandt, A. M. (1985). *No magic bullet: a social history of venereal disease in the United States since 1880*. Oxford University Press, New York.

Brunham, R. C. (1990). Sexually transmitted diseases in pregnancy. In *Sexually transmitted diseases*, 2nd edn, (ed. K. K. Holmes, P.-A. Mårdh, P. F. Sparling, P. J. Wiesner, W. Cates, Jr, S. M. Lemon, and W. E. Stamm), pp. 771–802. McGraw-Hill, New York.

Brunham, R. C. (1991). The concept of core and its relevance to the epidemiology and control of sexually transmitted diseases. *Sexually Transmitted Diseases*, **18**, 67–68.

Brunham, R. C., Maclean, I. W., Binns, B., and Peeling, R. W. (1985). *Chlamydia trachomatis*: its role in tubal infertility. *Journal of Infectious Diseases*, **152**, 1275–82.

Cates, W., Jr (1990). Sexually transmitted diseases: the scale of the problem in the developed and developing world. In *Public health and sexual transmission of diseases: directions for future research and health policy*. (ed. N. Job-Spira, B. Spencer, J. P. Moatti, and E. Bouvet), pp. 26–32. John Libbey Company, Paris.

Cates, W., Jr and Alexander, E. R. (1988). STD and the fetus: a continuing challenge. In *Impact on the fetus of parental sexually transmitted disease*, (ed. R. B. Kundsin, L. Falk, S. S. Hipp), pp. 1–16. New York Academy of Sciences, New York.

Cates, W., Jr and Hinman, A. R. (1992). AIDS and absolutism: the demand for perfection in prevention. *New England Journal of Medicine*, **327**, 492–4.

Cates, W., Jr. and Holmes, K. K. (1991). Sexually transmitted diseases. In *Maxcy-Rosenau's public health and preventive medicine*, (13th edn), (ed. J. Last and R. B. Wallace), pp. 99–114. Appleton and Lange, East Norwalk.

Cates, W., Jr and Stone, K. M. (1992). Family planning, sexually transmitted diseases, and contraceptive choice: a literature update. *Family Planning Perspectives*, **24**, 75–84.

Cates, W., Jr and Wasserheit, J. N. (1991). Genital chlamydial infection: epidemiology and reproductive sequelae. *American Journal of Obstetrics and Gynecology*, **164**, 1771–81.

Cates, W., Jr, Farley, T. M. M., Rowe, P. H., and the WHO Task Force on Infertility (1985). Worldwide patterns of infertility: is Africa different? *Lancet*, **ii**, 596–8.

Cates, W., Jr, Rolfs, R. T., Jr, and Aral, S. O. (1990). Sexually transmitted diseases, pelvic inflammatory disease, and infertility: an epidemiologic update. *Epidemiology Reviews*, **12**, 199–220.

Cates, W., Jr, Rothenberg, R. B., and Blount, J. H. (in press). Public health measures for syphilis control. In *Syphilis*, (ed. E. W. Hook, III and S. A. Lukehart). Blackwell Scientific Publications, Cambridge. (In press.)

Centers for Disease Control (1988). Policy guidelines for the prevention and control of congenital syphilis. *Morbidity and Mortality Weekly Report*, **37** (Suppl. 1), 1–13.

Centers for Disease Control (1993). 1993 sexually transmitted diseases treatment guidelines. *Morbidity and Mortality Weekly Report*, **42** (No. RR-14): 1–102.

Centers for Disease Control (1992). Ectopic pregnancy—United States, 1988–1989. *Morbidity and Mortality Weekly Report*, **41** (No. 32), 591–4.

Chow, W.-H., Daling, J. R., Cates, W., Jr, and Greenberg, R. S. (1987). Epidemiology of ectopic pregnancy. *Epidemiologic Reviews*, **9**, 70–94.

Cramer, D. W., Goldman, M. B., Schiff, I., Belisle, S., Albrecht, B., Stadel, B., *et al.* (1987). The relationship of tubal infertility to barrier method and oral contraceptive use. *Journal of the American Medical Association*, **257**, 2446–50.

Division of STD/HIV Prevention (1994). *1993 annual report*. Centers for Disease Control and Prevention, Atlanta.

Eschenbach, D. A., Hillier, S., Critchlow, C., Stevens, C., DeRouen, P., and Holmes, K. K. (1988). Diagnosis and clinical manifestations of bacterial vaginosis. *American Journal of Obstetrics and Gynecology*, **158**, 819–28.

Farley, T. M. M., Rosenberg, M. J., Rowe, P. J., Chen, J.-H., and Meirik, O. (1992). Intrauterine devices and pelvic inflammatory disease: an international perspective. *Lancet*, **339**, 785–8.

Forrest, K. A., Washington, A. E., Daling, J. R., and Sweet, R. L. (1989). Vaginal douching as a possible risk factor for pelvic inflammatory disease. *Journal of the National Medical Association*, **81**, 159–65.

Gerber, A. R., King, L. C., Dunleavy, G. J., and Novick, L. F. (1989). An outbreak of syphilis on an Indian reservation: descriptive epidemiology and disease-control measures. *American Journal of Public Health*, **79**, 83–5.

Hart, G. (1980). Epidemiologic treatment for syphilis and gonorrhea. *Sexually Transmitted Diseases*, **7**, 149–60.

Hart, G., Adler, M. W., Stapinski, A., Mroczkowski, T. F., and Wiesner, P. J. (1990). Evaluation of sexually transmitted diseases control programs in industrialized countries. In *Sexually transmitted diseases*, (2nd edn), (ed. K. K. Holmes, P.-A. Mårdh, P. F. Sparling, P. J. Wiesner, W. Cates, Jr, S. M. Lemon, and W. E. Stamm), pp. 1031–40. McGraw-Hill, New York.

Holmes, K. K., Mårdh, P.-A., Sparling, P. F., Wiesner, P. J., Cates, W., Jr, Lemon, S. M., and Stamm, W. E. (ed.) (1990). *Sexually transmitted diseases*, (2nd edn). McGraw-Hill, New York.

Johnson R. E., Nahmias, A. J., Magder, L. S., Lee, F. K., Brooks, C. A., and Snowden, C. B. (1989). A seroepidemiologic survey of the prevalence of herpes simplex virus type 2 infection in the United States. *New England Journal of Medicine*, **321**, 7–12.

Kahn, J. G., Walker, C. K., Washington, A. E., Landers, D. V., and Sweet, R. L. (1991). Diagnosing pelvic inflammatory disease. *Journal of the American Medical Association*, **266**, 2594–604.

Kaufman, R. E., Blount, J. H., and Jones, O. G. (1974). Current trends in syphilis. *Public Health Reviews*, **3**, 175–96.

Koutsky, L. A., Stevens, C. E., Holmes, K. K., Ashley, R. L., Kiviat, N. B., Critchlow, C. W., *et al.* (1992). Underdiagnoses of genital herpes by current clinical and viral-isolation procedures. *New England Journal of Medicine*, **326**, 1533–9.

Meheus, A., Schulz, K. F., and Cates, W., Jr (1990). Development of prevention and control programs for sexually transmitted diseases in developing countries. In *Sexually transmitted diseases*, (2nd edn), (ed. K. K. Holmes, P.-A. Mårdh, P. F. Sparling, P. J. Wiesner, W. Cates, Jr, S. M. Lemon, and W. E. Stamm), pp. 1041–6. McGraw-Hill, New York.

Mellinger, A. K., Goldberg, M., Wade, A., Brown, P. Y., Hughes, G. A., Lutz, J. P., *et al.* (1991). Alternative case-finding in a crack-related syphilis epidemic—Philadelphia. *Morbidity and Mortality Weekly Report*, **40**, 77–80.

Moore, D. E. and Cates, W., Jr (1990). Sexually transmitted diseases and infertility. In *Sexually transmitted diseases*, (2nd edn), (ed. K. K. Holmes, P.-A. Mårdh, P. F. Sparling, P. J. Wiesner, W. Cates, Jr., S. M. Lemon, and W. E. Stamm), pp. 763–9. McGraw-Hill, New York.

Mosher, W. E. (1985). Reproductive impairments in the United States, 1965–1982. *Demography*, **22**, 415–30.

Novack, D. H., Detering, B. J., Arnold, R., Farrow, L., Ladinsky, M., and Pezzullo, J. C. (1989). Physicans' attitudes toward using deception to resolve difficult ethical problems. *Journal of the American Medical Association*, **261**, 2980–5.

Osser, S., Persson, K., and Liedholm, P. (1989). Tubal infertility and silent chlamydial salpingitis. *Human Reproduction*, **4**, 280–4.

Parra, W. C. and Cates, W. Jr. (1985). Progress towards meeting the 1990 objectives for sexually transmitted diseases: The good news and the bad *Public Health Reports*, **100(3)**: 261–9.

Paavonen, J., Lehtinen, M., Lehto, M., Laine, S., Aine, R., Rasanen L, *et al.* (1989*a*). Concentrations of tumor-associated trypsin inhibitor and C-reactive protein in serum in acute pelvic inflammatory disease. *Clinical Chemistry*, **35**, 869–71.

Paavonen, J., Miettinen, A., Heinonen, P. K., Aaran, R. K., Teisala, K., Aine, R., *et al.* (1989*b*). Serum CA-125 in acute pelvic inflammatory disease. *British Journal of Obstetrics and Gynaecology*, **96**, 574–9.

Patton, D. L., Moore, D. E., Spadoni, L. R., Soules, M. R., Halbert, S. A., and Wang, S. P. (1989). A comparison of the fallopian tube's response to overt and silent salpingitis. *Obstetrics and Gynecology*, **74**, 622–30.

Quinn, T. C. and Cates, W., Jr (1992). Epidemiology of sexually transmitted diseases in the 1990s. In *Advances in host defense mechanisms: sexually transmitted diseases*, Vol. 8, (ed. T. C. Quinn, J. I. Gallin, and A. S. Fauci), pp. 1–37. Raven Press, New York.

Rando, R. F. (1988). Human papillomavirus: implications for clinical medicine. *Annals of Internal Medicine*, **108**, 628–31.

Rothenberg, R. B. (1990). Analytic approaches to the epidemiology of sexually transmitted diseases. In *Sexually transmitted diseases*, (2nd edn), (ed. K. K. Holmes, P.-A. Mårdh, P. F. Sparling, P. J. Wiesner, W. Cates, Jr, S. M. Lemon, and W. E. Stamm), pp. 37–42. McGraw-Hill, New York.

Rothenberg, R. B. and Potterat, J. J. (1990). Strategies for management of sex partners. In *Sexually transmitted diseases*, (2nd edn), (ed. K. K. Holmes, P.-A. Mårdh, P. F. Sparling, P. J. Wiesner, W. Cates, Jr, S. M. Lemon, and W. E. Stamm), pp. 1081–6. McGraw-Hill, New York.

Scott, G. B., Hutto, C., Makuch, R. W., Mastrucci, M. T., O'Connor, T., Mitchell, C. D., *et al.* (1989). Survival in children with perinatally acquired human immunodeficiency virus type 1 infection. *New England Journal of Medicine*, **321**, 1791–6.

Shafer, M. A. and Sweet, R. L. (1989). Pelvic inflammatory disease in adolescent females: epidemiology, pathogenesis, diagnosis, treatment, and sequelae. *Pediatric Clinics of North America*, **36**, 513–32.

Stamm, W. E., Guinan, M. E., Johnson, C., Starcher, T., Holmes, K. K., and McCormack, W. M. (1984). Effect of treatment regimens for *Neisseria gonorrhoeae* on simultaneous infection with *Chlamydia trachomatis*. *New England Journal of Medicine*, **310**, 545–51.

Turner, C. F., Miller, H. G., and Moses, L. E. (ed.) (1989). *AIDS: sexual behavior and intravenous drug use*. National Academy Press, Washington, D. C.

Wasserheit, J. N. (1989). The significance and scope of reproductive tract infections among third world women. *International Journal of Gynecology and Obstetrics*, **27** (Suppl 3), 145–68.

WHO (1989). *Changing patterns of STD: global epidemiology*. Presented at the Consultation on Development of Effective STD Treatment Strategies, 4 September. World Health Organization, Geneva.

5 AIDS in women

Deborah Cotton

In the USA, the acquired immunedeficiency syndrome (AIDS) was the fifth leading cause of death in women of childbearing age in 1990 (Chu *et al.* 1990*a*), and almost 80 000 women were estimated to be infected (Gwinn *et al.* 1991). World-wide the specter of AIDS is even more sobering, with estimates that 20–50 million women may be infected by the year 2000 (Mann *et al.* 1992). Despite the enormity of the problem, until recently little attention has been paid to the unique aspects of HIV infection in women, and there are inadequate data on the natural history of the disease in women. Few AIDS-related programs are gender specific in their approach to disease detection or management, and women as a group have had less access than men to state-of-the-art therapies and experimental drug trials.

In addition, it has been suggested that gender-specific manifestations of HIV infection (such as cervical carcinoma, severe pelvic inflammatory disease, and vaginal candidiasis) may produce significant morbidity and mortality in women and may represent the first or indeed the only manifestation of HIV infection. However, these manifestations are currently not included in standard definitions of the disease. As a consequence, many HIV-infected women are unable to benefit from social programs tied to case definitions (American Public Health Assocation 1991)

AIDS is increasing in women at a time when serious concerns are being voiced about societal neglect of the health problems of women in general. Questions have been raised as to possible gender-specific differences in drug efficacy and toxicity in several diseases, and gender-based differences in medical care have been documented (Ayanian and Epstein 1991). Long standing policies excluding women of childbearing age from clinical trials are being modified (Kirschstein 1991).

The majority of women with HIV infection are young, poor, and faced with a myriad of social problems which often pose more of an immediate threat to their well-being and that of their families than HIV. It is perhaps not too simplistic to say that AIDS in women represents a wholly different epidemic and that approaches to virtually all aspects of its control should ideally be gender specific.

This chapter will attempt to approach these challenges by summarizing current information about HIV infection in women and by outlining policy issues of current importance.

The epidemiology of AIDS in women

Risk factors for HIV infection in women have been reasonably well characterized. World-wide, the vast majority of women with HIV infection have acquired it through infected semen during vaginal intercourse. Genital ulceration in women, caused by several sexually transmitted diseases, appears to increase the risk of infection (Holmberg *et al.* 1989). Intercourse during menses may also increase risk, as may the use of oral contraceptives, perhaps by producing cervical erosion (Plummer *et al.* 1988). Rectal intercourse is significantly more likely to transmit infection than vaginal intercourse (Padian *et al.* 1987), probably because of increased trauma to the rectal mucosa. It is important to note that a significant percentage of couples in one US study were found to engage in rectal intercourse at least some of the time. It is more difficult for a woman to transmit the infection to a man than vice versa (Padian *et al.* 1991). While HIV can be recovered from cervical secretions (Wofsy *et al.* 1986) the infectivity of these secretions is probably less than that of semen.

Several anecdotal cases of female to female transmission have been reported (Monzon and Capellen 1987). Although this mode of transmission appears uncommon (Chu *et al.* 1990*b*), data on lesbian sexual activity has not been sought on CDC AIDS case-report forms, making it impossible to fully assess its role in transmitting infection.

In some industrialized countries such as the USA, transmission of HIV through intravenous drug use is a major cause of infection in women (Guinan and Hardy 1987; Gayle *et al.* 1990) Roughly half of all HIV-infected women in the USA are current or past intravenous drug users (Centers for Disease Control 1991). Moreover, intravenous drug-using women are also at risk for sexual transmission from partners who have acquired their own infection from intravenous drug use (Brown and Primm 1988). Drug use (including alcohol intoxication) may also contribute to infection through its disinhibiting effects, leading to unprotected sex, or through exchange of sex for drug money (DesJarlais and Friedman 1988).

Transfusion, often administered for obstetric indications, was a significant risk factor among women before the widespread screening of blood began in the mid-1980s in industrialized countries; today, transfusion remains a real risk in many parts of the world. Finally, health care workers are at risk—albeit at a relatively low level—and most are women.

The natural history of HIV infection in women

There is a paucity of data on possible gender-related differences in the manifestations of HIV. Early in the epidemic, the predominance of cases among gay men and the unknown nature of the illness led to the recruitment of many gay men to long-term longitudinal studies to assess both risk factors for infection and characteristics of the disease. The largest and best known of these is the so-called MACS (Multicity AIDS cohort study) in the USA which began in 1983 and has produced many important results from its follow-up of over 1800 infected men (MacDonell *et al.* 1990). Until recently, however, there have been few studies following groups of infected women over time (cohort studies) to assess the risk of development of full-blown AIDS, survival time, and possible differences in disease manifestation. The lack of such studies came about in part because women were not perceived to be at risk when the earliest studies began, and because greater emphasis has been placed on the role of women in transmitting infection to sexual partners and fetuses than on the impact of disease on the woman herself.

As a result, conclusions regarding the natural history of HIV in women, as well as health policy, have often been based on small case series and anecdotal reports. While there is now greater interest in recruiting and following larger groups of women to gain a more accurate assessment of these issues, current budgetary constraints in the USA may limit such studies. Moreover, even if well funded, well designed cohort studies were initiated today, it would be many years before definitive data would be available, given the likely long incubation period of the disease (estimated in men to be on the order of 10 years between infection and the development of full-blown AIDS).

There have been conflicting data from small studies as to possible gender-related differences in disease progression and survival (Rothenberg *et al.* 1987; Ellerbrock *et al.* 1991; Lifson *et al.* 1992). Some studies have been confounded by inclusion of Kaposi's sarcoma, which both occurs more frequently in gay/bisexual men and has a better prognosis than other initial AIDS-defining conditions. Several studies have demonstrated that women have had less access to routine HIV care and to state-of-the-art therapies for HIV infection than men, confounding any assessment of any possible biological differences (Moore *et al.* 1991; Stein *et al.* 1991). There does not appear to be a significant acceleration of disease in women, although in the absence of large studies and with known differences in access, such differences could exist without having been detected.

The pattern of opportunistic infection and other complications in women may differ from that in men. There are some data to suggest that esophageal candidiasis is more common in women (Berkelman 1991; Carpenter *et al.* 1991). Moreover, the pronounced sex difference in the occurrence of Kaposi's sarcoma is well known. Recent reports of Kaposi's sarcoma in gay men who are HIV-negative (Saltzman *et al.* 1992) support the view that the etiology of Kaposi's may be separate from that of HIV infection, and one study suggests that women who have acquired HIV from a bisexual partner are significantly more likely to have Kaposi's than women infected through other means, giving credence to this theory (Beral *et al.* 1990).

The possible occurrence of female-specific gynecologic manifestations of HIV infection is an area of even greater interest and current debate. Small studies have concluded that cervical dysplasia, carcinoma *in situ* and overt cervical carcinoma are more common and more aggressive in women with HIV infection (Byrne *et al.* 1989; Henry *et al.* 1989; Schrager *et al.* 1989; Maiman *et al.* 1990). In addition, there are anecdotal reports that HIV-infected women have more frequent or severe pelvic inflammatory diseases. Finally, infection of the mouth with the fungus *Candida albicans* has been known for many years to indicate progressive immune destruction in men with HIV infection. Some have suggested that vaginal infection with *Candida*—an extremely common affliction in HIV-negative women—may be more severe and more refractory to treatment in HIV-infected women and may occur earlier than oral candidiasis. This raises the possibility that it can serve as an early marker of disease progression in women (Rhoads *et al.* 1987). In the absence of large cohort studies, however, especially ones which include both HIV-infected and demographically matched non-infected women, it has been difficult to demonstrate a causal relationship between HIV and these conditions (Centers for Disease Control 1990; Minkoff and Dettovitz 1991).

Cervical carcinoma has been linked to human papilloma virus (Aurelian 1983; Vermund and Kelly 1990), and epidemiologically it is more likely to occur in women who have sex at an early age and with multiple partners (Munoz and Bosch 1989), supporting the view that it is due to the acquisition of an infectious agent. Women who have early sex and multiple partners are also more likely to acquire HIV infection, and thus the occurrence and progression of cervical disease in an individual woman may simply indicate dual infection with both agents rather than a causal role for HIV.

Despite this, female renal transplant recipients and women immunosuppressed from cancer therapy have been reported to have a greater incidence of—and a more aggressive course with—cervical carcinoma (Halpert *et al.* 1986; Katz *et al.* 1987). Finally, the occurrence of cervical dysplasia in HIV-infected women is correlated with advanced disease (Maiman *et al.* 1991; Vermund *et al.* 1991) lending biological plausibility to HIV acting either as a potentiator of human papilloma virus or independently to cause cervical carcinoma.

Determination of a causal role for HIV in the occurrence of pelvic inflammatory disease (PID) is even more difficult. Like human papilloma virus infection, PID is linked with early and multiple sex partners and is caused by a number of different infectious agents; therefore, suggestions about the precise role, if any, of HIV in its occurrence and virulence are currently based on uncontrolled studies (Hoegsberg *et al.* 1990; Safrin *et al.* 1990).

The scientific debate over female-specific manifestations of HIV infection has been hampered not only by inadequate cohort studies but also by the fact that in the USA, the provision of medical and social benefits for people with HIV infection is linked to the Centers for Disease Control (CDC) definition of AIDS (Levine and Stein 1991). Initially, these definitions, designed for epidemiologic surveillance, did not include female-specific conditions, and advocates for women with HIV argued that many women had significant morbidity and even died from complications without ever fulfilling the CDC AIDS definition (AIDS Coalition to Unleash Power, unpublished). These advocates have lobbied actively for an expanded definition of AIDS which would include cervical dysplasia and carcinoma, pelvic inflammatory disease, and perhaps vaginal candidiasis.

The CDC has now expanded its definition to include invasive cervical carcinoma. In addition, pelvic inflammatory disease and vaginal candidiasis have been included in a list of conditions which, while not AIDS-defining, are considered to occur more commonly in association with HIV infection, or to have altered diagnosis or treatment in the presence of HIV infection.

The epidemiology of HIV infection in pregnancy

In the USA and some other Western countries, HIV infection in women occurs predominately in poor women of color, who are of childbearing age, and is directly or indirectly related to intravenous drug use. These demographics are reflected in the profile of pregnant women with HIV infection. Studies in the USA have for the most part demonstrated that knowledge about HIV infection does not seem to influence decision making regarding birth control and pregnancy termination; that is, infected women appear to have the same reasons and rates of abortion as demographically matched uninfected women (Selwyn *et al.* 1989; Sunderland *et al.* 1992).

Reported rates of transmission of HIV to the fetus (vertical transmission) vary, and the overall rate is still not known with certainty. Early estimates of a vertical transmission rate of over 60 per cent were clearly too high. This is probably because the women reported in these studies had been identified because they had already borne an infected child, and they may thus have been more likely to transmit infection in subsequent pregnancies. More recent estimates suggest rates of 12–30 per cent (Blanche *et al.* 1989; Goedert *et al.* 1989; European Collaborative Study 1991). Some data suggest that women with more advanced disease (as manifested by lowered CD4 cell numbers or symptomatic disease) may be more likely to transmit infection to their fetus (Ryder *et al.* 1989).

The timing of fetal infection during pregnancy also remains unclear. While fetal malformations ascribed to infection were reported early in the epidemic, later studies have failed to demonstrate phenotypic abnormalities in infected children. Virus has been isolated from fetuses early in gestation (Sprecher *et al.* 1986), but the role of the virus in producing infertility or fetal loss is unknown. Recent studies in twins have demonstrated that the first twin born has a higher rate of infection with HIV; this finding suggests that the intrapartum period may represent a time of especially efficient viral transfer (Goedert *et al.* 1991). Some early studies demonstrated that babies born by elective cesarean section could still become infected, but the relative risks and benefits of this approach and of vaginal delivery remain unknown.

Prenatal diagnosis is currently not available for HIV infection. Even if appropriate testing could be developed, its utility may be limited by the possibility of accidentally contaminating an uninfected fetus with virus-laden maternal blood during fetal blood sampling.

Diagnosis of HIV infection in babies and young children in the absence of definitive illness is currently difficult. Maternal antibody is passively transferred to the infant before and during birth, and a positive antibody test is therefore a reliable sign that the child is infected only past the age of about 15–18 months, by which time maternal antibody would have disappeared. Attempts at earlier diagnosis through such tests as polymerase chain reaction (PCR), antibody testing, and viral culture appear promising, however (Johnson *et al.* 1989; Martin *et al.* 1991; Quinn *et al.* 1991; Rogers *et al.* 1991; Comeau *et al.* 1992).

The precise impact of pregnancy on the course of HIV infection in the woman herself is currently unknown. Early reports of maternal death associated with the development during pregnancy of *Pneumocysitis carinii* pneumonia (PCP), a common AIDS-related infection (Minkoff *et al.* 19xx; Goedert *et al.* 1990), generated concern that pregnancy might have a significant impact on maternal morbidity and mortality and led some clinicians to advice pregnancy termination for maternal indications. However, the majority of HIV-infected women in the USA still have CD4 counts above the range at which PCP is generally seen. With time and in the absence of development of effective antiviral therapies, though, more and more pregnant women will unfortunately be in the later stages of infection. Even for such women, however, current data are too limited to determine whether the course of their disease is accelerated during—let alone because of—pregnancy (Feinkind and Minkoff 1988; Koonin *et al.* 1989).

Advances in prophylaxis and therapy for PCP (the most common AIDS-defining opportunistic infection), more aggressive therapies for many other AIDS complications, and effective antiviral therapy may improve the chances for maternal survival enough to preclude a deleterious effect of pregnancy even in women with advanced disease. The greatest danger may in fact occur in pregnant women whose HIV infection is undetected or in women known to be HIV-infected but who receive inadequate prenatal or routine HIV care. These situations are unfortunately quite common in many countries, including the USA.

The impact of AIDS on women's health care

Women with HIV infection often have poor access to appropriate medical care, either because they live in countries with few services or because they are members of a socio-economic group which must rely on clinics or emergency rooms with long waiting times and poor continuity of care. When pregnant, they may receive late or even no prenatal care. Thus, programs which link preventive counselling, disease detection, and medical intervention solely to settings such as family planning or prenatal clinics may miss many women at risk of or already infected with HIV.

Moreovers because in some Western countries AIDS is commonly perceived as a male disease, practitioners may neglect to consider this diagnosis in women even in the face of symptoms or signs which would prompt HIV testing in a male patient. In addition, since women are more likely to be unaware of past infection, they may deny risk even if questioned. Finally, women of reproductive age often use obstetrician–gynecologists as their primary care providers, and such practitioners may have had less direct experience with HIV infection than internists or family practitioners, and so may attribute their patients' complaints to other causes.

Women with HIV-infected or at-risk infants are likely to attend pediatric AIDS clinics, and the time it takes to access appropriate care for their children may mean they cannot find time for their own care as well. This has led to suggestions that care for HIV-infected women and their children be integrated at one site. There are several pragmatic obstacles to such care, however. In most cities, tertiary-care children's hospitals provide the bulk of care for infected children, and these are often separate and even geographically distant from adult hospitals and clinics specializing in HIV. Few sites could afford or attract full-time HIV doctors specializing in care of the other population. Thus, adult practitioners would need to be brought in from the outside for sessions at a children's hospital, or vice versa. Even if this were successful for routine out-patient visits, referral would still have to be made for specialized testing and for in-patient care. An alternative is to have a partnership between adult and pediatric sites with good communication but separate systems of care; however, this still has the disadvantage of requiring a woman to make separate appointments and travel to two sites. None the less, these are models of care for women which appear viable, and they need to be studied and adapted (Kloser *et al.* 1990; Gregonis *et al.* 1992; Muther *et al.* 1992).

Additional issues are raised in trying to provide women with access to experimental therapies (Levine 1990). As of the end of 1990, fewer than 7 per cent of participants in federally sponsored HIV clinical trials sponsored by the AIDS Clinical Trials Group (ACTG) had been women. Early on, as has traditionally been the case in other diseases, women were in some cases categorically barred from such protocols largely because of concerns over possible teratogenic effects of experimental drugs. While all ACTG trials now permit the entry of non-pregnant women, accrual of women still lags compared to their representation among all cases of AIDS in the USA. Studies have documented that relative to the entire population of women with AIDS, women entering ACTG trials are more likely to be White and less likely to have ever used intravenous drugs. However, with time, the demographic characteristics of women participating in these trials has come closer to that of all women with the disease (Cotton *et al.* 1991). A separate Women's Health Committee has been established within the ACTG to attempt to improve accrual of women to trials as well as to design trials which will study possible female-specific manifestations of the disease, such as cervical carcinoma and pelvic inflammatory disease.

Often, sites providing experimental drug protocols require that patients have a separate primary care provider. If a woman with HIV is already bringing a child to a pediatric site, it is extremely burdensome for her to obtain her own care at two additional sites. Moreover, few experimental sites are equipped with the kinds of support services needed by women to successfully participate in drug trials. Transportation and childcare are rarely included in the budgets of such programs. In the USA, activists have called for increased funding for such services to improve participation of women in trials; however, the National Institutes of Health has argued that provision of such services is not in the mandate of the NIH and is properly addressed by agencies such as the Health Resource Services Administration and the Health Care Financing Administration. These agencies, in turn, have declined to provide such services because of the experimental nature of the therapies given. Thus, attempts at integrated care for women and children have run into bureaucratic obstacles at the institutional, local, state, and federal levels.

The problems in providing care to women with HIV infection have not been experienced to the same degree with other life-threatening diseases. In part this is because women with HIV tend to be poorer and have fewer social supports than women with other diseases such as breast cancer or end-stage renal disease. Unlike other women, they may not be able to rely on informal networks of support such as family, neighbors, or church volunteers to care for them and their children during a life-threatening illness. Moreover, HIV infection is relatively unique in being sexually acquired and vertically transmitted, creating whole families with infection. When women are responsible for others, their own needs are often relegated to last place. The AIDS epidemic has demonstrated that modern Western societies are poorly equipped to provide care for such a disease.

Long-term care of children of infected mothers is another area where AIDS provides particular stresses. In the USA, women with AIDS are often single mothers with little or no ongoing relationship to the fathers of their children and without financial support from them. When they are too ill to continue to care for their children, and after their death, the care of children often falls to the foster care system of large financially beleaguered cities. Grandmothers, sisters, and other relatives often become the guardians of such children, financially supported through the foster care system. While many such caregivers have been enormously successful in providing care to these children, others are poorly equipped to take on this burden because of poverty, age, intravenous drug use, or even their own HIV infection. Health care providers who work with women with HIV have noted that concern over what will happen to their children is their patients' greatest source of fear and depression as death approaches.

Increasing numbers of children are actually or effectively orphaned by AIDS, and a growing number are in the care of the state. The plight of these AIDS orphans is unheard of in modern American life. Some of these children are infected and sick themselves. Others are asymptomatic carriers but unlikely to be adopted because of both their HIV and their minority status. Other uninfected siblings are often difficult to place as well because of public misconceptions about their risk of transmitting infection.

The dramatically higher rates of infection among women of childbearing age in African countries portend even greater disaster (Mann *et al*. 1992). While in Africa the extended family has remained strong, a society that loses its young parents and workers in large numbers is at great jeopardy (DeCock *et al*. 1990). The very fabric of African society is at risk of being torn apart by HIV. Recent advances in improving infant mortality are being reversed. Progress in limiting family size may be halted as families replace the children lost to AIDS with additional children who tragically are also likely to be infected.

Ethical dilemmas in caring for women with HIV

There is growing awareness in the USA that the health problems of women have not been adequately addressed (Healy 1991). Research concerning such problems as breast cancer, osteoporosis, and connective tissue disease, which are all more far common in women than men, has been inadequately funded; and studies of diseases common to both sexes, such as heart disease and other forms of cancer, have included few women. The National Institutes of Health (NIH) has announced a large-scale Women's Health Initiative which will seek to address pressing health care problems in American women (Palca 1991). The NIH has also formulated new guidelines intended to require that women be included in all research studies including protocols of experimental drugs, in numbers proportional to their representation among people with the disease concerned.

Many specific issues relating to optimal methods of research, treatment, and prevention of disease in women are yet to be resolved, however. For example, should women of childbearing age with life-threatening diseases be included in drug studies where the risk of benefit is low and the teratogenic effects of the drugs unknown? When an experimental protocol seeks to prevent a disease *in utero*, who is the patient—mother, fetus, or both? How are the risks and benefits to each to be determined? Should women be represented in a drug trial in numbers which reflect the proportion of people with the disease who are women? Alternatively, should they be over-represented in order to have sufficient statistical power to address possible gender differences in drug efficacy or toxicity?

Because AIDS is a disease in which new therapies are being tested rapidly and there are no therapies which are curative or even provide long-lasting benefit, AIDS research is likely to become the arena where many of these ethical and scientific issues are debated and, hopefully, resolved.

The issue of inclusion of pregnant women in clinical trials has proven to be especially controversial in AIDS. Women of childbearing age were categorically excluded from early reflecting the standard practice in most drug trials. However, since women were likely to receive these drugs if they proved effective and were licensed, it was argued that possible gender-related side-effects or differences in drug efficacy should be detected at the earliest possible time and under the most controlled conditions possible.

AIDS has caused a profound shift in the way clinical trials are viewed. As recently as 10 years ago, they were viewed as experiments in which there was little chance of personal benefit and in which the main intent was to provide knowledge which might benefit future patients (National Commission for the Protection of Human Subjects of Biomedical and Behavioral Research 1978). Recently, however, people with AIDS and their advocates have argued that in a life-threatening disease with no effective therapies, clinical trials are healthcare, too. Therefore, they argue, everyone should have the right to access to trials. However, while non-pregnant women are now eligible to enter most trials, issues of liability have yet to be resolved, and debate continues over the appropriateness of inclusion of pregnant women, especially in phase I testing of both drugs and vaccines (in which the chance of benefit is viewed as extremely low).

AIDS is unusual in that an infected mother may or may not infect the fetus she is carrying. Thus, drugs given to the mother will not only have risks and benefits for her, but also risks and perhaps benefit for the fetus. Many now argue that it would be safer to include pregnant women in trials where they can be more closely monitored, and where teratogenic effects can be identified as early as possible.

Recently a clinical trial (ACTG #076) was designed to look at the possible benefit of zidovudine—the first antiviral drug demonstrated to be of benefit in AIDS—in preventing vertical transmission of HIV. In this trial, sponsored by the National Institutes of Allergy and Infectious Diseases, pregnant women with AIDS or asymptomatic HIV infection were to be randomized to receive either placebo or zidovudine. At birth their infants would continue to receive whichever drug the mother had been receiving until 6 weeks of age. This trial was criticized for several different reasons, resulting in a delay of almost 2 years before its initiation.

Critics noted that zidovudine was considered standard care for persons with AIDS and for symptomatic infected persons with fewer than 500 CD4 cells, especially those with symptoms, or very low CD4 cell counts. Thus, it was argued that women in that CD4 range enrolled in this trial would be denied standard therapy in order to assess the effect of the drug on transmission to the fetus. In effect, the care of women was being subordinated to the fetuses they were carrying: they were routinely denied access to trials designed to look at possible benefit for themselves, and entered into trials in which their own well-being was being ignored in order to attempt to study the fetus. Ultimately, this trial was redesigned to exclude women for whom zidovudine had become standard care even during pregnancy—those with symptomatic disease or fewer than 200 CD4 cells. In late February, 1994, trial was stopped when a planned data review indicated a highly statistically significant benefit of zidovudine in reducing perinatal transmission (25 per cent, transmission in women receiving placebos, 8 per cent in women receiving zidovudine).

Prevention of HIV infection in women

Programs to prevent HIV infection have for the most part been male oriented, focusing on the use of condoms and voluntary change of sexual behaviors. Women face a more complex set of challenges in AIDS prevention. First, it is easier for them to become infected, and thus the use of a condom for each act of intercourse is essential. However, a woman often does not control the decision to use a condom, as she is often the less powerful partner in the relationship and may suffer if she demands its use. Her partner may leave her, question her own background, or accuse her of questioning his. He may force her to have sex without a condom anyway, or may physically abuse her in other ways.

The development and recent licensure of the 'female condom' is promising. It is a vaginal sheath designed to serve both as a contraceptive and as a safer sex device that a woman controls. However, because of the urgency of the epidemic, the female condom was contraception or safe sex. Thus, it remains to be seen if it will be useful (Washington Post 1991).

A recent study (Kreiss *et al.* 1992) demonstrated an increase in acquisition of HIV in a trial of vaginal spermicide in African prostitutes. This disappointing result points up the difficulty in making recommendations on contraception and prevention of infection to women at risk for HIV. Innovative programs to increase the empowerment of women at risk for HIV, are essential.

Screening for HIV antibody is especially critical for women, who may be unaware of being placed at risk for infection through the behaviors of their partners. However, as has often been the case in AIDS, much of the discussion has focused on prenatal testing. Proponents have argued that such information is so vital to women's reproductive decision making that testing should be mandatory. In addition, pediatricians have argued for routine prenatal testing, on the theory that, in the absence of definitive tests of infection in young infants, all children at risk of HIV infection should be identified as soon as possible so that optimal medical care can be provided.

Overall, however, the population of pregnant women in the USA is at very low risk for HIV, and the benefits of testing in this population may be outweighed by potential negative consequences, such as a false-positive test leading to pregnancy termination, avoidance of future pregnancy, and possible discrimination in housing, employment, and even healthcare (Field 1990). In addition, women at highest risk are also most likely to receive poor, late, or even no prenatal care, which severely limits the benefits of a prenatal testing program.

A committee of the National Institute of Medicine (1991) concluded that mandatory prenatal testing was inappropriate. Since 1991, however, the use of prenatal HIV testing has increased and it is now used widely in a voluntary but routine manner. While it is difficult to predict future trends, the increasing use of prophylactic therapy for *Pneumocystis carinii* prenmonia in infants with HIV-positive mothers makes it more likely that a policy will be adopted of mandatory, or at least aggressive routine, testing of pregnant women perceived to be at increased risk.

The ability to significantly reduce vertical transmission of HIV with AZT has escalated the debate on routine HIV testing during pregnancy. At this writing, mandatory testing of pregnant women has not become law in any state in the United States, and the extent to which women even in high prevalence areas are routinely being offered such testing is known. Further, whether testing will result in increased prescription of AZT to identified women and reduced rates of neonatal infection remains to be seen.

Conclusion

AIDS in women differs from the disease in men in virtually all respects. Women have a more diverse set of risk factors than men and are less likely to be aware of the source of their infection. They are more likely to be poor, young, and from an ethnic minority. They are often members of families where others, including their own children, have AIDS. As a group, they have less knowledge concerning AIDS and far less access to health care and experimental drug trials. They may have additional manifestations of the infection and may have a different pattern and incidence of some opportunistic diseases than men. Drugs they receive are unlikely to have been previously tested in women. If they become pregnant, only limited information is available to them to guide choices about pregnancy termination and future family planning, and there is little published literature to guide their treatment. Their ability to avoid infection may be severely limited because of their low societal status.

For all these reasons, HIV infection in women may be best approached in a targeted and gender-specific fashion. While the delay in recognizing the enormity of the problem of HIV infection in women in tragic, it is heartening that interest in this problem is increasing, as evinced by the inclusion of many sessions on HIV infection in women at the recent International Conferences on AIDS. There is hope that this challenge can be met.

References

American Public Health Association (1991). *Women and HIV disease*, a report of the special initiative on AIDS. APHA, Washington DC.

Aurelian, L. (1983). Evidence of viral etiology of squamous cell carcinoma of the cervix. *Gynecologic Oncology*, **1**, 62.

Ayanian, J. Z. and Epstein, A. M. (1991). Differences in the use of procedures between men and women hospitalized for coronary heart disease. *New England Journal of Medicine*, **325**, 221–5.

Beral, V. Peterman, T. A., Berkelnau, R. L., and Jaffe, H. W. (1990). Kaposils sarcoma among persons with AIDS: a sexually-transmitted infection? *Lancet*, **335**, 123–8.

Berkelman, R. (1991). *AIDS indicator disease among men and women, United States*, 1988–89. Centers for Disease Control data presented at the National Conference on Women and HIV, 12–13 December, Washington DC.

Blanche S., Rouzioux, C., and Mascato, M. G. (1989). A prospective study of infants born to women seropositive for human immunodeficiency virus type I. *New England Journal of Medicine*, **320**, 1643–8.

Brown, L. S. and Primm, B. J. (1988). Sexual contacts of intravenous drug abusers: implications for the next spread of the AIDS epidemic. *Journal of the National Medical Association*, **80**, 651–6.

Byrne, M. A., Taylor-Robinson, D., Mundy, P. E., and Harris, J. R. (1989). The common occurrence of human papillomavirus infection and intraepithelial neoplasia in women infected by HIV. *AIDS*, **3**, 379–82.

Carpenter, C. C. J., Mayer, K. H., Stein, M. D., Leibman, B. D., and Fisher, A. (1991). HIV infection in North American women: experience with 200 cases and a review of the literature. *Medicine*, **70**, 307–25.

Centers for Disease Control (1990). Risk for cervical disease in HIV-infected women—New York City. *MMWR*, **39**, (47), 846–49.

Centers for Disease Control (1991). *HIV/AIDS Surveillance Report*, December, p. 10.

Centres for Disease Control (1993). Revised classification system for HIV infection and expanded surveillance case definition for addescents and adults. *MMWR*, **41**, 1–19.

Chu, S., Buehler, J. W., and Berkelman, R. L. (1990*a*). Impact of the human immunodeficiency virus epidemic on mortality of women of reproductive age, United States. *Journal of the American Medical Association*, **264**, 225–9.

Chu, S., Buehler, J. W., Fleming, P. L., Berkelman, R. L. (1990*b*). Epidemiology of reported cases of AIDS in lesbians, United States 1980–1989. *American Journal of Public Health*, **80**, 1380–1.

Comeau, A. M., Harris, J. A., McIntosh, K., Weiblen, B. J., and Hoff, R. (1992). Polymerase chain reaction in detecting HIV infection among seropositive infants: relation to clinical status and age and to results of other assays. *Journal of the Acquired Immune Deficiency Syndrome*, **5**, 271–8.

Cotton, D., Feinberg, J., and Finkelstein, D. (1991). Participation of women in a large multicenter HIV/AIDS clinical trials program in the United States. In *Proceedings of the VII International Conference on AIDS*, p. 87.

Cotton, D. J., Finkelstein, D. M., He, W., and Feinberg, J. (1993). Determinants of accrual of women to a large multicenter clinical trial program of HIV infection. *Journal of Acquired Immune Deficiency Syndrome*, **6**, 1322–8.

DeCock, K. M., Barrere, B., Diaby, L., Lafontaine, M. F., Gnaore, E., Porter A., *et al.* (1990). AIDS—the leading cause of adult death in the West African city of Abidjan, Ivory Coast. *Science*, **17**, 793–6. DesJarlais, D. C. and Friedman, S. R. (1988). Intravenous cocaine, crack, and AIDS risk reduction. *Journal of the American Medical Association*, **259**, 1945–6.

Ellerbrock, T., Lieg, S., James, D., Rogers, M., Harrington, P., and Bush, T. (1990). Sexual practices and reproductive choices of HIV+ and HIV− pregnant women in a rural community with a high HIV seroprevalence in the United States. In *Proceedings of the VI International Conference on AIDS*, Vol. 6, p. 230.

European Collaborative Study (1992). Risk Factors for mother-to-child transmission. *Lancet*, **339**, 1007–12.

Feinkind, L. and Minkoff, H. (1988). HIV in pregnancy. *Clinics in Perinatology*, **15**, 189–202.

Field, M. A. (1990). Testing for AIDS: uses and abuses. *American Journal of Law and Medicine*, **16**, 33–106.

Gayle, J. A., *et al.* (1990). Surveillance for AIDS and HIV Infection among black and Hispanic children and women of childbearing age, 1981–9. *Morbidity and Mortality Weekly Report*, **38**, SS-3, 23–30.

Goedert, J. J., Mendez, H., Drummond, J. E., Robert-Guroff, M., Minkoff, H., Hiolnan, S., *et al.* (1989). Mother-to-infant transmission of human immunodeficiency virus type 1: association with prematurity or low anti-pg120. *Lancet*, **ii**, 1351–54.

Goedert, J. J, Landesman, S. H. (1990). Serious infections during pregnancy among women with advanced human immunodeficiency virus infection. *American Journal of Obstetrics and Gynecology*, **162**, 30–4.

Goedert, J. J., Duliege, A. M., Amos, C. T., Felton, S., and Biggar, R. J. (1991). High risk of HIV-1 infection for first-born twins. *Lancet*, **338**, 1471–5.

Gregonis, S., Tedaldi, E., and Treston, C. (1992). Providing health care to families in a pediatric hospital. In *Proceedings of the VIII International Conference on AIDS*, p. PoD 5539.

Guinan, M. E. and Hardy, A. (1987). Epidemiology of AIDS in women in the United States: 1981 through 1986. *Journal of the American Medical Association*, **257**, 2039–42.

Gwinn, M., Pappaioanou, M., George, J. R., Hannon, W. H., Wasser, S. C., Redus, M. A., *et al.* (1991). Prevalence of HIV infection in childbearing women in the United States. *Journal of the American Medical Association*, **265**, 1704–8.

Halpert, R. Fruchter, R., Sedis, A., Butt, K. Boyce, J., and Sillman, F. (1986), Human papillomavirus, and lower genital neoplasia in renal transplant patients. *Obstetrics and Gynecology*, **68**, 251–8.

Healy, B. B. (1991). Women's health, public welfare. *Journal of the American Medical Association*, **266**, 566–88.

Henry, M. J., Stanley, M. W., Cruikshank, S., and Carson, L. (1989). Association of human immunodeficiency virus-induced immunosuppression with human papillomavirus infection and cervical intrepithelial neoplasia. *American Journal of Obstetrics and Gynecology*, **160**, 52–3.

Hoegsberg, B., Abulafia, O., Sedlis, A., Feldman, J., DesJarlais, D., Landesman, S., *et al.* (1990). Sexually transmitted disease and human immunodeficiency virus infection among women with pelvic inflammatory disease. *American Journal of Obstetrics and Gynecology*, **163**, 1135–9.

Holmberg, S. D., Horsburgh, C. R., Ward, J. W., and Jaffe, H. W. (1989). Biologic factors in the sexual transmission of human immunodeficiency virus. *Journal of Infectious Diseases*, **160**, 116–25.

Johnson, J. P., Nair, P., Hines, S. E., Seiden, S. W., Alkger, L., Revie, D. R., *et al.* (1989). Natural history and serologic diagnosis of infants born to human immunodeficiency virus-infected women. *American Journal of Diseases of Childhood*, **143**, 1147–53.

Katz, R. L., Veanattukalathil, S., and Weiss, K. M. (1987). Human papillomavirus infection and neoplasia of the cervix and anogenital region in women with Hodgkin's disease. *Acta Cytologiea*, **31**, 845.

Kloser, P., Pinto, R. C., Lombardo, J., Bais, P., Lyunch, A., and Gibson, C. (1990). Women's clinic: a full service clinic for women with HIV disease. In *Proceedings of VI International Conference on AIDS*, Vol. 6, p. 294.

Koonin, L. M., Ellerbrock, T. W., Atrash, H. K., Roger, M. F., Smith, J. C., Hogue C. J., *et al.* (1989). Pregnancy-associated deaths due to AIDS in the United States. *Journal of the American Medical Association*, **261**, 9.

Kirschstein R. L. (1991). Research on women's health. *American Journal of Public Health*, **81**, 291–3.

Kreiss, J. K. *et al.* (1992). Efficacy of nonoxynol-9 contraceptive sponge use in preventing heterosexual acquisition of HIV in Nairobi prostitutes. *Journal of the American Medical Association*, **268**, 477–82.

Levine, C. (1990). Women and HIV/AIDS research: the barriers to equity. *Evaluation Review*, **14**, 447–63.

Levine, C. and Stein, G. L. (1991). What's in a name? The policy implications of the CDC definition of AIDS. *Law, Medicine and Healthcare*, **19**, 278–90.

MacDonell, K. B., Chmiel, J. S., Poggensee, L., Wu, S., Phair, J. P. (1990). Predicting progression to AIDS: combined usefulness of CD4 lymphocytes and p24 antigenemia. *American Journal of Medicine*, **89**, 706–12.

Maiman, M., Fruchter, R. G., Serur, E., Remy, J. C., Feuer, G., and Boya, J. (1990). Human immunodeficiency virus infection and cervical neoplasia. *Gynecologic Oncology*, **38**, 377–82.

Maiman, M., Tarricons, N., Viera, J., Suarez, J., Serur, E., and Boyce, J. G. (1991). Colposcopic evaluation of human immunodeficiency virus seropositive women. *Obstetrics and Gynecology*, **78**, 84–8.

Mann, J., Tarantola, D. J. M., and Netter, T. W. (ed.) (1992). *AIDS in the World*. Harvard University Press, Cambridge.

Martin, N. L., Levy, J. A., Legg, H., Weintrub, P. S., Cowan, M. J., and Wara, D. W. (1991). Detection of infection with human immunodeficiency virus (HIV) type 1 in infants by an anti-HIV immunoglobulin A assay using recombinant proteins. *Journal of Pediatrics*, **118**, 354–8.

Minkoff, H. L., and DeHovitz, J. A. (1991). Care of women infected with the human immunodeficiency virus. *Journal of the American Medical Association*, **266**, 2253–8.

Minkoff, H. L., Willoughby, A., Mendez, H., Moroso, G., Holman, S., Goedert, J. J., *et al.* (XXXX). Serious infections during pregnancy in women with advanced HIV infection. *American Journal of Obstetrics and Gynecology*, **162**, 30–4.

Monzon, O. and Capellan, J. M. (1987). Female to female transmission of human immunodeficiency virus. *Annals of Internal Medicine*, **105**, 969.

Moore, R. D., Hidalgo, J., Sugland, B. W., and Chaisson, R. E. (1991). Zidovudine and the natural history of the acquired immune deficiency syndrome. *New England Journal of Medicine*, **20**, 1412–6.

Munoz, N. and Bosch F. X. (1989). Epidemiology of cervical cancer. In *Human Papillomavirus and Cervical Cancer* (ed. N. Munoz, F. X. Bosch, and O. M. Jenson), pp. 9–39. International Agency for Research on Cancer, Lyon.

Muther, J., Keen, P., Klein, E., Nesbein, S., Sawyer, M., Pratt-Palmore, M. (1992). Family clinic: a model for delivery of comprehensive services to HIV positive children and their parents. In *Proceedings of VIII International Conference on AIDS*.

National Commission for the Protection of Human Subjects of Biomedical and Behavioral Research (1978). *The Belmont report: ethical principles and guidelines for the protection of human subjects of research*. Department of Health and Human Services, Washington, DC.

National Institute of Medicine. (1991). *HIV screening of pregnant women and newborns. National Academy Press, Washington DC.*

Padian, N., Marquis, L., Francis, D. P., Anderson, R. E., Rutherford, G. W., O'Malley, P. M., *et al.* (1987). Male-to-female transmission of human immunodeficiency virus. *Journal of the American Medical Association*, **258**, 780–90.

Padian, N. S., Shiboski, S. C., and Jewell, N. P. (1991). Female-to-male transmission of human immunodeficiency virus. *Journal of the American Medical Association*, **25**, 1664–7.

Palca, J. (1991). NIH unveils plan for a women's health project. *Science*, **254**, 792.

Plummer, F., Simonsen, J. N., Cameron, D. W., Ndinya-Achola, J. O., Kreiss, J. K., Gakinya, M. N., *et al.* (1988). Co-factors in male-female transmission of HIV. In *Proceedings of IV International Conference on AIDS*, Vol. 2, p. 200.

Quinn, T. C., Kline, R. L., Halsey, N., Hutton, N., Ruff, A., Butz, A., *et al.* (1991). Early diagnosis of perinatal HIV infection by detection of viral specific IgA antibodies. *Journal of the American Medical Association*, **266**, 3439–42.

Rhoads, J. L., Wright, D. C., Redfield, R. R., and Burke, D. S. (1987). Chronic vaginal candidiasis in women with human immunodeficiency virus infection. *Journal of the American Medical Association*, **257**, 3105–7.

Rogers, M. F., Ou, C. Y., Rayfield, M., Thomas, P. A., Schoenbaum, E. E., Abrams, E., *et al* (1991). Use of the polymerase chain reaction for early detection of the proviral sequence of HIV in infants born to seropositive mothers. *New England Journal of Medicine*, **320**, 1649–54.

Rothenberg, R., Woefel, M., Stoneburner, R., Milberg, J. Parker, R., and Truman, B. (1987). Survival will be acquired immunodeficiency syndrome. *New England Journal of Medicine*, **317**, 1297–302.

Ryder, R. W., Nsa, W., Hassig, S. E., Behets, F., and Rayfield, M. (1989). Perinatal transmission of the human immunodeficiency virus type 1 to infants of seropositive women in Zaire. *New England Journal of Medicine*, **320**, 1637–42.

Safrin, S., Dattel, B. J., Haver, L., and Sweer, R. L., (1990). Seroprevalence and epidemiologic correlation of infection in women with acute pelvic inlfammatory disease. *Obstetrics and Gynecology*, **75**, 666–70.

Schrager, L. K., Friedland, G. H., and Maude, D. (1989). Cervical and vaginal squamous cell abnormalities in women infected with human immunodeficiency virus. *Journal of AIDS*, **2**, 570–5.

Selwyn, P. A. *et al.* (1989). Prospective study of human immunodeficiency virus infection and pregnancy outcomes in intravenous drug users. *Journal of the American Medical Association*, **261**, 1289–94.

Selwyn, P. A. *et al.* (1989). Knowledge of HIV antibody status and decisions to continue or terminate pregnancy among intravenous drug users. *Journal of the American Medical Association*, **261**, 3567–71.

Sprecher, S., Soumenhoff, G., Puissant, F., and De gueldre, M. (1986). Vertical transmission of HIV in a 15-week fetus (letter). *Lancet*, **2**, 288–9.

Stein, M. D., Piette, J., Mor, V., Wachtel, T. J., Fleishman, J., May, K. H., *et al.* (1991). Differences in access to zidovudine (AZT) among symptomatic HIV-infected persons. *Journal of General Internal Medicine*, **6**, 35–40.

Sunderland, A., Minkoff, H. L., Hante, J., Moros, G., and Landesman, S. (1992). The impact of HIV serostatus on reproduction decisions for women *Obstetrics and Gynecology*, **6**, 1027–3.

Vermund, S. H. and Kelley, K. F. (1990). Human papillomavirus in women: methodolgic issues and role of immunosuppression. In *Reproductive and Perinatal Epidemiology* (ed. M. Kiely), CRC Press, Boca Raton.

Vermund, S. H., Kelly, K. F., Klein, R. S., Feingold, A. M., Schreber, K., Munk, G., *et al.* (1991). High risk of human papillomavirus infection and cervical squamous intrepithelial lesions among women with symptomatic human immunodeficiency virus infection. *American Journal of Obstetrics and Gynecology*, **165**, 392–400.

Washington Post. (1991). February 1, P. 1.

Wofsy, C. B., Cohen, J. B., Hauer, L. B., Padian, N. S., Michaelis, B. A., Evans, L. A., *et al.* (1986). Isolation of AIDS-associated retrovirus from genital secretions of women with antibodies to the virus. *Lancet*, **i** 527–9.

6 Screening for cancer in women

Jonathan Niloff and Jocelyn Chamberlain

The purpose of screening for cancer is to interrupt the natural history of development of a cancer by detecting and removing the affected cells at an early stage, usually before they have given rise to any symptoms. The reason for believing that this will be an effective measure is based on the common clinical experience that asymptomatic cancers diagnosed at an early stage are frequently curable, whereas those diagnosed at a late stage are not.

It cannot necessarily be assumed that screen-detected cancers will behave in exactly the same way as symptomatic disease and one cannot infer that simply by detecting early disease one has improved prognosis. It is first necessary to find out by research what proportion of women can be helped by screening, before offering it to all women as a means of reducing their risk. As in all forms of preventive medicine which offer a service to well people (as opposed to patients), there is a particular ethical responsibility on the health care providers to be certain that the benefits of screening outweigh the disadvantages (Fig. 6.1).

Potential benefits of screening

The benefits of screening depend principally on curing cases of disease which would otherwise go on to advanced stages or death. The natural history of cancer can be portrayed as a triangular passage (Fig. 6.2). Above the triangle is the vast majority of people who are free from any sign of the cancer concerned; at the top of the passage are people whose epithelial cells show a hint of mild abnormality, which is not in itself harmful, but indicates a slight risk of subsequent cancerous change. Then come people with more severe cellular abnormality. The next stage is cancerous cells which have not yet invaded through the epithelium (intra epithelial neoplasia), then early invasive cancer. This advances to secondary spread and finally death. Only a small minority of

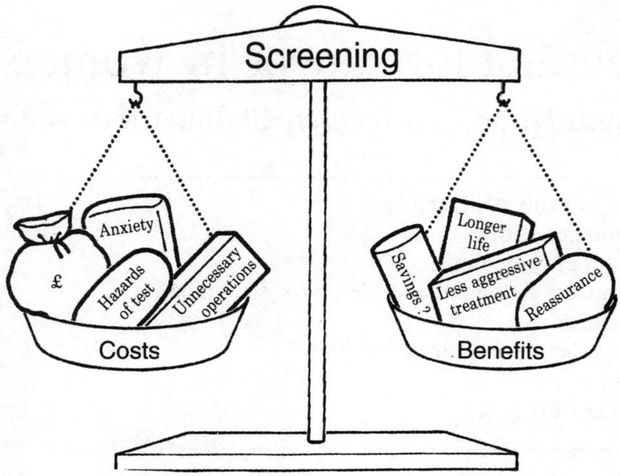

Fig. 6.1 The balance of benefits and costs.

the people with the early changes will eventually progress to more advanced disease. Moreover, cancers of any site have variable progression rates, some being so indolent that it may take decades for them to progress to invasion at which time they are still curable; while others are highly malignant and will go through the various stages in a matter of weeks. Screening is unnecessary for the former group and ineffectual for the latter; it is for cases between these two extremes that it may be helpful.

The point in this natural history at which it is possible to intervene depends on which screening tests are available. Some tests, such as the cervical smear, are aimed at detecting and removing severe epithelial abnormality (point A). Others, such as mammography, are not as sensitive for preinvasive disease and are aimed at detecting early invasive disease (point B). The benefit of screening

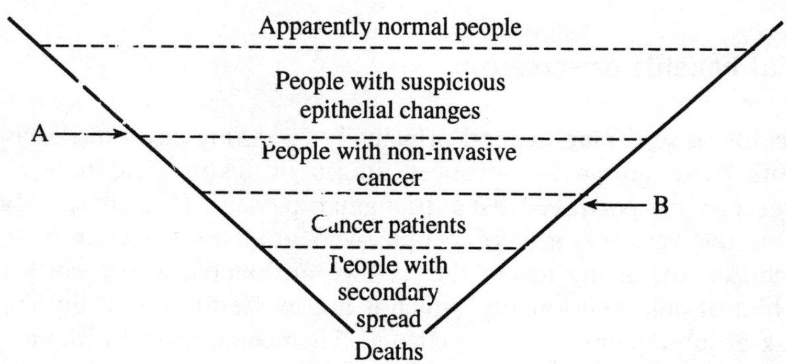

Fig. 6.2 The cut-off point for screening. Model of progression of precancerous and cancerous changes in a population.

at point A is that removal of abnormalities at this stage prevents the woman from developing invasive cancer, with all it entails in morbidity and expensive treatment, and cure can normally be achieved by an inexpensive and simple treatment. Screening at point B, however, entails somewhat greater morbidity and more complicated treatment; it does not prevent invasive cancer but can prevent death. Thus, the benefits of screening are judged either by a reduction in cases of invasive disease (reduced incidence) or a reduction in deaths (reduced mortality).

Disadvantages of screening

The price for detecting very early warning signs of subsequent cancer (point A) is that many women who would never go on to develop cancer in their lifetime are labeled as 'positive' by the test. There is currently no method for dividing borderline cases into those that will progress and those that will not, and so all have to be treated as though they will, leading to the psychological and physical harm of over-diagnosis and overtreatment. But screening at the early invasive stage has the converse disadvantage that some of the cases detected may have seeded off microscopic secondary deposits in other organs and hence will already be incurable. Therefore, among patients with cancers and precancers detected by screening, some suffer because they are overtreated for a non-progressive lesion, and others suffer because they are told of their cancer diagnosis sooner and have to endure the morbidity of treatment for longer than they otherwise would, without any compensating improvement in prognosis.

There is also a risk that some people will be harmed because of the deficiencies of the screening test. The ideal screening test will tell the truth, the whole truth, and nothing but the truth. But in practice, no test meets these absolute criteria of perfect sensitivity (no false-negative results in women with cancer) and perfect specificity (no false-positive results in women without cancer). So some women who have cancer may suffer because the test gives a false-negative result and their diagnosis and treatment are therefore delayed and so their disease becomes incurable. Alternatively, some non-diseased women may suffer because they have a false-positive diagnosis and have to go through the anxiety and physical morbidity of further diagnostic tests, sometimes requiring a biopsy operation, only to find that they do not, in fact, have cancer. The sensitivity and specificity of a test balance against one another and depend on the cut-off point (reference value) between what is designated a positive result and what is designated negative. Hence the test can be made more sensitive by including the merest suspicion of abnormality as a positive result, but this will make the test less specific and give many false positives; on the other hand, using a stricter definition of what constitutes a positive will improve specificity and reduce the number of false positives, but only at the price of reducing sensitivity and missing some cancers.

Because the incidence of any cancer is quite low (typically affecting less than one woman in 1000 each year), many more women are exposed to the risk of a false-positive result than the risk of a false-negative result. Although the adverse consequences of a false positive tend to be minor, the sheer volume of this minor morbidity needs to be considered against the magnitude of any improvement in prognosis for the true positives, in deciding whether or not screening does more good than harm, and in setting the cut-off point between a positive and a negative screening test result.

Most practicing physicians providing screening are much more concerned with sensitivity because they are fearful of missing a case—not least because of the threat of litigation—and hence tend to have a high index of suspicion and often argue for extending the screening test to include additional investigations. While this approach is entirely correct for diagnosing a complaint in a symptomatic patient, it may be inappropriate for screening both because of the accompanying fall in specificity and because of its costs. It is important that women themselves should also appreciate that screening tests are not perfect and do not provide an absolute diagnosis.

The final, and probably the major, disadvantage of cancer screening is its resource cost. Even with the simplest test, screening is an expensive and inefficient form of medical care, because the number of people who need to be screened, investigated, and treated in order to prevent one cancer death commonly runs into tens of thousands. Another problem is that a single negative test does not imply lifelong protection from the disease. It only indicates that the person is probably free from disease at that time, but further routine screening is still necessary at intervals thereafter.

Evaluation of screening

Research to measure the proportion of potential cancer patients whose prognosis is improved by screening is more complicated than it may at first appear. We have already seen that the value of screening cannot be judged just by the number of cancers or precancers it detects because some of the cancers might not progress, some might be curable even if left until they presented with symptoms, and, at the other end of the natural history spectrum, some might already be incurable.

Nor can any conclusion be drawn by comparing the survival of patients with screen-detected cancers with those with symptomatic cancers. Survival is expressed as the proportion of people with cancer who are alive at a set time (for example, 5 years) after diagnosis. Because screening advances the date of diagnosis, a screen-detected case will always appear to have a longer survival than a comparable symptomatic case even if their dates of death are identical. Moreover screening tends to differentially pick out slower-growing good prognosis cases because such cases spend a longer time progressing through the stage when they are detectable but not yet symptomatic than do fast-growing more aggressive cases. So the case-mix of screen-detected cancers is biased toward those with a good prognosis, and may contain some which would never progress within the woman's lifetime. A further bias is that the sort of women who avail themselves of screening tend to be health aware, with a positive attitude towards the curability of cancer. Therefore, even in the absence of screening, they would be likely to have a longer survival than the fatalistic sort of women who reject screening because they prefer not to know and, whether or not a screening service is available, defer seeking medical care until it is too late.

The only way of overcoming these methodological difficulties is to compare the number of cancer deaths (or invasive cancers if the test is screening for preinvasive disease) in a whole population of women for whom screening has been available, with the number of these endpoints in a comparable 'control' population for whom it has not. The size of population which needs to be studied in this way, and the length of time before the comparison is likely to show a statistically significant difference, typically runs into tens of thousands of women studied over seven years or more. Ideally, the study should be a prospective trial in which women in a set population are identified and then randomly allocated either to be offered screening or to be in the control group. Such trials are long, laborious, and expensive, and so far have only been completed for two cancer sites: lung cancer, for which screening has been shown to be of no value; and breast cancer, for which it has been shown to be of limited value.

Retrospective comparisons of the number of endpoints before and after introduction of screening into a population without a control group can also give useful information. However, they do not obviate the need for screening to have been provided for a large population over many years, and do not give such statistically precise estimates of the level of benefit.

In population-based comparisons, it is important to include the number of deaths not only among women whose disease was detected by screening, but also among women who did not take up the offer of screening, and in women who developed cancers after a negative test. There are two reasons for this. First, those deaths from cancers not detected by screening have their counterparts in the control group, and therefore the comparison would be invalid if they were excluded. Second, from the viewpoint of a public health authority considering the introduction of screening, the estimate of mortality reduction in the entire population—taking into account the uptake of screening and the sensitivity of the test—is the figure required for judgments as to whether screening is worthwhile.

But the inclusion of deaths among women who did not take up the offer of screening clearly dilutes the estimate of level of benefit to an individual screened woman. In prospective trials, the proportion of women who do not accept screening is known, and their mortality rate can be compared with that in the control group. From these two figures, the reduction among women who have been screened can be calculated.

In contrast to research trying to measure the benefit of screening, comparatively little has been done to evaluate its disadvantages and costs. Some disadvantages, such as the number of false-positive test results, can be included in information systems for routine monitoring of the performance of the screening program. But the psychological and physical effects which false positives have on quality of life can only be measured by sample surveys and there have been few of these. Similarly, there have been very few economic studies of the resource costs of screening. It is important to realize that it is not merely the costs of the test itself which affect the costs of screening compared with no screening. The costs of investigating women with positive results are also attributable to the screening program, as well as the costs of treating the cancers found. An estimate of all these costs needs to be set against the costs of diagnosing and treating these cancers if there were no screening program, to give the net cost resulting from screening. It is sometimes postulated that, because treatment of early cancer is generally less expensive than that of late cancer, there may actually be a saving. In practice, however, the large number of cases detected at the start of a screening program means that the volume of early cases needing treatment outweighs any saving from having to treat fewer advanced cases in later years.

Having obtained the best available information on both benefits and costs, a decision must be made on whether screening is worthwhile. Such decisions are made both by women themselves and by health policy makers. In either case, unquantifiable value judgments—personal for each woman, political for the policy makers—play a large part. In trying to help policy makers decide whether to use resources on a cancer screening program or on some alternative public service, economists express the cost-effectiveness of each alternative in terms of the net cost for each year of life gained, with an allowance for the quality of life—the QUALY, or quality-adjusted life year. The number of years of life gained can be estimated from the reduction in deaths shown in research trials of the effectiveness of screening, but the adjustment for quality is currently based on very crude estimates which include many untested assumptions. Similarly, current estimates of net costs of screening programs are usually based on 'guesstimates' rather than on laboriously collected real data. There are a variety of computer simulation models of the cost-effectiveness of the different screening programs, but because of the untested assumptions these contain they should be regarded with extreme caution.

Which cancers should be considered for screening?

The first criterion used in decisions on screening is that the condition sought should be an important health problem. The relative importance of different cancers can be gauged from their incidence rates (number of new cases diagnosed each year) and their mortality rates (number of deaths each year). The frequency of cancers of different sites varies in different parts of the world, but the pattern is similar in most developed countries, which are also those most likely to be able to afford screening programs.

Table 6.1 shows the incidence and mortality rates from the most common cancer sites in women in the European Community during the 1980s. Breast and large bowel top the list for both incidence and mortality. It should be noted that although the incidence of lung cancer is low, compared with other sites, it ranks third with stomach cancer as a cause of death. Conversely, the mortality from endometrial cancer is low, which puts it at a low priority for screening. Skin cancer is omitted from this table; non-melanoma skin cancer is common in

Table 6.1 Most common cancers in women in Western Europe

	Number of new cases per 100 000 women per year	Number of deaths per 100 000 women per year
Breast	56.8	21.4
Large bowel	22.4	12.5
Stomach	11.1	8.2
Ovary	11.0	6.2
Cervix	10.4	5.1
Endometrium	9.7	2.5
Lung	8.2	8.2

elderly women but is almost always completely curable so it is not a candidate for screening. Melanoma of the skin, however, is an important problem because although its incidence (4.9 per 100 000 women) and mortality (1.0 per 100 000 women) are still relatively low, they are both increasing year by year. In the following sections, current evidence on the benefits and costs of screening for different cancers is reviewed.

Breast cancer

For the past 20 years, breast cancer has been the most common female cancer world-wide, and the incidence rate (the number of new cases per 1000 women per year) is continuing to increase. Breast cancer is a disease of affluence, and its known predisposing factors are associated with the socially desirable goals of adequate nutrition and control of family size. Hence, incidence rates are highest in Western societies but it is inevitable that they will continue to rise in the developing world. There have been some advances in treatment by use of drugs to control systemic disease, in addition to surgery and radiotherapy for control of local disease in the breast. The main determinant of prognosis, however, remains the stage at which the cancer is diagnosed. This has led to great hopes that screening could have a major impact in reducing the number of deaths from breast cancer.

Effectiveness of screening

More research has been done to evaluate screening for breast cancer than for any other cancer. Six prospective trials, comparing populations offered screening with control populations, have so far been published and others are under way. All have used mammography as the screening test, in some cases in combination with physical examination of the breast by a doctor or nurse. Although not all the studies had statistically significant results, they were remarkably consistent in concluding that screening is of benefit.

Among a population of women aged 50–74 years when first screened, the risk of dying from breast cancer over the ensuing 10 years is reduced by about 25 per cent (ranging from a low of 9 per cent in one trial to a high of 40 per cent in another). This is the estimate of benefit to the whole population; in fact, the benefit to an individual screened woman is greater and has been estimated from the combined trials to average 39 per cent. Only the earliest trial, started in New York in the late 1960s, has so far analysed results beyond 10 years and has found that the reduction in mortality persisted, albeit at a slightly lower proportion, up to at least 18 years. Given the very high mortality rates from breast cancer in women in the sixth, seventh, and eighth decades, even the limited reduction achieved by screening means it is possible to prevent tens of thousands of breast cancer deaths internationally. Within the UK, it is hoped that screening for breast cancer will lead to 1000–1500 fewer deaths each year.

Another consistent result of the trials has been the lack of any convincing reduction in mortality among women aged less than 50 when first invited for screening. One reason for this is that mammography and physical examination are much less sensitive in premenopausal breasts because of the greater density of breast tissue. Another contributing factor is that none of the trials had sufficient statistical power to prove or disprove a mortality reduction because they included too few women in this age group. Further trials are now under way. Until they are concluded, however, the value of screening women under 50 remains unproven.

As screening is known to have some disadvantages and has not been proven to have any benefit in this age group, firm recommendations to screen women under 50 cannot be made. Possible exceptions are women whose mothers or sisters have developed breast cancer when premenopausal. These women are at particularly high risk, and although there is no evidence that screening can alter their prognosis, the reassurance given by a negative screening test (accompanied by the proviso about its imperfect sensitivity) may justify regular mammograms for these women.

Sensitivity of screening

Mammography is a reasonably sensitive screening test in women over 50. It detects approximately 85 per cent of cancers, in contrast to physical examination, which can only pick up 60–70 per cent. Moreover lesions detected by mammography tend to be smaller, many of them being impalpable. The effectiveness of physical examination on its own has never been tested, which is unfortunate for women in developing countries which have neither the resources nor the skills for mammography screening. Similarly, the effectiveness of breast self-examination is unproven, although one large trial has shown no difference in mortality between populations who were or were not exposed to an intensive education campaign about self-examination. Further research is needed, but the present position can be summed up by saying that education campaigns in a population are probably ineffective, but breast self-examination by an individual woman might be effective.

Frequency of screening

Related to sensitivity is the frequency with which routine screening is repeated. The largest mammography trial, in Sweden, found that screening every 3 years using just a single X-ray view of each breast led to a 40 per cent reduction in mortality in women aged 50 or more. But many radiologists, for fear of missing a cancer, advocate screening every 2 years, or even annually. In deciding on screening policy, it is desirable to estimate how many extra lives are saved by this more intensive screening, so that the additional cost per death avoided is known. Current research is addressing this issue.

Disadvantages of screening

The postulated disadvantages of screening are the hazards of mammography, its lack of specificity, the possibility of overdiagnosis (false-positive test), and the costs of the whole screening process. Mammography involves compression of the breast against an X-ray plate so that all the breast tissue appears on the X-ray image. This is uncomfortable for many women, and painful for a few, but since the compression only lasts for a few seconds this is not a major drawback.

Much more concern has been expressed in the past about whether the dose of radiation given by mammography could itself cause breast cancer to develop in the future. But the doses of radiation given by modern techniques are so tiny that this risk—if it exists at all—is minuscule compared with the level of protection against death from breast cancer given by screening. Hence, provided that the radiological equipment and the exposure dose of a mammogram are regularly and adequately monitored, this putative danger can safely be discounted.

Mammography does not have a very high specificity. Between 3 and 7 per cent of women without cancer have a suspicion on their X-ray which requires further investigation. However, using a diagnostic approach which combines further X-rays, physical examination, ultrasound investigation, and, in some cases, aspiration of cells from the suspicious area, the proportion of women who progress to have an excision biopsy with a benign diagnosis is now very small—around one in 200 screened women. Anxiety levels after being referred for investigation of a suspicious mammogram have been found to be temporarily raised, but are less than in symptomatic women, and do not persist.

The rate of diagnosis of non-progressive disease for breast screening programs is still unknown. In the first trial, conducted in the 1960s when mammography was less sensitive, the cumulative number of breast cancers in the screened group was no greater than that in the control group, so there was no overdiagnosis. But with the greater sensitivity of modern mammography, later trials have found more than expected number of cancers, particularly ductal *in situ* cancers, whose rates of progression to invasive cancer are unknown. Around 20 per cent of lesions detected on first screening are ductal carcinomas *in situ*, but on routine rescreening, the proportion of *in situ* lesions is much lower.

Probably the greatest constraint to implementation of breast screening by mammography is its resource cost. Obviously, this varies according to different health care systems but, whether it is provided from public or private funds, it still requires considerable financial expenditure for a fairly limited probability of benefit. The potential saving in treatment costs of advanced disease which might result from screening has not yet been quantified, but is unlikely to be substantial compared with the costs associated with screening.

Verdict

The decision about whether the likely benefit justifies the expenditure and other disadvantages depends on the value judgments of the decision makers, be they health policy makers or individual women. The fact that so many developed countries now have policies providing or promoting mammography screening for women aged 50 and over indicates a broad consensus view that its benefits justify its costs.

Cancer of the uterine cervix

World-wide, cancer of the cervix ranks second in frequency to breast cancer but its geographical distribution is very different. Eighty per cent of cases occur in developing countries, where it is the leading cause of cancer death; in the developed world, it is much less frequent. It is tempting to ascribe the lower incidence in developed countries to their screening programs, but it is possible that a more important reason is a lower exposure to the etiological agent(s).

In the USA in 1991, there were approximately 13 000 new cases of invasive carcinoma of the cervix and approximately 4500 deaths attributable to it (Boring *et al.* 1991). Known risk factors include early age at first intercourse and multiple sexual partners. A male consort who in turn has had intercourse with multiple women also confers a significant risk. Carcinoma of the cervix is more common in women who smoke. Barrier contraceptives are protective, but the role of oral contraceptives remains controversial. Carcinoma of the cervix is more common in women who are immunosuppressed, especially those who have undergone renal transplantation; this may be mediated by the human papilloma virus. HIV infection may increase a woman's risk for cervical neoplasia.

Natural history of cervical intraepithelial neoplasia

Cervical cancer has a well defined precursor lesion. It has been referred to as dysplasia which develops into carcinoma *in situ* and then progresses to invasion. More modern terminology refers to dysplasia and carcinoma *in situ* as cervical intraepithelial neoplasia (CIN). The recognition that carcinoma *in situ* of the cervix (CIN III), could progress to invasive cervical cancer arose from Papanicolaou's original observation of women with this abnormality who were untreated and who subsequently developed cancer. Approximately 50–60 per cent of CIN III cases will progress to invasion. It has been estimated that dysplasia precedes carcinoma *in situ* by at least 7 years and carcinoma *in situ* precedes invasion by 8–30 years. The proportion of lesser grades of CIN which progress is less, and the average duration before they do so longer. The peak age for carcinoma *in situ* is between 25 and 35 years. Invasive carcinomas are typically found in women over 40 but are now being diagnosed increasingly in younger women.

Human papilloma virus

Human papilloma virus (HPV) is a common sexually transmitted disease. It typically manifests itself as condylomata (genital warts). The annual incidence of HPV in the USA is increasing and has been estimated to be as high as 500 000 to 1 000 000 cases per annum (Campion 1989). Over the past two decades an increased prevalence of CIN has been observed in the USA and Western Europe. There were more than 1 500 000 cases of CIN in the USA in 1989; 50 000 were CIN III (Acs *et al.* 1989). Strong laboratory evidence suggests that HPV is associated with the development of cervical cancer. However, two large cross-sectional epidemiological studies failed to detect a significant association between this virus and cervical cancer (Kjaer *et al.* 1988; Acs *et al.* 1989). In contrast, a case-control study suggested that HPV does significantly increase the relative risk for developing cervical cancer (Reeves *et al.* 1989).

If HPV infection is indeed a significant risk factor for cervical cancer, its prevalence in the female population is important in risk assessment and in forming screening strategies. The most sensitive test for detecting HPV is the polymerase chain reaction (PCR). Using this technique, HPV was demonstrated in 33 per cent of students attending an American college (Bauer *et al.* 1991) and in 22 per cent of the general population aged 16–60 in the Netherlands (van der Brule *et al.* 1989). The expression of HPV is episodic however. Therefore, these numbers may underestimate the actual prevalence of HPV infection.

Effectiveness of screening

Screening by cervical cytology was the forerunner of cancer screening programs and was widely introduced in the 1960s on the basis of Papanicolaou's demonstration of a preclinical phase, and the fact that it was feasible to apply the test to large numbers of women. At that time no one appreciated the need to conduct a randomized controlled trial to quantify the reduction in incidence and mortality, and in most countries screening developed in a haphazard fashion with no consistent policy.

Pap smear screening has a specificity of approximately 99 per cent. It is better for high grade and invasive lesions. The test is less specific for low grade CIN. Over-diagnosis of these lesions is common, and is in part due to the test's inability to distinguish low-grade CIN from HPV infection. The sensitivity of Pap smear screening has been reported to range from 40 to 70 per cent. The generally accepted false-negative rate is 15–25 per cent. Due to the long latent period associated with the precursor lesion (CIN), this false-negative rate does not compromise screening strategies as long as smears are performed frequently enough.

Over the course of about 20 years evidence has accumulated to show that regular screening could reduce the incidence of invasive cervical cancer by a substantial amount. The best evidence comes from a retrospective comparison of various Scandinavian countries with different screening policies. Finland, Sweden, and Iceland all set up, in the mid-1960s, highly organized screening programs whereby all women of the target age range were personally invited to be screened at regular intervals. More than 80 per cent accepted. By contrast, Norway had an organized program in just one county which covered only 5 per cent of the national population. All four countries had a very similar incidence of cervical cancer in 1960, which is not surprising given the homogeneity of their populations. However, over the ensuing 20 years the incidence of invasive cervical cancer in Norway hardly altered, whereas in the other three countries it fell by close to 50 per cent. Consequently, mortality from cervical cancer followed the same pattern (Johannesson *et al.* 1978).

In British Columbia, Canada, the incidence of cervical cancer fell by 85 per cent from 24.8 per 100 000 in 1955 to 4.2 per 100 000 in 1988 (Benedet *et al.* 1992). There was a similar 80 per cent decrease in mortality: it fell from 11.4 per 100 000 in 1955 to 2.3 per 100 000 in 1988. The decrease in mortality attributable to cervical cancer has been correlated with the intensity of Pap smear screening (Worth 1984).

Need for an organized program

A patient who presents with invasive cervical carcinoma is a failure of the Pap smear screening program. This may be attributable to failure at one of several steps: lack of participation in the screening program, inadequate performance of the Pap smear, inaccurate interpretation of the cytology slide, or failure to appropriately follow up or evaluate an abnormal smear. In the UK, screening in the National Health Service was available from the mid-1960s, but over the next 20 years incidence and mortality were unchanged, despite the fact that sufficient screening tests were performed to cover all women aged 20–64 every 5 years (the interval used in Finland). The main reason for the failure of the UK program to match the achievements of its Scandinavian counterparts was the fact that its performance was neither organized nor monitored. The result was that young, well-educated, low-risk women were being screened frequently while older women at greater risk were not participating. A survey of women who developed invasive cervical cancer found that two-thirds of them had never been screened and a further 10 per cent had lapsed from regular screening, 15 per cent had had a mildly abnormal smear which had not been adequately investigated, and 9 per cent had developed cancer within 5 years of a negative smear (Fig. 6.3).

Anderson *et al.* (1992) evaluated 437 patients presenting with invasive carcinoma of the cervix in British Columbia from 1985 to 1988. Forty-nine per cent

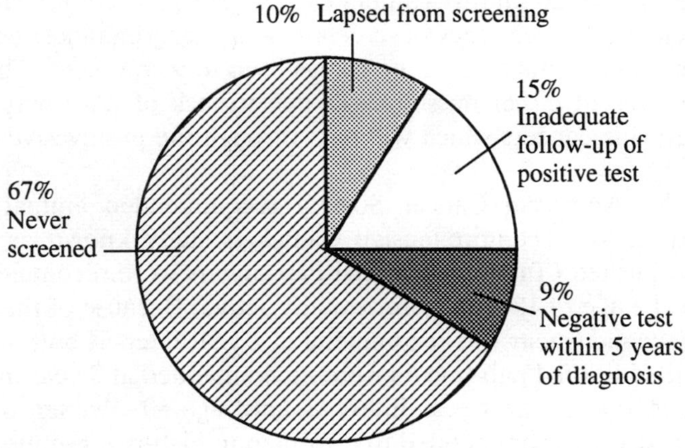

Fig. 6.3 Reasons why women developed invasive cervical cancer.

had either never been screened or had not had a Pap smear in the prior 5 years. Fifteen per cent of the patients who had had a prior cytology had abnormal cells missed or undercalled.

These experience indicate that a high priority should be to achieve universal screening. A 1989 survey indicated that more than one-third of American women were not having Pap smears at either 1 or 3 year intervals. Studies in the USA and Canada have identified the geographic distribution and socio-economic factors associated with non-participation in screening and higher mortality from cervical cancer. Studies should be undertaken in each geographic area to define the demographics of non-participation in the local screening program. Population-specific outreach strategies should then be developed to bring these women into the detection program. Programs are required to educate primary care physicians how to perform optimal screening. The full benefit of cervical screening will only be realized when a set policy is established, followed, and carefully monitored.

Frequency of routine screening

The appropriate interval between one screen with a negative result and the next routine screen depends on the time it takes for a potential cancer patient to progress from negative to invasive cancer. This, in turn, may be influenced by epidemiologic and personal risk factors. By studying previously screened women who have later developed invasive cancer and comparing them with control women without cancer, useful information has been obtained about the probability of progression in different intervals. From this the protection against invasive cancer given by screening at different intervals can be derived. The frequency of screening is also influenced by the sensitivity of the test. Making certain assumptions about the underlying incidence of cancer, it has been estimated that in Western countries screening a woman every 5 years between the ages of 20 and 64 confers 84 per cent protection against invasive cancer. Increasing the frequency of screening to 3-yearly enhances her protection to 91 per cent, and annual screening brings it up to 93 per cent. The remaining 7 per cent represent either missed cases due to lack of sensitivity of the test, or rapidly growing cancers which will pass through the preinvasive stage within 1 year.

Initially, the American Cancer Society recommended annual Pap smear screening. In 1976, a comprehensive Canadian study known as the Walton report was published (Table 6.2). Initial Pap smears were recommended for all women over the age of 18 who were sexually active. Because of the risk of false negatives, a second smear was recommended 1 year later. If both initial smears were normal, additional pap smears were recommended at 3 year intervals until age 35 and, thereafter, at 5 year intervals until age 60. Women over 60 were not screened. It was recommended that women in high-risk groups be screened more frequently.

The American Cancer Society, in 1980, recommended a similar screening strategy. After two initial negative Pap smears, further screening was recommended at 3 year intervals until age 65. Again, more frequent screening was recommended for patients considered to be at high risk. The American College of Obsetricians and Gynecologists (ACOG) has always recommended annual screening. In 1984, the Canadian recommendations were modified and annual Pap smear screening was recommended for all sexually active women between 18 and 35 years of age (Worth 1984). This was based on mathematical models and European studies suggesting that a 4–5 a year screening interval was too long.

Disagreement remains concerning the optimal screening interval. There are many problems with screening less than annually. As Pap smears have a false-negative rate of 15–25 per cent, an interval of 3 or more years could lead to a new lesion remaining undetected for a decade. Some lesions progress rapidly and lesions at risk for rapid progression cannot be predicted. Richart and Barron (1981) suggested that 5 per cent of cases of CIN III will progress to invasion in less than 3 years. In another study, similar progression was calculated to occur in less than 1 year in 4 per cent of cases (Albert 1981). Dunn *et al.* (1984) reported that 33 per cent of their patients with invasive carcioma of the cervix had had normal Pap smears 1–5 years earlier. The average interval from the normal smear was 2.6 years.

Despite the known epidemiologic risk factors, it is difficult to select high-risk women for more frequent screening. Ninety per cent of women enrolled in a DES (Diethylstilbestrol) screening program (the DESAD project) aged 35 years or younger had had first sexual intercourse at less than 20 years of age or had had more than two partners. HPV infection is very prevalent in Western countries and its potential for significantly increasing the risk of cervical neoplasia and the rate of progression of CIN must be considered; these factors would argue for erring on the side of a rigorous screening schedule. The American population is highly mobile and women have poor knowledge of their prior Pap smears. Annual screening fosters both physician and patient compliance with the program.

Table 6.2 Pap smear screening recommendations

Report	Begin	Age 18–35	Age 36–60	Over age 60
Walton Report Canada (1976)	Sexually active, over age 18	Every 3 years after two consecutive annual normal Paps More frequently if high high risk	Every 5 years	Stop if prior normal Paps
Canadian Task Force (1982)	Sexually active, over 18	Annually if sexually active	Every 5 years if two prior negative Paps More frequently if high risk	Stop if prior normal Paps
American Cancer Society (1980)	Age 20 or when sexually active	Every 3 years after two consecutive normal Paps More frequently if high risk	Every 3 years More frequently if high risk	Every 3 years More frequently if high risk
American College of Obstetricians and Gynecologists (1980)	Age 18 or when sexually active	Annually	Annually	Annually

There is no general agreement on the appropriate screening for elderly women. ACOG recommends continuing annual screening indefinitely. In one study, 6 per cent of patients with invasive carcinoma of the cervix were over the age of 60 and had prior normal Pap smears (Anderson *et al.* 1992). In another study, 25 per cent of patients over the age of 65 had never had Pap smears (Mandelblatt *et al.* 1986). There were 16 abnormal smears per 1000 cervices at risk. Abnormal smears after the menopause, especially in patients not previously screened, are more commonly associated with invasive tumors.

While instinctively it may appear obvious to opt for the maximum protection, the marginal balance between benefit and cost is a good illustration of the law of diminishing returns. For the population of England and Wales it has been calculated that the cost (1987 prices) to the National Health Service of universal screening every 5 years (the current maximum interval recommended by the Department of Health) would be £34 000 000, representing £8500 per invasive cancer prevented. Changing the frequency to every 3 years would prevent an additional 300 cancers but would cost an additional £21 000 000, giving a marginal cost per cancer prevented of £70 000. Changing from triennial to annual screening would only prevent a further 100 cases at a marginal cost of more than £1 000 000 each.

Such estimates are clearly of interest to public health authorities who must assess the relative priorities of the many different demands on their finite resources. However, although the aggregate cost is large, many women would consider the expense of an annual Pap smear small to decrease their risk of dying from cervical cancer. Ultimately the trade-off is between cost and preventable death. Less frequent screening intervals and restriction of screening to young women will result in increased mortality from cervical cancer. It is difficult to determine the tolerable number of such excess deaths balanced against the extra cost of more rigorous screening.

Problems with screening

The strategy employed to manage women with abnormal Pap smears is a major secondary determinant of the cost of screening in terms of money and resources, as well as patient morbidity and anxiety. Depending on the cytology laboratory, 10–30 per cent of women can be expected to have abnormal smears (Benedet *et al.* 1992). More than half of these will regress or represent HPV. About 80 per cent of abnormal tests are atypical and low-grade smears. Evaluation of such a large number of abnormal smears, many of which do not reflect a significant neoplastic potential, is very costly and places a large burden on medical resources. The British Columbia strategy mandates the evaluation only of high-grade or persistent abnormal Pap smears. In the USA, a more aggressive philosophy is more commonly followed. The most appropriate, safe, and cost-effective management program for patients with low-grade atypical Pap smears must be defined because clearly the strategy selected to manage the large number of low-grade lesions identified by screening will have a major influence on the cost effectiveness of the program.

Pap smear failure studies indicate that quality control in some cytology laboratories is a significant problem. Yobs *et al.* (1985) administered on-site proficiency tests using 'normed' samples. The target diagnosis was made in only 64 per cent of samples. The false-negative rate was 7.5 per cent and the false-positive rate was 9 per cent. Using actual laboratory output, the false-negative rate was 5–11 per cent and the false-positive rate was 3 per cent. The need for educational programs and supervision is clear. The US federal government has set limits on the number of slides that a cytotechnologist can evaluate per day. Efforts are currently being directed toward developing new technologies for evaluating cytology slides. These should remove the subjectivity associated with cytologic evaluation and therefore increase accuracy. In the future, automation may permit more rapid evaluation at significantly lower cost.

Ovarian cancer

There are approximately 21 000 new cases of ovarian cancer in the USA annually (Boring *et al.* 1991). About 13 000 women in the USA and 3700 women in the UK succumb to this malignancy each year. As yet, there are no screening tests that can recognize a premalignant lesion for ovarian cancer. Therefore, the goal is to identify patients who have stage I tumors. Because ovarian cancer is very difficult to diagnose, it has a high death-to-case ratio. Early symptoms are typically subtle or absent, and most patients therefore present with advanced disease in which the tumor has already spread extensively beyond the ovaries. Advances in the management of ovarian cancer, including more aggressive surgery and new chemotherapy agents, have improved the short-term survival of patients with ovarian cancer. However, despite these innovations, there has not been a significant improvement in the long-term survival or cure rates for this malignancy over the last 30 years.

Survival among patients with ovarian cancer is closely related to the stage (extent of tumor) at the time of diagnosis. Women with stage I disease (tumor confined to the ovary) have a 5-year survival of about 70 per cent. Women whose tumors have spread beyond the ovary have 5 year survival on the order of 12 per cent. The high proportion of patients presenting with advanced disease accounts for the overall poor outcome associated with this tumor. Given the significantly more favorable prognosis associated with early stage disease, it is intuitive that a screening test that could identify tumors when they were still confined to the ovary, and therefore still surgically curable, would improve the overall survival for the malignancy.

Specificity is a particularly important parameter of a screening test for ovarian cancer. The diagnosis of this tumor can only be made surgically. Therefore, a test with a poor specificity (high false-positive rate) would result in a large number of unnecessary surgical procedures, with their attendant morbidity and cost. This is especially problematic because the women at greatest risk for ovarian cancer are of advanced age and therefore often have illnesses that place them at increased risk for surgery. Informing a woman that she has a positive screening test will cause undesirable anxiety for her and her family until it is determined that her test was a false positive.

The specificity of a screening test is influenced by the prevalence of the disease concerned in the population being screened. The more common the tumor, the greater the specificity. The incidence of ovarian cancer rises with age. It is less than 15 per 100 000 in women below the age of 40, but rises to 25 per 100 000 for women aged 45, and 50 per 100 000 for women aged 70 (OPCS Monitor 1981). Given this age distribution it is predictable that some modalities of screening will be more efficiacious in older (postmenopausal) women.

Familial ovarian cancer

One to three per cent of ovarian cancer cases are hereditary in origin. Three syndromes have been identified: ovarian cancer alone, ovarian cancer and breast cancer, and the Lynch II syndrome, which includes cancers of the ovary, breast, endometrium, and colon. Predisposition to these cancers are transmitted in an autosomal dominant pattern. The lifetime risk of ovarian cancer in the general population is approximately 1.4 per cent. Among women belonging to ovarian cancer families, the risk may be as high as 50 per cent. Familial ovarian cancer typically occurs at an early age. The tumors are histologically indistinguishable from non-familial cases, but they are typically aggressive, present as advanced-stage tumors, and carry a poor prognosis. There are no specific physical stigmata associated with women belonging to such families, and genetic markers are not currently routinely available although genetic research gives optimism that the gene may soon be identified. At the moment, women are best identified by studying their family pedigree (Lynch 1992).

Screening modalities

Three modalities have been proposed as screening techniques for ovarian cancer: pelvic examination, ultrasound, and tumor markers. Pelvic examination is a very insensitive and inefficient method and will not have a significant impact on the early detection rate for ovarian cancer. Although firm data are not available, it has been estimated that ovarian cancer is detected in women of all ages only once in approximately 10 000 examinations. This is not to suggest, however, that women should not have annual gynecologic examinations.

A number of studies have evaluated both transabdominal and transvaginal ultrasound as screening techniques for ovarian cancer (Table 6.3), but none of them have been population based and all have been flawed by selection biases. Such biases included self-referral of patients, no exclusion or varying criteria for family history, and inclusion of patients with palpable masses. Campbell *et al.* (1989) performed abdominal ultrasounds on 5479 self-referred asymptomatic women. The false-positive rate was 3.5 per cent; only one in 67 patients with an abnormal ultrasound had ovarian cancer. In a subsequent analysis of this population using more refined ultrasound criteria the false-positive rate was 1.6 per cent and the odds of finding a primary ovarian cancer were still only one in

Table 6.3 Screening with sonography

Modality	Number of women screened	Population	False positive rate (%)	Chances of finding primary ovarian cancer	Reference
Abdominal ultrasound	5479*	Self-referred	3.5	1 : 67	Campbell (1989)
Abdominal ultrasound	5479*	Self-referred	1.6	1 : 50	Campbell (1990)
Vaginal ultrasound	1000	Asymptomatic Age > 40 years Positive family history 7%	3.1	None detected in study	van Nagell (1990)
Vaginal ultrasound	776	Asymptomatic One first- or second-degree relative with ovarian cancer	5.2	1 : 13	Bourne (1991)

*Same study population: different sonographic criteria

50 (Campbell *et al.* 1990). Abdominal ultrasound has inadequate sensitivity to be used as a screening modality for ovarian cancer.

Transvaginal ultrasound permits more precise visualization of the ovaries. An advantage of transvaginal ultrasound is that the bladder need not be filled; however, the transvaginal probe is less acceptable to some patients. Van Nagell *et al.* (1990) reported on 1000 asymptomatic women over the age of 40 who underwent transvaginal ultrasound. Seven per cent of this population had a positive family history for ovarian cancer. In 3.1 per cent of the patients (9.2 per cent of the premenopausal and 2.3 per cent of the postmenopausal women), the scans were abnormal, but none of the patients turned out to have primary ovarian tumors. This false-positive rate is not acceptable for widespread screening.

Tumor markers

Tumor markers are substances which can be measured in the blood and which suggest or confirm the presence of a tumor in the body. Tests for tumor markers are typically easy to perform and, when done in large numbers, should be inexpensive. The best-studied tumor marker for ovarian cancer is CA125. The sensitivity of the assay for CA125 in a screened population has yet to be defined, but is likely to be substantially less than 50 per cent. Jacobs and Bast (1989) reviewed the literature and concluded that only half of patients with stage I ovarian cancer had elevated CA125 levels. Even this figure is probably unrealistically high, because patients were included who were not from a screened population but who had presented with pelvic masses or symptoms of ovarian cancer. This is not very encouraging.

Einhorn *et al.* (1992) evaluated the specificity of the CA125 assay in a screened population in Sweden consisting of 5550 women aged 40 or older. In 9.3 per cent of women younger than 50 and in 3 per cent of women older than 50, CA125 levels exceeded what were considered to be normal values. Altogether, elevated levels were detected in 175 of the women. They were followed with serial measurements of CA125 levels, physical examinations, and ultrasonography as clinically indicated. Ovarian cancer was subsequently detected in six women, all of whom were over 50 years of age; however, only two of these patients had stage I tumors. After serial measurements of CA125 levels and clinical investigations, the odds of finding ovarian cancer in women of all ages was only one in 29 of the women with high CA125 levels. Among women over the age of 50, the odds of finding ovarian cancer was one in 17. This study suggests that a menopausal population is better suited to screening with CA125. Nevertheless, the specificity of the assay is less than optimal and it is discouraging that only two of the six cancers detected were stage I. Appropriate population-based study is required to assess the potential benefits of this screening modality.

A number of strategies have been attempted to increase screening specificity. These involve the use of multiple tests either in combination or sequentially. Jacobs *et al.* (1988) screened 1000 postmenopausal women primarily with CA125 levels and vaginal examinations. If the initial screen was positive, secondary screening with an abdominal ultrasound was performed. If the ultrasound was abnormal, surgery was recommended. If the ultrasound was negative, patients were followed with serial ultrasounds and physical examinations at 3 month intervals for 1 year. Ultrasound was designated to be a secondary screen because it cost more than the CA125 assay. In this series, screening did not identify any case of ovarian cancer that was not detectable by physical examination alone. Three per cent of the population had elevated CA125 levels and therefore required further evaluation.

Jacobs and colleagues (1992) presented data suggesting that the use of multiple tumor markers in combination could improve screening specificity. However, the compromise in sensitivity was not assessed. The use of the color doppler as a second modality is another possible way of improving specificity (Bourne *et al.* 1989). It requires further study.

Current status of screening for ovarian cancer

Neither the CA125 assay nor ultrasound, used either alone or in combination, has sufficient sensitivity or specificity to screen the general population. The false-positive rate would generate a large number of unnecessary surgical procedures. Creasman and DiSaia (1991) estimated that if all 43 million women in the USA over the age of 45 were annually screened with sonographic examination ($275) and CA125 evaluation ($45), the total cost would exceed $13 billion per year. Then, follow-up for each woman with a positive screening test would undoubtably incur several billion dollars more. All these procedures would place a significant demand on medical resources.

Westhoff and Randall (1991) estimated the potential effect on mortality of screening for ovarian cancer in the USA. If a screening test were available with a sensitivity of 80 per cent, and if universal annual screening of women aged 45–74 were performed, 5000 additional 5 year survivors from ovarian cancer could be predicted annually. This is an overly optimistic estimation of sensitivity, and universal screening is an unreasonable expectation. The number of women likely to benefit from a screening program for ovarian cancer which used presently available tests would certainly be substantially less.

Routine screening of the general population for ovarian cancer thus cannot be recommended at present, although there is a case for trials of its effectiveness. Screening with serial CA125 levels and ultrasonography may be appropriate in selected populations who have a high incidence of ovarian cancer, such as women with a familial risk for ovarian cancer in whom the chance of developing this tumor may be as high as 50 per cent. However, assignment of women to this high-risk group should be based on strict criteria. They should have at least two first-degree relatives who had ovarian cancer or have pedigrees that are clearly consistent with one of the three known syndromes. The most appropriate screening interval for these women is yet to be defined, but 6 months has been suggested. This strategy is appropriate for women who wish to remain fertile.

Because the efficacy of screening this population has not been clearly demonstrated, once childbearing is completed, prophylactic removal of the ovaries should be recommended. These interventions may have an important impact among women belonging to ovarian cancer families; however, as only 1–3 per cent of ovarian cancers are familial in origin, screening such individuals will not have a major impact on the overall survival from ovarian cancer.

Other sites of cancer

Lung cancer

Lung cancer is increasing rapidly among women in the developed world, as a direct consequence of the rise 30–40 years ago in cigarette smoking among women. Although the number of cases of lung cancer is considerably less than that of breast cancer, the fatality rate is much higher (only 5 per cent surviving for 5 years) and in the USA and Scotland, lung cancer has already overtaken breast cancer as the leading cause of cancer death in women.

There have been a number of trials of screening for lung cancer in men by means of chest X-rays and sputum cytology. Despite promising early results in terms of a high yield of operable lung cancers and greater survival of screen-detected cases, there is no difference in the number of lung cancer deaths between a screened group and a control group. The most likely explanation is that progressive lung cancer is so aggressive that screening, even repeated as often as every 4 months, cannot halt it in time; the main effect of screening is to detect non-progressive disease which would not have harmed the person if left undetected. Although this research only looked at men, there is no reason to suppose that screening women would be any more effective. Clearly the only hope of stemming the increase in lung cancer deaths is to halt cigarette smoking.

Large bowel cancer

Cancers of the colon and rectum are also extremely common in both women and men in the developed world, and rank second or third as causes of cancer death in women in many countries. It is thought that most large bowel cancers arise from premalignant adenomas, so that detection and removal of the latter could reduce the incidence of subsequent cancer. Tests which detect occult blood in faeces are reasonably sensitive for cancer but less so for adenoma. Large randomized controlled trials are in progress and should give an answer within a few years about the extent of reduction (if any) in incidence and mortality which could result from screening. Sigmoidoscopy is a more sensitive method which might confer greater protection, but its acceptability to well people is doubtful and its value still unproven.

Stomach cancer

World-wide the incidence of stomach cancer in both sexes is falling, probably due to greater consumption of fresh fruit and vegetables. However, Japan has had a particularly high incidence, and screening by double contrast barium X-ray of the stomach has been employed there for several years. It has not been evaluated by research and, although mortality is falling, it is difficult to disentangle the effect of dietary change from the possible effect of screening.

Malignant melanoma of the skin

Sunburn, indicating acute damage of the skin by ultraviolet irradiation, is thought to be the cause malignant melanoma, which is the most malignant variety of skin cancer. Its incidence is rising rapidly in fair-skinned people, probably because of the increasing tendency for holidays in the sun. Depletion of the ozone layer may also play a part. Mortality is also rising, more rapidly in men than in women. Protection of the skin against sunlight is the best method of prevention, but 'self-screening' by looking for the early signs might help to reduce mortality. Research is under way to evaluate the effectiveness of health education campaigns promoting early detection.

General conclusions

Despite its inherent appeal, the potential for screening to reduce the burden of cancer in women is limited. So far, it is only of proven value for two sites: the cervix for all adult women and the breast only for women aged 50 and over. For societies wealthy enough to afford them, organized screening programs with careful quality control are certainly desirable for these two cancers and should make a measurable impact on morbidity and mortality, without causing an excess number of undersirable side-effects. But for all other cancers, screening is of unproven value and should be restricted to research trials.

From a public health perspective, the optimal balance between benefit and cost is achieved by a tightly controlled screening program which organizes screening for all eligible women at set intervals, and maintains quality assurance both of the screening process itself and of follow-up investigation of positives. The most important aspects of quality are a high participation rate and high levels of sensitivity and specificity. If screening is allowed to develop in an unsystematic way, resources will certainly be squandered on too frequent screening of women who are least at risk. This confers little or no benefit and may increase the chances of false positives and over-diagnosis, and will waste money.

Women who believe in the value of screening may question why they should be discouraged from being screened very frequently, particularly if they are prepared to pay for it themselves. Clearly they have this right, but it is also desirable that they should be aware of the marginal benefits and costs of so doing. The same applies to doctors who recommend screening at unnecessarily frequent intervals.

It is important that both the providers and recipients of cancer screening should familiarize themselves with its evaluation and should make their decisions on the balance of evidence on benefits and costs.

References

Acs, J., Hildesheim, A., Reeves, W. C., Brenes, M., Brinton, L., Lavery, C. *et al.* (1989). Regional distribution of human papilloma virus DNA and other risk factors for invasive cervical cancer in Panama. *Cancer Research*, **49**, 5725–9.

Albert, A. (1981). Estimated cervical cancer disease state incidence and transition rates. *Journal of the National Cancer Institute*, **67**, 571–6.

American Cancer Society (1980). Report on cancer-related health check-up: cancer of the cervix. *Cancer*, **30**, 215–23.

American Cancer Society (1989). *Cancer Facts and Figures: 1989*. American Cancer Society, Chicago.

American College of Obstetricians and gynecologists (1980). *ACOG statement of policy: periodic cancer screening for women*.

Anderson, G. H., Benedet, J. L., LeRiche, J. C., Matisic, J. P., and Thompson, J. E. (1992). Invasive cancer of the cervix in British Columbia: a review of the demography and screening histories of 437 cases seen from 1985–1988. *Obstetrics and Gynecology*, **80**, 1–4.

Bauer, H. M., Ting, Y., Greer, C. E., Chambers, J. C., Tashiro, C. J., Chimera, J. *et al.* (1991). Genital human papilloma virus infection in female university students as determined by a PCR-based method. *Journal of the American Medical Association*, **265**, 472–7.

Benedet, J. L., Anderson, G. H., and Matisic, J. P. (1992). A comprehensive program for cervical cancer detection and management. *American Journal of Obstetrics and Gynecology*, **166**, 1254–9.

Boring, C. C., Squires, T. S., and Tong T. (1991). Cancer statistics, 1991. *Cancer Journal for Clinicians*, **41**, 19–36.

Bourne, T., Campbell, S., Steer, C., Whitehead, M. I., Collins, W. P. (1989). Transvaginal colour flow imaging: a possible new screening technique for ovarian cancer. *British Medical Journal*, **299**, 1367–70.

Bourne, T. H., Whitehead, M. I., Campbell, S., Royston, P., Bhan, V., and Collins, W. P. (1991). Ultrasound screening for familial ovarian cancer. *Gynecologic Oncology*, **43**, 92–7.

Campbell, S., Bhan, V., Royston, P., Whitehead, M. I., and Collins, W. P. (1989). Transabdominal ultrasound screening for early ovarian cancer. *British Medical Journal*, **299**, 1363–7.

Campbell, S., Royston, P., Bhan, V., Whitehead, M. I., and Collins, W. P. (1990). Novel screening strategies for early ovarian cancer by transabdominal ultrasonography. *British Journal of Obstetrics and Gynecology*, **97**, 304–11.

Campion, M. J. (1989). Human cervival papillomavirus infection: a clinical perspective. *IARC Scientific Publications*, **94**, 41–65.

Creasman, W. T., and DiSaia, P. J. (1991). Screening in ovarian cancer. *American Journal of Obstetrics and Gynecology*, **165**, 7–10.

Dunn, J. E., Crocker, D. W., Rube, I. F., Erickson, C. C., and Coleman, S. A. (1984). Cervical cancer occurrence in Memphis and Shelby County, Tennessee, during 25 years of its cervical cytology screening program. *American Journal of Obstetrics and Gynecology*, **150**, 861–4.

Einhorn, N., Sjovall, K., Knapp, R. C., Hall, P., Scully, R. E., Bast, R. C., Jr *et al.* (1992). Prospective evaluation of serum CA125 levels for early detection of ovarian cancer. *Obstetrics and Gynecology*, **80**, 14–8.

Jacobs, I. and Bast, R. C. Jr. (1989). The CA125 tumour-associated antigen: a review of the literature. *Human Reproduction*, **4**, 1–12.

Jacobs, I. S., Oram, D. H., and Bast, R. C. Jr (1992). Strategies for improving the specificity of screening for ovarian cancer with tumor-associated antigens CA125, CA15-3, and TAG 72.3. *Obstetrics and Gynecology*, **80**, (3) 396–9.

Jacobs, I., Stabile, I., Bridges, J., Kemsley, P., and Reynolds, C. (1988). Multimodal approach to screening for ovarian cancer. *Lancet* **i**, 1(8580) 268–71.

Johannesson, G., Geinsson, G., and Day, N. (1978). The effect of mass screening in Iceland 1965–74 on the incidence and mortality of cervical cancer. *International Journal of Cancer*, **21**, 418.

Kjaer, S. K., de Villiers, E-M., Haugaard, B. J., Christensen, R. B., Teison, C., Mouerka, *et al.* (1988). Human papilloma virus, herpes simplex virus and cervical cancer incidence in Greenland and Denmark: a population-based cross-sectional study. *International Journal of Cancer*, **41**, 518–24.

Lynch, H. T. (1992). Genetic risk in ovarian cancer. *Gynecologic Oncology*, **46**, 1–2.

Mandelblatt, J., Gopaul, I., and Wistreich, M. (1986). Gynecological care of elderly women: another look at Papanicolaou smear testing. *Journal of the American Medical* Association, **256**, 367–71.

OPCS (Office of Population Census and Surveys (1981). Deaths by case. *OPCS Monitor*.

Reeves, W. C., Brinton, L. A., Barcia, M., Brnes, M. M., Herrero, R., Gaitan, E. *et al.* (1989). Human papilloma virus infection and cervical cancer in Latin America. *New England Journal of Medicine*, **320**, 1437–41.

Richart, R. M. and Barron, B. A. (1981). Screening strategies for cervical cancer and cervical intraepithelial neoplasia. *Cancer*, **47**, 1176.

van der Brule, A., Claas, E., Main, M., Melchers, W. S., Helmerhorst, T. Quins, W. G. *et al*. (1989). Use of anticontamination primers in the polymerase chain reation for the detection of human papilloma virus genotypes in cervical scrapes and biopsies. *Journal of Medical Virology*, **29**, 17–20.

van Nagell, J. R., Jr, Higgins, R. V., Donaldson, E. S., Gallion, H. H., Powell, D. E., Paulik, E. S. *et al*. (1990). Transvaginal sonography as a screening method for ovarian cancer: a report of the first 1000 cases screened. *Cancer*, **65**, 573–7.

Walton, R. J. (1982). Cervical cancer screening programs: summary of the 1982 Canadian task force report. *Canadian Medical Association Journal*, **127**, 581–9.

Walton, R. J., Blanche, T. M., Boyes, D. A. *et al*. (1976). Cervical cancer screening programs (Department of National Health and Welfare Task Force Report). *Canadian Medical Association Journal*, **114**, 1003–12.

Westhoff, C. and Randall, M. C. (1991). Ovarian cancer screening: potential effect on mortality. *American Journal of Obstetrics and Gynecology*, **165**, 502–5.

Worth, A. J. (1984). The Walton report and its subsequent impact on cervical cancer screening programs in Canada. *Obstetrics and Gynecology*, **63**, 135–9.

Yobs, A. R., Swanson, R. A., and Lamotte, L. C., Jr (1985). Laboratory reliability of the Papanicolaou smear. 65, 235–44.

7 Benign gynecological conditions: changing indications for surgery

David Chapin

Epidemiology, indications, mortality, and complications of hysterectomy
Alternatives to hysterectomy
Future developments

The field of gynecologic surgery includes procedures of two types: those that deal with the treatment of life-threatening diseases such as cancer or obstetrical catastrophe, and those that deal with improving the quality of life by treating conditions such as menstrual disturbances, infections, infertility, incontinence, and less serious complications of pregnancy. Here we will discuss those quality-of-life procedures, which include dilatation and curettage, laparoscopy, and hysterectomy. These widely performed procedures are surrounded by an atmosphere of tradition, emotion, and controversy, with very little documentation of their effectiveness, safety, or cost-to-benefit ratio. I will consider the epidemiology, history, and current understanding of these procedures, review what little literature exists, discuss the interplay between societal forces and medical practice, predict future directions, and suggest areas of future research.

Hysterectomy—surgical removal of the uterus—is the second most common major operation performed in the USA, averaging 650 000 cases annually (Bachmann 1990). Other developed countries also perform large numbers of hysterectomies. The rates vary from country to country, county to county, and hospital to hospital, and considerable controversy has arisen throughout the world about the appropriate indications for hysterectomy.

Although the lay public often believes that hysterectomy means removal of all the internal reproductive organs, it actually means only the removal of the uterus and cervix. Removal of the ovaries is a separate procedure, called oophorectomy, which is sometimes carried out at the same time as hysterectomy, but must be separately described. Oophorectomy before menopause brings on immediate cessation of estrogen secretion (surgical menopause). If estrogen replacement therapy is not instituted promptly, the woman will have annoying symptoms of hot flushes and vaginal atrophy, and the long-term sequelae of osteoporosis and coronary artery disease will begin to develop.

Epidemiology, indications, mortality, and complications of hysterectomy

When one considers that only half the population is eligible to receive this operation, and that the only operation performed more often is cesarean section, also pertinent only to women, one must pause to consider the epidemiological, cultural, and political implications behind the facts and figures. Access to health care, financing of health care, sexist attitudes of health care providers, and feminist attitudes toward health care providers contribute to the controversy surrounding this issue. A discussion of the epidemiology, indications, mortality, complications, techniques, alternatives, and the future of hysterectomy is worth undertaking in view of these current controversies.

Epidemiology

Removal of the uterus was first described in ancient Greece (Bachmann 1990), but of course the operation was not practical until the late nineteenth century when sterile surgical techniques and anesthesia became available. Following these developments, the popularity of hysterectomy rose steadily through the middle part of the twentieth century. The largest number of procedures performed in 1 year in the USA was 725 000 in 1975. Since then the number of cases has decreased to average about 650 000 per year. The rate has decreased even more, as the population of women has increased. Other English speaking countries—New Zealand, Australia, the UK, South Africa—also perform large numbers of hysterectomies. In New Zealand, the chance of having a hysterectomy by the age of 85 is 39 per cent (Macintosh 1987) and in the UK the chance of having one by age 55 is 20 per cent (Vessey *et al.* 1992). Continental European rates vary as well: They are low in France, with a hysterectomy rate of 5.8 per cent of all women, and higher in Italy, where the rate is 15.5 per cent. Naylor (1984) in South Africa reported having personally performed 2901 procedures; Gitsch (1991) in Austria reported on 9967 hysterectomies performed at one hospital within a 30 year period. Although country-wide rates of hysterectomy are not available for South Africa or Austria, these large personal series document the popularity of the procedure.

A striking epidemiological finding is that the rate of hysterectomy varies in different parts of the USA (Bachmann 1990). The highest rate of hysterectomy is found in the south and southeast and the lowest rate is in the northeast (Dicker *et al.* 1982*a*; Easterday *et al.* 1983). The Roos (1984) study in Canada evaluated variations within a single province and documented that certain characteristics of the patient and of the doctor are important ingredients in the decision-making process. The patient's attitudes toward hysterectomy and sexuality, as well as education, cultural values, and medical background, all play an important role. For example, wives of physicians are more likely to have hysterectomies than other women. Physician characteristics that appear to be important include medical training, upbringing, religious attitudes, and gender. For example, female gynecologists perform fewer hysterectomies than males. The training of primary care physicians also enters into determining whether hysterectomy will be performed: the Canadian study showed that the rate is higher for patients whose primary care physician was a gynecologist than if he or she was a general practitioner.

Recently, efforts have been made to contain costs by lowering the rate of hysterectomy through second opinion programs, precertification programs, and strong quality assurance programs. However, in one second opinion program, the second physician's opinion had no effect on the surgical rate (Finkel 1990). Some quality assurance efforts have been more successful (Gambone *et al.* 1990*b*).

The feminist movement has also taken notice of the large number of hysterectomies performed, and various writings have appeared alleging that medical professionals, mostly men, use hysterectomy to enhance their control over women patients.

> Supported by conventional views of women in society, trained to intervene surgically, and motivated by professional and economic pressures, obstetrician–gynecologists may be inclined to remove a women's uterus in the absence of clear-cut indications to do so. The patients become unwitting conspirators in this process by allowing their knowledge to be gleaned only from the physician's input and by not taking advantage of other educational opportunities (Kasper 1985).

Patients occasionally echo these views in discussing the necessity for hysterectomy.

Indications

The indications for hysterectomy have changed so rapidly over the past few years that they are difficult to delineate in the absence of consensus (Easterday *et al.* 1983; Bachmann 1990). The five most common reasons cited for hysterectomy are fibroids (leiomyomata), uterovaginal prolapse, endometriosis, carcinoma, and endometrial hyperplasia (Dicker *et al.* 1982; Bachmann 1990). Other indications are abnormal bleeding, pelvic pain, and complications of pregnancy. In recent years, the number of vaginal hysterectomies performed for prolapse has increased because this condition occurs more frequently in elderly women and the numbers of elderly women are increasing. Documentation of the incidence of prolapse and how it may have changed with time is lacking. Elective hysterectomy is not given much credence as a legitimate indication, despite at least one study that found gains in life expectancy and quality of life outweighed its risks and expense (Sandberg *et al.* 1985). Hysterectomy for sterilization can no longer be justified, because simpler, less risky, and less expensive methods, such as vasectomy and tubal ligation by laparoscopy have become readily available (Amerikia 1979; Bachmann 1990). The removal of asymptomatic fibroids is no longer considered a legitimate indication unless they are very large, and even in those cases there is some debate (Reiter *et al.* 1992). Prophylaxis of cancer by hysterectomy is no longer considered a legitimate indication, although it was until recently (Bachmann 1990).

Mortality

Mortality from hysterectomy when performed vaginally was about 2.5 per cent in the early part of this century, and had fallen by 1980 to about 2.5 per 10 000 cases. Similarly, mortality from abdominal hysterectomy, which had an approximate mortality of 3 per cent in the early twentieth century had fallen to 12 per 10 000 by 1980 (Bachmann 1990). When operations unassociated with cancer or obstetrical emergencies are considered separately, the mortality is only six per 10 000 for abdominal hysterectomies, and lower for those performed vaginally (Wingo *et al*. 1985) but, since there are so many hysterectomies, there are still more than 500 deaths per year in the USA so they must be taken seriously (Bachmann 1990). The lower mortality rate for vaginal procedures than for abdominal procedures may be due to inherent characteristics of the techniques, but it is also likely to reflect the fact that difficult hysterectomies for cancer, endometriosis, and obstetrical emergency are never performed vaginally (Dicker *et al*. 1982*b*; Bachmann 1990).

Complications

Understanding and quantifying the complications of hysterectomy are difficult tasks because the literature is replete with varying definitions of complications. The two most common untoward events are post operative infection causing fever, and blood loss requiring transfusion. There have been suggestions that coronary artery disease (Centerwall 1981), premature ovarian failure (Siddle *et al*. 1987), and osteoarthritis (Spector *et al*. 1991) may be late complications of hysterectomy, even without oophorectomy, but the information is scant and fragmented and most of these studies are subject to considerable criticism.

The use of prophylactic antibiotics during the operation has been demonstrated to lower the risk of infection and to decrease hospital costs and length of stay for hysterectomy, and it should be a universal practice by now (Shapiro *et al*. 1983; Mercer *et al*. 1988; Hemsell *et al*. 1990; Matkaris *et al*. 1991).

The number of homologous (other donors') blood transfusions received by hysterectomy patients has been reduced by surgical techniques involving injection of vasoconstricting drugs into the tissues preoperatively, the use of new cautery and laser devices to reduce intraoperative blood loss, and the availability of autologous (the patient's own) blood for transfusion.

Anticoagulation by heparin in cancer patients and immobilized patients lowers the incidence of post operative thrombophlebitis and pulmonary embolism. However, the more unusual complications of ureteral injuries and prolapse of the vaginal vault following hysterectomy will probably continue to be with us in small numbers despite our efforts to reduce them.

Psychological complications are even more difficult to quantify and to describe. Sexual dysfunction following hysterectomy may be related to the alterations in anatomy (Zussman *et al*. 1981) and/or hormone changes (Dennerstein *et al*. 1980). More commonly, however, there was preoperative dysfunction or the patient had unrealistic expectations (Dennerstein *et al.* 1977). The general consensus of the literature is that when major mood disturbance occurs after hysterectomy it is usually in patients with pre-existing mood disturbance or in patients whose psychological, social and cultural ideas about hysterectomy were not fully explored, explained, and dealt with before the operation (Bachmann 1990).

The future

Evaluation of the history, epidemiology, indications, complications, and mortality is difficult because the literature is largely composed of retrospective, uncontrolled, unrandomized studies, rife with methodologic imperfections. However, the gynecologic, public health, and lay literatures do converge on one consensus: that there is little consensus about the proper indications for removal of the uterus. This lack of uniformity creates unusual variations in hysterectomy rates, and therefore *some* of the hysterectomies performed must be unnecessary. Cost-control efforts, quality assurance reviews, women's resistance, and educational endeavors will all contribute to lowering the hysterectomy rate in the future and provide the impetus to modify the surgical technique itself so as to minimize its physiologic effects.

Alternatives to hysterectomy

Alternatives to hysterectomy have been advanced in recent years for almost all of the traditional indications.

Abnormal uterine bleeding

Dilatation and curettage (D&C), a traditional gynecologic operation, has long been believed to ameliorate the symptoms of abnormal uterine bleeding, making hysterectomy unnecessary in most patients. Today, D&C itself is often replaced by an in-office biopsy of the endometrial surface (Grimes 1982; Smith and Schulman 1985; Speroff *et al.* 1989; Stovall *et al.* 1991*a*; Chambers and Chambers 1992) followed by progesterone therapy (Speroff *et al.* 1989) and/or by hysteroscopy performed either in the office or in the operating room. Hysteroscopy allows a view of the entire endometrium and specific lesions including fibroids and polyps can be visualized on a video screen and biopsied away or resected without resorting to removing the uterus (Books and Serdon 1988; Gimpelson and Rappold 1988). Hysteroscopic ablation of the entire endometrial surface obviates the need for hysterectomy in about half of the patients with persistent abnormal uterine bleeding. It can be carried out either with a laser or an electrocautery rollerball and can be performed as an out-patient procedure, occasionally under local anesthesia (Decherney *et al.* 1987; Serden and Brooks 1991). The procedure can be made more effective by pretreating the patient with a gonadotropin-releasing hormone analogue such as leuprolide depot (Books *et al.* 1991), given as a monthly injection. This creates a temporary menopausal state, causing the uterine surface to atrophy and become more easily ablated and less likely to regenerate.

Pelvic pain

Hysterectomy has ceased to be the major form of therapy for pelvic pain. Deeper understanding of chronic pelvic pain has led to the establishment of multidisciplinary pain management units, which employ more conservative therapies such as chiropractic manipulations, trigger point injections, nerve blocks, psychotherapy, biofeedback, and acupuncture (Kames *et al.* 1990).

Endometriosis

The advent of the gonadotropin-releasing hormone analogs has greatly increased our ability to provide patients with a tolerable medication for suppressing the disease before or instead of surgical therapy (Dlugi *et al.* 1990). Operative laparoscopy techniques and instruments for excision and/or ablation of endometriosis have so improved that hysterectomy is more often avoidable even for cases of severe endometriosis.

Leiomyomas (fibroids)

Myomectomy—removal of the fibroids from the uterus—is an alternative to hysterectomy for fibroids. A transabdominal approach is used to remove large fibroids or many fibroids; in cases where the fibroids are small or few in number, laparoscopic or hysteroscopic myomectomy can be performed. Shrinking the leiomyomas preoperatively with gonadotropin-releasing hormone agonists renders the procedures technically easier and less morbid (Friedman *et al.* 1989). Unfortunately, the fibroids are likely to recur unless the woman passes into menopause within a few years after the operation.

Cervical intraepithelial neoplasia (CIN)

This is a premalignant condition detected by Pap smear screening. Laser ablation of the cervical transformation zone and large loop electrocoagulation of the transformation zone have largely replaced hysterectomy in its treatment (Kolstad and Klem 1976; Weight *et al.* 1992). In fact, the traditional cold knife conization of lesser degrees of CIN is also becoming a technique of the past in the face of these newer modalities.

Utero vaginal prolapse

This is a condition in which the uterus and vaginal walls lose their supporting tissues and protrude through the vaginal opening, creating discomfort, embarrassment, and urinary difficulties. A plastic or rubber pessary can be inserted into the vagina to temporarily support the prolapsing tissues relatively well, but they require frequent medical attention and usually preclude sexual intercourse. New, inflatable pessaries that can be managed by the patient have been developed. Pelvic floor training exercises can be taught to the patient with the use of computer-generated biofeedback and can help patients control the degree of prolapse and any urinary incontinence (Jeter 1991). The Manchester procedure, in which the cervix is amputated and the uterus elevated in the pelvis by plication of the cardinal ligaments, can be used to repair prolapse without hysterectomy (Mattingly and Thompson 1985). For selected patients this operation, combined with vaginal wall repair, is apparently enjoying a resurgence in popularity among gynecologists, although it has scarcely been mentioned in the literature for 20 years and has traditionally been thought to have a higher failure rate than hysterectomy with repair.

Stress urinary incontinence

Hysterectomy is no longer advocated to accompany the urologic procedure unless there is co-existent uterine disease. Bladder neck suspension by needle (for example, the Raz or the Stamey procedure), abdominal bladder neck suspension by the Burch procedure, and paravaginal repair are now commonly performed for stress incontinence, and do not involve the uterus at all. Prolapse and incontinence are diseases more commonly found in the elderly than endometriosis or fibroids or abnormal bleeding, and as the population continues to age, treating them effectively will become a greater priority.

Future developments

Improved hysterectomy techniques

In addition to reducing the number of hysterectomies, effort has been directed at improving techniques to minimize undesired after-effects, both real and perceived. Subtotal hysterectomy, in which the uterus is removed but the cervix remains, has been advocated recently by certain women's publications, including, the book *Hysterectomy: before and after* (Cutler 1988). This recommendation is unfortunately largely based on only one study from Finland which unconvincingly purported to demonstrate a greater impact on libido and orgasm by total hysterectomy then subtotal hysterectomy (Killku *et al.* 1983). Subtotal hysterectomy may well be more suitable for certain conditions and should be more widely performed in some emergencies involving severe endometriosis, pelvic inflammatory disease, or obstetrical complication (Baker 1985).

Performing hysterectomy vaginally rather than abdominally appears to lower the risk and the complication rate and certainly lowers the length of stay (Dicker *et al.* 1982*b*; Browne and Frazer 1991). In fact the literature now demonstrates that ambulatory vaginal hysterectomy is a procedure of distinct possibility (Reiner 1988; Stovall *et al.* 1992). Even large fibroid uteri can be removed vaginally if the fibroids are first made smaller by gonadotropin-releasing hormone analogs (agonists) Friedman *et al.* 1987; Schneider *et al.* 1991; Stovall *et al.* 1991*b*). The development of laparoscopically assisted vaginal hysterectomy and even hysterectomy performed totally through the laparoscope also provides the opportunity of lessening the impact of hysterectomy on the patient's life by decreasing pain and the length of recovery (Reich *et al.* 1989). Compliance with third party payers' requirements for early discharge has demonstrated that the length of stay for abdominal hysterectomy can be much shorter then previously believed. In the 1970s a routine stay for abdominal hysterectomy was 7 or 8 days and now in the USA the average is 4–5 days—a considerable reduction. In addition, a preoperative stay is no longer allowed or necessary.

Quality assurance

The future also holds improvements in the quality assurance overview function of the medical profession, better educational efforts for physicians and patients, and better research. The work of Gambone and Reiter has spearheaded the effort to improve quality assurance. They have established a set of indications and diagnoses (see Table 7.1) applicable to all hysterectomies (Gambone *et al.* 1989). They require that one diagnosis be chosen preoperatively as the indication for hysterectomy and that the surgeon record whether or not pathologic confirmation should be expected. A careful documentation of the history and physical findings that indicate hysterectomy must appear in the record if no pathologic confirmation is expected. The indication can then be retrospectively verified by pathologic confirmation or validated by preoperative documentation by quality assurance reviewers (Gambone *et al.* 1990*a*; Reiter 1992). This tool has lowered the hysterectomy rate for several indications, especially chronic pelvic pain, recurrent uterine bleeding, cervical intraepithelial neoplasia, and severe infection (Gambone *et al.* 1990*b*). This type of quality control method will probably continue to gain popularity throughout the world, reducing the number of hysterectomies and more clearly delineating a consensus of indications making comparative studies more meaningful.

Patient education

The need for better preoperative teaching and truly informed consent is widely recognized. Physicians are urged to spend more time explaining as factually as possible what the patients should expect and should not expect from any operation, and engaging the patient in a discussion of the substantive risks. The public is demanding more information about hysterectomy, and we should willingly provide it. When hysterectomy becomes necessary, the consequences of oophorectomy with and without estrogen replacement must be understood by the patient in advance so that the decision to remove or conserve the ovaries is made rationally. Written material is very helpful in educating the patient. The American

Table 7.1 Hysterectomy Indication List

A.	Acute condition—to save life
A-1	Pregnancy catastrophe (eg, postpartum hemorrhage, ectopic, etc)
A-2	Severe infection (eg, ruptured tubo-ovarian abscess)
A-3	Operative complication (eg, uterine perforation)
B.	Benign disease (presumed)—to correct deformity or relieve suffering
B-1	Leiomyomata
a)	Symptomatic (eg, bleeding, discomfort, etc)
b)	Asymptomatic (eg, >12-week size and confuses adnexal evaluation)
B-2	Recurrent uterine bleeding (unresponsive to hormonal and surgical therapy)
B-3	Endometriosis
B-4	Adenomyosis
B-5	Chronic infection (eg, recurrent pelvic inflammation)
B-6	Adnexal mass (eg, ovarian neoplasm)
B-7	Other (operator-defined, criteria specified)
C.	Cancer or significant premalignant disease—to prolong life
C-1	Invasive disease
C-2	Preinvasive disease of the uterus
C-3	Cancer of adjacent or distant organ (GI, GU, or breast cancer)
D.	Discomfort (normal tissue expected)—to correct deformity or relieve suffering
D-1	Chronic pelvic pain
D-2	Pelvic relaxation
D-3	Stress urinary incontinence
D-4	Other (operator-defined, criteria specified)
E.	Extenuating circumstances (not indicated but may be justified in certain situations)
E-1	Sterilization
E-2	Cancer prophylaxis (eg, familial ovarian cancer)
E-3	Elective

GI = gastrointestinal; GU = genitourinary.

College of Obstetricians and Gynecologists (1991) has developed an information booklet, *Understanding hysterectomy*, to assist the physician in this task. Other agencies, health plans, and physicians have developed their own educational booklets and brochures as well, for example the Oregon Medical Association (Rose 1992). However, more comprehensive and constantly updated materials are needed. Currently, there are not enough even-handed and accurate trade books available in libraries and bookstores, although inaccurate and opinionated books (such as Cutler 1988) are readily available.

Research goals

Hysterectomy remains an extremely controversial topic of discussion among women, physicians, insurers, government health officials, and epidemiologists. It is amazing that such a common procedure has so little scientific foundation. In the coming years, current alternatives to hysterectomy will undoubtedly be joined by others. Conditions that now commonly lead to hysterectomy will be treated less drastically and there will be greater understanding by patients of their treatment. More research must be directed to the psychologic effects of hysterectomy in the context of the individual patient's culture and society. Investigation into the possible effects of hysterectomy on coronary artery disease, osteoarthritis, and premature ovarian failure is also needed. Although difficult to design, prospective studies in these areas are needed to enable us to determine if too many hysterectomies are being performed (or too few) and how to nudge the number in a more appropriate direction.

The future of D&C and operative laparoscopy

The future of two other gynecologic procedures must also be discussed: dilatation and curettage (D&C) and operative laparoscopy. These procedures—one old, one new—demonstrate that, unlike medications, surgical procedures can arrive on the scene and gain widespread popularity without monitored therapeutic trials or randomized studies of effectiveness and safety.

The popularity of D&C, the stock in trade for gynecologists for years, was established largely by tradition; its effectiveness as a diagnostic tool was never thoroughly evaluated and its therapeutic mechanism was overestimated (Grimes 1982; Sperott *et al.* 1989). The D&C is a blind procedure, performed essentially by feel. Only a fraction of the endometrial surface is actually removed and cure rates by D&C alone for abnormal uterine bleeding are not different from placebo (Grimes 1982), calling into question whether the operation has any therapeutic effectiveness at all. Endometrial biopsy has been shown to equal the curettage in diagnostic accuracy (Stovall *et al.* 1991*a*; Chambers and Chambers (1992). Hysteroscopy has increased the ability to locate polyps and myomas by direct visualization of the entire endometrial surface (Brooks and Serden 1988; Gimpelson and Rappold 1988). These lesions, often missed by D&C, can be removed by hysteroscopic resection using a resectoscope modified from those used by urologists in prostatic surgery (Gimpelson and Rappold 1988). We must conclude that the ever-popular D&C does not merit its current usage and when it is performed it should be accompanied by hysteroscopy for completeness and accuracy.

Operative laparoscopy has acquired widespread popularity in a short time. As surgeons have learned new skills, equipment manufacturers have developed more sophisticated and reliable instruments, and entrepreneurial physicians have developed a plethora of courses in which the new techniques are taught. A superabundance of experiential reports has appeared in the literature, but there have been few clinical trials demonstrating the effectiveness, safety and benefits of these techniques. Grimes' (1992) excellent review expresses the opinion that the literature supports a recommendation that operative laparoscopy be used in the treatment of ectopic pregnancy, ovarian biopsy and polycystic ovary syndrome. There is insufficient data of quality, however, to recommend the procedure for other uses advocated by the laparoscopic avante garde, such as adnexectomy, ovarian cystectomy, drainage of pelvic abscess, uterosacral nerve ablation, suspension of the uterus, myomectomy, and laparoscopically assisted vaginal hysterectomy. Grimes points out that the increase in procedures performed, instruments sold and courses offered has outpaced critical evaluation: 'that an operation can be done through a telescope does not imply that it should be'. His sentiments are echoed by Pitkin (1992), who implores gynecologic surgeons to critically evaluate this new surgical technique before declaring it the standard of care. None the less, gynecologists are performing operative laparoscopies in large numbers and there is no turning back the clock.

Quality assurance for operative laparoscopy is beginning to take shape in the form of credentialing guidelines recommended by, for instance, The American College of Obstetricians and Gynecologists (1992). Medical staff are encouraged to establish criteria for privileges to perform operative laparoscopy unsupervised. The ACOG guidelines require each physician to acquire didactic experience as well as to perform several procedures under the supervision of more experienced members of the staff. As surgeons gain increasing experience under proper supervision and proceed with more critical evaluation, operative laparoscopy will undoubtedly assume an appropriate role in the surgical world.

References

American College of obstetricians and Gynecologists (1991). *Understanding hysterectomy*, (2nd edn). ACOG, Washington DC.

American College of Obstetricians and Gynecologists, Committee on Gynecologic Practice. (1992). *Credentialing guidelines for operative laparoscopy*. Committee opinion No. 106, April 2.

Amirikia, H. and Evans, T. N. (1979). Ten year review of hysterectomies: trends, indications and risks. *American Journal of Obstetrics and Gynecology*, **134**, 431–4.

Bachmann, G. A. (1990). Hysterectomy: a critical review. *Journal of Reproductive Medicine*, **35**, 839–62.

Baker, H. W. (1985). Selective indications for subtotal abdominal hysterectomy. *Journal of the Kentucky Medical Association*, **83**, 355–8.

Brooks, P. G. and Serden, S. P. (1988). Hysteroscopic findings after unsuccessful dilatation and curettage for abnormal uterine bleeding. *American Journal of Obstetrics and Gynecology*, **158**, 1354–7.

Brooks, P. G., Serden, S. P., and Davos, I. (1991). Hormonal inhibition of the endometrium for resectoscopic endometrial ablation. *American Journal of Obstetrics and Gynecology*, **164**, 1601–8.

Browne, D. S. and Frazer, M. I. (1991). Hysterectomy revisited. *Australia and New Zealand Journal of Obstetrics and Gynecology*, **31**, 148.

Centerwall, B. S. (1981). Premenopausal hysterectomy and cardiovascular disease. *American Journal of Obstetrics and Gynecology*, **139**, 58–61.

Chambers, J. T. and Chambers, S. K. (1992). Endometrial sampling: when? where? why? with what? *Clinical Obstetrics and Gynecology*, **35**, 28–39.

Cutler, W. B. (1988). *Hysterectomy: before and after*. Harper and Row, New York.

DeCherney, A. H., Diamond, M. P., Lavy, G., and Polan, M. L. (1987). Endometrial ablation for intractable uterine bleeding: hysteroscopic resection. *Obstetrics and Gynecology*, **70**, 668–9.

Dennerstein, L., Wood, C., and Burrows, G. D. (1977). Sexual response following hysterectomy and oophorectomy. *Obstetrics and Gynecology*, **49**, 92.

Dennerstein, L., Burrows, G. D., Wood, C., and Hyman, G. (1980). Hormones and sexuality: effect of estrogen and progestogen. *Obstetrics and Gynecology*, **56**, 316–22.

Dicker, R. C., Scally, M. J., Greenspan, J. R., Layde, P. M., Ory, H. W., Maze, J. M., and Smith, J. C. (1982*a*). Hysterectomy among women of reproductive age: trends in the United States, 1970–1978. *Journal of the American Medical Association*, **248**, 323–7.

Dicker, R. C., Greenspan, J. R., Strauss, L. T., Cowart, M. R., Scally, M. J. Peterson, H. B. *et al.* (1982*b*). Complications of abdominal and vaginal hysterectomy among women of reproductive age in the United States. *American Journal of Obstetrics and Gynecology*, **144**, 841–8.

Dlugi, A. M., Miller, J. D., and Knittle, J. (1990). Leuprolide acetate for depot suspension in the treatment of endometriosis: a randomized placebo-controlled, double-blind study (Lupron Study Group). *Fertility and Sterility*, **54**, 419–27.

Easterday, C. L., Grimes, D. A., and Riggs, J. A. (1983). Hysterectomy in the United States. *Obstetrics and Gynecology*, **62**, 203–12.

Finkel, M. L. and Finkel, D. J. (1990). The effect of a second opinion program on hysterectomy performance. *Medical Care*, **28**, 776–83.

Friedman, A. J., Barbieri, R. L., Benacerraf, B. R., and Schiff, I. (1987). Treatment of leiomyomata with intranasal or subcutaneous leuprolide, a gonadotropin-releasing hormone agonist. *Fertility and Sterility Fertility and Sterlity*,**48**, 560–4.

Friedman, A. J., Rein, M. S., Harrison-Atlas, D., Gorfield, J. M. and Doubilet, P. M. (1989). A randomized, placebo-controlled, double-blind study evaluating leuprolide acetate depot treatment before myomectomy. *Fertility and Sterility*, **52**, 728–33.

Validation of hysterectomy indications and the quality assurance process. *Obstetrics and Gynecology*, **73**, 1045–9.

Gambone, J. C., Reiter, R. C., and Lench, J. B. (1990*a*). Quality assurance indicators and short-term outcome of hysterectomy. *Obstetrics and Gynecology*, **76**, 841–5.

Gambone, J. C., Reiter, R. C., Lench, X., and Moore, J. G. (1990*b*). The impact of a quality assurance process on the frequency and confirmation rate of hysterectomy. *American Journal of Obstetrics and Gynecology*, **163**, 545–50.

Gimpelson, R. J. and Rappold, H. O. (1988). A comparative study between hysteroscopy with directed biopsies and dilatation and curettage: a review of 276 cases. *American Journal of Obstetrics and Gynecology*, **158**, 489–92.

Grimes, D. A. (1982). Diagnostic dilatation and curettage: a reappraisal. *American Journal of Obstetrics and Gynecology*, **142**, 1–6.

Gitsch, G., Berger, E., and Tatra, G. (1991). Trends in thirty years of vaginal hysterectomy. *Surgical Gynecology and Obstetrics*, **172**, 207–10.

Grimes, D. A. (1992). Frontiers of operative laparoscopy: a review and critique of the evidence. *American Journal of Obstetrics and Gynecology*, **166**, 1062–71.

Hemsell, D. L., Johnson, E. R., Hemsell, P. G., Nobels, B. J., and Heard, M. C. (1990). Cefazolin for hysterectomy prophylaxis. *Obstetrics and Gynecology*, **76**, 603–6.

Jeter, K. F. (1991). Pelvic muscle exercises with and without biofeedback for the treatment of urinary incontinence. *Problems in Urology*, **5**, 72–84.

Kames, L. D., Rapkin, A. J., Naliboff, B. D., Afifi, S., and Ferrer-Brechner, T. (1990). Effectiveness of and interdisciplinary pain management program for the treatment of chronic pelvic pain. *Pain*, **41**, 41–6.

Kasper, A. S. (1985). Hysterectomy as social process. *Women and Health*, **10**, 109–27.

Killku, P., Gonroos, M., Hirvonen, T., and Rauramo L. (1983). Supravaginal amputation vs. hysterectomy: effects on libido and orgasm. *Acta Obstetrica & Gynecologica Scandinavica*, **62**, 147–52.

Kolstad, P. and Klem, V. (1976). Long term followup of 1121 cases of carcinoma in situ. *Obstetrics and Gynecology*, **48**, 125–9.

Macintosh, M. C. M. (1987). Incidence of hysterectomy in New Zealand. *New Zealand Medical Journal*, **100**, 345–7.

Matkaris, M., Markantes, K., Stayannis, K., Latrakis, G., Kourounis, G., and Tzingounis, V. (1991). Reduction of hospital cost and administration of prophylactic antibiotherapy in gynecological surgery. *Israeli Journal of Medical Science*, **27**, 134–6.

Mattingly, R. F. and Thompson, J. D. *TeLinde's operative gynecology*, (6th edn). Lippincott, Philadelphia.

Mercer, L. J., Murphy, H. J., Ismail, M. A., and Hajj, S. N. (1988). A comparison of cefonicid and cefoxitin for preventing infections after vaginal hysterectomy. *Journal of Reproductive Medicine*, **33**, 223–6.

Naylor, A. C., (1984). Hysterectomy—analysis of 2901 personally performed procedures. *South African Medical Journal*, **65**, 242–5.

Pitkin, R. M. (1992). Editorial: Operative laparoscopy: surgical advance or technical gimmick? *Obstetrics and Gynecologys*, **79**, 441–2.

Reich, H., DeCaprio, J., and McGlynn, F. (1989). Laparoscopic hysterectomy. *Journal of Gynecological*, Surgery, **5**, 213–5.

Reiner, I. J. (1988). Early discharge after vaginal hysterectomy. *Obstetrics and Gynecology*, **71**, 416–8.

Reiter, R. C., Wagner, P. L., and Gambone, J. C., (1992). Routine hysterectomy for large asymptomatic uterine leiomyomata: a reappraisal. *Obstetrics and Gynecology*, **79**, 481–4.

Reiter, R. C., Gambone, J. C., and Lench, J. B. (1992). Appropriateness of hysterectomies performed for multiple preoperative indications. *Obstetrics and Gynecology*, **80**, 902–5.

Roos, N. P. (1984). Hysterectomy: variations in rates across small areas and across physicians' practices. *American Journal of Public Health*, **74**, 327–35.

Rose, B.K. (1992). Informed consent and hysterectomy: enhancing the right to know. *American Journal of Public Health*, **82**, 609–10.

Sandberg, S. I., Barnes, B. A., Weinstein, M. C., and Braun, P. (1985). Elective hysterectomy: benefits risks and costs. *Medical Care*, **23**, 1067–85.

Schneider, D., Golan, A., Bukovsky, I., Pansky, M., and Caspi, E. (1991). GNRH analogue-induced uterine shrinkage enabling a vaginal hysterectomy in large leiomyomatous uteri. *Obstet NCS and Gynecology*, **78**, 540–1.

Serden, S. P. and Brooks, P. G. (1991). Treatment of abnormal uterine bleeding with the gynecologic resectoscope. *Journal of Reproductive Medicine*, **36**, 697–9.

Shapiro, M., Schoenbaum, S. C., Tager, I. B., *et al.* (1983). Benefit–cost analysis of antimicrobial prophylaxis in abdominal and vigial hysterectomy.*Journal of the American Medical Association*, **249**, 1290–4.

Siddle, N., Sarrel, P., and Whitehead, M. (1987). The effect of hysterectomy on the age of ovarian failure: identification of a subgroup of women with premature loss of ovarian function and literature review. *Fertility and Sterility*, **47**, 94–100.

Smith, J. J. and Schulman, H. (1985). Current dilatation and curettage practice: a need for revision. *Obstetrics and Gynecology*, **65**, 516–8.

Spector, T. D., Hart, D. J., Brown, P., Almeyda, J., Dacre, J. E., Doyle, D. V., and Silman, P. J. Frequency of osteoarthritis in hysterectomized women. *Journal of Rheumatology*, **18**, 1877–83.

Speroff, L., Glass, R. H., and Kase, N. G. (1989). *Clinical gynecologic endocrinology and infertility*, (4th edn.) pp. 147, 276–281. Williams and Wilkins, Baltimore.

Stovall, T. G., Photopulos, G. J., Poston, W. M., Ling, F. W., and Sandles, L. G. (1991*a*). Pipelle endometrial sampling in patients with known endometrial carcinoma. *Obstetrics and Gynecology*, **77**, 954–6.

Stovall, T. G., Ling, F. W., Henry, L. C., and Woodruff, M. R. (1991*b*). A randomized trial evaluating leuprolide acetate before hysterectomy as treatment for leiomyomas. *American Journal of obstetrics and Gynecology*, **164**, 1420–5.

Stovall, T. G., Summitt, R. L. Jr, Bran D. F., and Ling, F. W. (1992). Outpatient vaginal hysterectomy: a pilot study. *Obstetrics and Gynecology*, **80**, 145–9.

Vessey, M. P., Villard-Mackintosh, L., McPherson, K., *et al.* (1992). The epidemiology of hysterectomy: findings in a large cohort study. *British Journal of Obstetrics and Gynaecology*, **99**, 402–7.

Wingo, P. A., Huezo, C. M., Rubin, G. L., Ory, H. W., and Peterson, H. B. (1985). The mortality risk associated with hysterectomy. *American Journal of Obstetrics and Gynaecology*, **152**, 803–8.

Wright, T. C. Jr, Gagnon, S., Richart, R. M. and Ferenczy, A. (1992). Treatment of cervical intraepithelial neoplasia using the loop electrosurgical excision procedure. *Obstetrics and Gynecology*, **79**, 173–8.

Zussman, L., Zussman, S., Sunley, R., and Bjornson, E. (1981) Sexual response after hysterectomy—oophorectomy: recent studies and reconsideration of psychogenesis. *American Journal of Obstetrics and Gynecology*, **140**, 725.

II Family Planning and Fertility

8 Contraception

Luigi Mastroianni Jr

History of contraception

Methods designed to prevent pregnancy have been the subject of intense social and religious scrutiny. Although the earliest medical writings refer to efforts to control reproduction, debate did not intensify until methods became available that were at least somewhat effective. Firm positions were taken based on an evolving religious dogma relating to sexuality and the family. There continue to be widely diverging opinions on the appropriateness of contraception. Earlier, perhaps because of a need to increase the population and because of high infant mortality, the position against contraception was almost universal. This nearly unanimous position has been supplanted by a more liberal stance that takes into account the effect of uncontrolled population growth on quality of life and survival on an increasingly crowded planet.

In primitive societies, the connection between sexual intercourse and procreation was not recognized. Fertility was consummately desired and was supported by magic and prayer. Out of these efforts came amulets, concoctions, and various gadgets designed to cure infertility and others to prevent pregnancy. Some early medical and philosophical writings contain records of contraceptives. The use of pessaries is recorded in Egyptian papyri as early as the eighteenth century BC (Robertson 1989). Medicated tampons to absorb semen were also described. There are records of the use of sheaths for the penis made from a variety of animal materials. A variety of products to be taken by mouth were used. These were, of course, ineffective and in many cases unsafe.

In the Old Testament, recognition of the relationship between ejaculation and pregnancy is clearly documented. Coitus interruptus was practiced by Onan as a contraceptive measure when he was obliged to perform 'the duty of a husband' for his deceased brother's wife. The marriage laws required that a man have children by his deceased brother's wife and raise them in his brother's name. The story of Onan has been used as an argument against masturbation and contraception. Onan's sin has also been interpreted as a sinful and uncharitable unwillingness to produce a pregnancy in his deceased brother's wife.

Aristotle commented on contraception and advised that the probability of pregnancy could be reduced by the use of cedar oil or olive oil mixed with either lead or frankincense. Occlusive pessaries, vaginal plugs of wool, and various other substances are all described in the Greek literature of the second century. It was thought that the most fertile period in the cycle occurred immediately before or after menstruation. This fallacy was probably related to the fact that when some animals are in heat and therefore fertile, they present a bloody discharge. It persisted until the mysteries of the ovulatory cycle were unraveled (Hartman 1962). Pills and pessaries are described in Islamic literature. Methods of contraception are also documented in Indian erotic literature and by the Chinese.

During the Middle Ages, there was virtually no progress in birth control development. Gabriele Fallopius, after whom the fallopian tube is named, described a condom in the medical literature in 1564. It was recommended not for contraception but for protection against syphilis. The condom engendered a great deal of controversy, but it was more than a century before spermatozoa were discovered and described by Anton van Leeuwenhoek. From then on, efforts were made to observe and immobilize spermatozoa with various agents. Birth control became much more feasible and was the subject of intense scrutiny and debate. In the eighteenth century, some suggested birth control as a way of reducing poverty and Thomas Malthus introduced his theory that population would soon outgrow available resources.

During the nineteenth century, controversy heightened. Efforts to suppress family planning were highlighted in the USA by the activities of Anthony Comstock. He established a Society for the Suppression of Vice which successfully sponsored a law in New York making dissemination of knowledge about contraception a punishable crime. Comstock opined that obscenity and atheism 'occupy the same bed' and that birth control was the work of the devil. At about the same time, the theory of Malthus was popularized and movements were organized to promote family planning throughout Europe. The diaphragm had been developed and clinics were established for its distribution.

In the United States, the birth control movement was led by Margaret Sanger (1883–1966), who established the first clinic in New York City (1916). A few days after it was opened, it was raided by the vice squad and closed. She was jailed, but out of her efforts eventually came the formation of the Planned Parenthood Federation. Similar ups and downs were experienced throughout Europe, although contraception became legal in most European countries by the 1930s. In the USA, it was still a criminal offense to prescribe contraception in Connecticut as late as 1965, when the law was declared unconstitutional by the Supreme Court (Griswold V. Connecticut 1965). The condom was distributed legally for disease prevention but not for contraception. Those who could afford private care received family planning advice, which at the time consisted mainly of diaphragm fitting and use of spermicides. Until the Connecticut law was repealed, there were no public family planning clinics. When I worked at Yale University between 1955 and 1962, it was clear that contraception was prescribed only for those who could afford private medical care. The concept that family planning is an integral part of general health care is not universally accepted even today. The Connecticut law was challenged by Professor C. Lee Buxton, Chairman of Obstetrics and Gynecology at Yale University, who was briefly jailed for his position. He was incensed by the inequities in the system and finally succeeded in establishing contraception as a right for all women in the USA.

Development of the Pill

As the law in Connecticut was being challenged three decades ago, a new approach to contraception was in its early phases of development. Paradoxically, the law was challenged through an illegal diaphragm fitting, while at the same time a method that would essentially require no medical intervention except for a prescription was being initiated. The development of the Pill would do more to revolutionize contraceptive practice than anything that had happened in millennia.

The history of the Pill has been written many times from a variety of perspectives. Of particular interest was the motivation of those who fostered and financed its development (Mchanghlin 1962). Mrs Robert R. McCormick, heir to a Chicago fortune, was an avowed feminist. She was also an admirer and confidant of Margaret Sanger. Their purpose was to empower women so that they could control their own reproductive destinies. When approached by Gregory Pincus and John Rock to help to finance the early phases of Pill research, Mrs McCormick jumped at the opportunity and it was her early financial backing that supported the initial phases of oral contraceptive development. Her interest in family planning persisted until her death. She bequeathed a substantial legacy to the Alan Guttmacher Institute in New York, which continues to have a major impact on issues of family planning and abortion.

A 1965 national fertility study from the Office of Population Research at Princeton University showed that there was still widespread ignorance concerning basic issues of reproduction (Ryder and Westoff 1971). Not unexpectedly, there was a wide discrepancy in knowledge between the socially advantaged and the disadvantaged population. Only 50 per cent of White and 22 per cent of African American women were correctly informed and this correlated with level of education. These investigators found that most American women were in favor of fertility control. An additional 10 per cent approved only of what was then called the rhythm method. The study documented a rapidly disappearing objection to contraception among Roman Catholic women. Although not stated, it is obvious that the availability of the Pill had a substantial influence on this changing attitude.

By 1965, the Pill was the single most popular method of family planning, with the condom a close second. In the under-30 age group, 20 per cent were using condoms and 43 per cent the Pill. Increasing numbers of younger Catholic women chose the Pill over the rhythm method. In 1968, the Papal encyclical *Humanae vitae* condemned the use of all artificial contraception including the Pill. Yet when Westoff and Ryder (1969) reviewed the impact of the encyclical on contraceptive choice among Roman Catholics, it appeared to have had no effect. The methods that were replaced by the Pill were the rhythm method, the diaphragm, and the condom. At about that time, US Senate hearings resulted in a great deal of adverse publicity for the Pill. Early side-effects, including thromboembolic disease, were reported and there was concern over safety. Woman began to discontinue Pill use, substituting the older, less effective methods once again. This was an early demonstration of the importance of the press and its influence on acceptance of one method over another. Controversy surrounding Pill use has continued and the effect of adverse publicity on discontinuation rates has been documented (Grimes 1989).

Feminist groups have approached the Pill use with caution. Early on, they focused attention on risks and side-effects and pointed to the fact that the Pill-taking woman is asked to bear the entire responsibility of contraception. They took a position very different from that of Sanger and McCormick, who felt that it was a woman's solemn right to control her own reproductive destiny. Margaret Sanger encouraged use of the diaphragm, which placed control directly in the hands of the woman. This must be examined within the context of a society in which legal and safe abortion was not available. As evidence emerged that the Pill might be associated with some risk, feminist groups pushed in the direction of the safer barrier methods. They failed to consider fully the substantial failure rate associated with diaphragm and condom use, at a time when abortion was not available except to save the life of the mother. As Pill use dropped off, the rate of unintended pregnancies increased.

Sterilization

Sterilization has engendered a great deal of controversy. In 1965, about 8 per cent of women 18–39 years old used sterilization for contraception. This was an increase by 3 percentage points over the 1960 rate. Five per cent had had tubal ligations and 3 per cent had partners who had had vasectomies. Contraceptive sterilizations were carried out mainly in the older age group and only after childbearing was completed. The ratio between tubal sterilization and vasectomy was very different in different groups. Among African American couples, vasectomy was virtually non-existent. Among White couples, who were generally in a higher socio-economic group, tubal ligation and vasectomy were equally represented. These racial differences have now been largely erased.

One of the factors behind the increasing tendency toward permanent sterilization has been a changed social attitude. The American College of Obstetricians and Gynecologists (1969) published guidelines with criteria for tubal sterilization. These state, 'Since there are important emotional problems relating to sterilization, it is essential that consultation be obtained before the operation is performed. In a few hospitals, committee review, like that for therapeutic abortion, is required; but in most, the permission of two senior obstetrician–gynecologists is all that is necessary. As with therapeutic abortion, the properly signed consultation forms should be completed before the patient is taken to the operating room. In 1965, the incidence of sterilization operations was much higher on the West Coast of the USA than in other regions of the country, attesting to a slightly more permissive attitude toward contraceptive practice generally. Outside the West Coast, the vast majority of operations were carried out on older women with at least three children. Attitudes were judgmental and the wishes of the patient were given very limited consideration. Consent of the husband was usually required. When the husband could not be located or was unwilling to sign the consent form, the sterilization was withheld.

The sterilization was carried out by a primary abdominal operative procedure or at the time of cesarean section. Most sterilizations were done on women who were having their third or more cesarean section, and in many centers the procedure was withheld until the woman had had at least three cesarean births, unless there were compelling health reasons to terminate childbearing. These rules and regulations led to a great deal of subterfuge, and ways were found to circumvent them. For example, a woman might elect to have a vaginal hysterectomy to terminate her childbearing potential. Large numbers of such operations were carried out. The exact incidence of hysterectomy for sterilization is undocumented but remains one of the dark issues in contraceptive history.

Attitudes toward sterilization have changed dramatically. In 1990 in the USA one-third of all couples using contraception have had permanent sterilization, almost equally divided between male and female methods (Mastroianni *et al.* 1990).

The increased popularity of sterilization in the past decade is probably related to the availability of less cumbersome methods (See Chapter 9). Development of laparoscopic tubal coagulation has played a major role.

The influence of effectiveness on choice

In the US national fertility study by Ryder and Westoff (1965), the failure rate for each method was analyzed. The failure rate associated with use of the Pill over 1 year was 5 per cent, with the intrauterine device (IUD), 8 per cent with the diaphragm, 18 per cent, the condom, 19 per cent, withdrawal, 23 per cent, rhythm, 30 per cent, and foam, 32 per cent. Not unexpectedly, sterilization failure was substantially lower than for any of the other methods. These failure rates occurred at a time when legal elective abortion was unavailable and so they resulted either in a risky abortion or an unplanned, often unwanted baby. The survey also classified pregnancies as to whether or not they were planned or unplanned and births as to whether or not they were desired. One-third of women surveyed had at least one unintended child. Of those who desired the last child that they had, more than half had previously suffered a contraceptive failure or had become pregnant at a time when pregnancy was not desired. Overall, 64 per cent of women had at least one failure of pregnancy timing.

Then, by and large, family planning was not practiced in a successful way except by a small number of women. Success in avoiding unwanted pregnancy was much higher among highly educated couples than among the less well educated, with little difference between Catholics and non-Catholics, influenced in part by the fact that the Catholics of the time seemed to desire larger families.

The impact of these failure rates on overall population growth was significant. In the absence of legal abortion, the majority of pregnancies were allowed to proceed to delivery. Between 1960 and 1965, 20 per cent of births were unplanned, resulting in the birth of 4.7 million children in the USA (Trussel and Kost 1987). Obviously, increased availability of more effective methods of family planning would have influenced the rate of population growth significantly.

The intrauterine device: political and ethical considerations

Intrauterine devices (IUDs)—the Grafenberg ring in Germany and the Ota ring in Japan—had been used in the late 1920s and 1930s, but failed to gain wide popularity, possibly because of pressure in these countries then to have large families. The availability of malleable plastic resulted in there introduction of a number of IUD configurations in the early 1960s. Under the influence of the Population Council in New York City, IUD development was fostered and encouraged.

In the USA, it became immediately popular and in Ryder and Westoff's survey (1965), 8 per cent of couples using contraception used this method. IUD use increased further and then fell off sharply after the late 1970s, when the Dalkon Shield was shown to be associated with a high incidence of pelvic inflammatory disease because of design defects. This device, in fact, was introduced before FDA approval was required, and the manufacturer continued to in 1975 distribute the product long after the reports of complications surfaced. It was finally withdrawn from production, in 1974, but even then the company did not recommend that women with devices in place should have them removed until 1980. Several deaths were associated with Dalkon Shield use. The net result was hundreds of millions of dollars in lawsuits.

These events created a legal climate in the USA that caused the pharmaceutical industry to reconsider the introduction of other IUDs. Although the other IUDs that were available were never shown to be defective, all of the major manufacturers withdrew their products from the market in the USA. Unfortunately, this concern over litigation influenced attitudes on contraceptive development (Mastroianni *et al.* 1990). A copper-containing IUD is now being distributed there by a smaller company, but, with each insertion, an elaborate informed consent form must be completed. Even though the IUD is in widespread use in other countries, it still constitutes but a small percentage of contraceptives in use in the USA.

Debate on the relationship between IUD use and pelvic infection continues. There is increasing evidence that the modern IUD is not associated with pelvic inflammatory disease except in women who are at greater risk (that is, those with multiple sexual partners). There may be a slightly increased risk of infection in the first 20 days after insertion (Farley *et al.* 1992). IUD infections can be correlated with the increased incidence of sexually transmitted diseases, particularly *Chlamydia trachomatis* infection. Although IUD use is very limited in the USA, there has been a rapid increase world-wide. More than 90 million woman are now using IUDs. Because of its extensive use in China—country with the world's largest population—the IUD has become the most widely used method overall. Of the IUDs in use, approximately 25 million are copper-releasing devices.

The WHO's Special Programme of Research Development and Research Training in Human Reproduction continues to evaluate newer configurations of IUDs. The programme's long-term term studies on two copper IUDs showed an annual risk of accidental pregnancy of approximately 0.5–1 per cent. In 1991, the US Food and Drug Administration increased the recommended duration of use for the newer copper-containing devices from 6–8 years. Thus, we have available a method that requires one insertion only and provides protection for up to 8 years. The WHO has also provided extensive data on the relationship between IUD use and pelvic infection and confirms the impression that the risk is extremely low.

The IUD, then, has had a varied history from one culture to another. In China, where the incidence of sexually transmitted disease is much lower than in many developed countries, complications are rare. The history of IUD use in the USA reflects a vastly changing pattern. In the 1970s, four in ten married women viewed IUDs favorably, whereas in 1991 women were much more likely to have a very unfavorable attitude (Forrest 1992). In spite of the availability of very safe and effective IUDs, their use in the USA has not risen since 1988. The satisfaction rate among those who do use the IUD remains high—in fact, higher than for any other method.

Another factor that has influenced attitudes toward the IUD is its mechanism of action. It was largely assumed that the IUD worked by preventing implantation of the embryo into the endometrium. Implantation occurs on the sixth to seventh day after fertilization and would certainly be influenced adversely by any alterations in uterine environment. The local foreign body reaction of the uterine wall was thought to play a role and has been shown to affect implantation in laboratory animals. However, extensive observations in Santiago, Chile, involving ovum and embryo recovery from the human reproductive tract have failed to establish a relationship between expulsion of fertilized eggs and the presence of the IUD (Croxatto 1992). On the contrary, the rate of recovery of eggs from the fallopian tube in IUD users was significantly lower than in control women. No eggs were found in the uterine cavity at all. This suggests that there is a rapid delivery of the egg into the uterus and expulsion before fertilization. Attempts have also been made to detect the presence of an early pregnancy by assaying for human chorionic gonadotropin (hCG), the hormone produced by the embryo (Alvarez *et al.* 1988). These efforts have provided further assurance that early embroys are not routinely aborted in IUD users and that the main mode of action of IUDs is not the loss of viable embroys but rather an effect that occurs before fertilization.

IUD use in Latin America is influenced by a number of social factors (Faundes 1992). There is still a perception that the IUD causes a monthly abortion and that there is a high risk of infection and a much lower effectiveness than with other methods. The major factors, however, are the lack of properly trained workers to insert IUDs, and the unwillingness or inability of the health care system to provide the infrastructure for training and supply. This has fostered an inappropriately high use of premature surgical sterilization.

There has been a steady increase in IUD use in North Africa (Shaaban 1992). Anxieties over the possibility that the IUD is an abortifacient have been alleviated. Because women in the region start their reproductive career very early, there is need for a method with long-term effectiveness and this is especially important among women who have already had the number of children they desire at a young age. The incidence of sexually transmitted disease is still relatively low. The method is particularly useful among lactating women in Egypt, where breast feeding is the rule rather than the exception. Finally, perhaps the major factor there is the excellent cost: benefit ratio, particularly important in countries with limited capacity for medical care. The IUD is clearly not an acceptable method in much of subsaharan Africa where the incidence of pelvic inflammatory disease (gonorrhea and clamydia) is already high and climing and AIDS has become pandemic.

The development and the use of the IUD has been greatly influenced by social and religious factors. As the device has been refined and as more accurate knowledge of the mechanism of action has become available, some of the early reservations have been put to rest. In the USA, the major factors limiting IUD use are attitudinal and influenced largely by realities of practice, including an unfavorable medico-legal climate. IUD insertion is still looked upon as a high-risk activity by US physicians, although the facts do not support this concern.

Development of Norplant

Norplant is the only other method which acts for several years following its insertion. The development of Norplant was a long and arduous task. In 1966, Sheldon Segal of the Population Council introduced the concept that steroids could be released slowly from subdermal implant. He spreadheaded its initial development in collaboration with Horatio Croxatto. They studied the steroid-releasing properties of silastic and were able to demonstrate a slow and steady release of progestogens in laboratory animals. In the next 3–4 years, the concept was taken from the laboratory to the patient (Segal 1987). Clinical development was supported by foundations and the public sector. The final product was evaluated in several countries and has been tested extensively in more than half a million women, who received Norplant under careful surveillance.

The system involves placing six subdermal capsules beneath the skin in a minor surgical procedure. The lifespan of Norplant is about 5 years. Its long-term effectiveness has been particularly good, and the incidence of side-effects has been relatively low, consisting principally of irregular and unpredictable vaginal bleeding. Norplant has now been introduced in several countries and has attained wide popularity. In the USA, Wyeth-Ayerst, the manufacturer of the progestogen in Norplant, began to market the method in January 1990. They felt initially that it would be suitable for a relatively small market niche in the USA, principally among women in late reproductive years who were considering sterilization but were not quite ready to decide on a permanent method. To the surprise of many, Norplant proved popular among others, including young women who wish to postpone childbearing for at least 4 or 5 years (Polaneczki *et al.*, 1994).

Not unlike the IUD, one of the early questions concerned the mechanism of action of Norplant. By and large, it works by inhibiting ovulation; hence, no egg, no fertilization. However, Norplant's effectiveness in inhibiting ovulation is not consistent, so there was a theoretical possibility that conception could occur. Studies have confirmed that Norplant does not work after fertilization (Segal *et al.* 1991). However, it does exert a secondary effect on the cervical mucus, which becomes tacky and less receptive to spermatozoa, interfering with their migration to the site of fertilization.

Norplant has raised a number of issues in the realms of informed consent and coercion. In most societies, the woman is in control when she accepts the method. However, once Norplant is inserted, technical skill is required to remove it. In that sense, the method is similar to the IUD. If a woman makes the decision to discontinue contraception, she must have available to her a family planning agency that will acquiesce to its removal. When population pressures are paramount, there could easily be reluctance to remove the implant.

Such issues have been the subject of intensive debate among advocates for women's health. Given its reliability and long duration of action, Norplant use has been considered when, for social reasons, an additional pregnancy would be unwise. In the USA, it has even been suggested that the method be used to prevent pregnancies among mothers who have been convicted of child abuse. It has also been suggested that the sentence for an offense be modified if the woman is willing to prevent a future pregnancy. Fortunately, the voice of reason has prevailed.

In the USA, it has also been suggested that women who are in the welfare system and who clearly cannot support an additional child on their own be given a financial incentive to use the method. This, again, raises issues of choice and coercion and has been the subject of intense public debate. The medical profession, by and large, has taken the position that it will not be party to a coercive act of pregnancy prevention. Issues of individual rights versus the rights of society and the rights of a child which is not yet conceived continue to be the focus of spirited discussion.

Another issue that surfaced as Norplant was introduced is expense. The method is initially rather costly, although when measured in terms of long-term effectiveness, the cost is less formidable. The availability of Norplant in the developing world has been assured through an arrangement between the pharmaceutical companies that manufacture it and the Population Council, which developed it. In the USA, willingness of government to pay for Norplant varies from one state to another. Most reason that it is less costly to provide even an expensive contraceptive than to support an unplanned child. There are still those, however, who take the position that contraception is a private matter and should not be provided with public tax dollars. Wyeth-Ayerst Company, the manufacturer of Norplant in the USA, has established a mechanism for supplying it to those who have fallen between the cracks in the health care system. This is less of an issue in other developed countries where health care is a basic right. Norplant has refocused attention on the issue of whether the availability of contraception is also a basic human right.

Depo-medroxyprogesterone acetate (Depo-Provera)

A long-acting injectable progestogen agent, depo-medroxyprogesterone acetate (Depo-Provera) has been available more than two decades. An injection at 3 monthly intervals can result in complete suppression of ovulation. Although Depo-Provera has been used in the USA for the treatment of endometrial cancer and occasionally for the treatment of endometriosis for several years, it was only approved for use as a contraceptive in 1993. Preliminary laboratory testing of Depo-Provera in beagle dogs during the 1960s revealed an increased incidence of breast nodules and tumors, raising the fear that it could cause breast cancer in women. However, clinical studies at the time failed to establish a relationship between breast cancer and Depo-Provera.

A more recent multinational study on the long-term safety of Depo-Provera showed no increased incidence of cancer of the breast even among women who use it for a long time (WHO 1991). Meanwhile, the beagle dog has been discarded by the FDA as subject for steroid evaluation.

Depo-Provera is available in many parts of the world and is among the most popular methods in some of the lesser developed countries. Its contraceptive efficacy is very high, although there are side-effects such as irregular bleeding and vaginal dryness.

Hormonal contraception: safety issues

The long-term effects of contraceptive use in young women must be continuously scrutinized. One can extrapolate only to a degree from experiments in animals. Subhuman primates were suggested as a reasonable model for evaluating the overall effects of a contraceptive agent on the reproductive tract and on overall bodily physiology, but these studies are very expensive and impractical. Something as serious as carcinoma of the breast might develop only after prolonged exposure. Only now has sufficient evidence accured on long-term effects of oral contraception. With the exception of a small group of long-term users who displayed a very slightly increased incidence of breast cancer, there is no associated risk (Thomas 1991). Evidence strongly supports the conclusion that use of the Pill results in a significant overall reduction in the incidence of ovarian tumors (Rory 1992). This effect has been confirmed in a number of large studies. Pill use is also associated with a lower incidence of endometrial carcinoma (Cancer and Steroid Hormone Study 1987). Progesterone modulates the influence of estrogen on endometrial growth. This mechanism has served as the basis for the medical management of carcinoma of the endometrium, for which Depo-Provera is sometimes prescribed.

The previously reported relationship between oral contraceptives and cardiovascular diseases, such as stroke, venous thromboembolism, and myocardial infarction, was observed among women taking the high-dose Pills. The early Pills contained ten times as much hormone as their present-day counterparts. Variability in the overall incidence of cardiovascular disease between developed and developing countries makes it difficult to extrapolate from one study to another. In a multicenter international reassessment of the effect and safety of low dose triphasic and monophasic oral contraceptive pills, published in 1993 (Dunson *et al.*), there were no associated major medical complications. The only reported side effects were mild headaches and dizziness. Cycle control and contraceptive effectiveness were excellent.

There are other positive health benefits. (Peterson and Lee 1989). Because there is less menstrual flow with oral contraceptives, there is less iron loss, and so they have a protective effect against iron-deficiency anemia. This is an especially important benefit in countries where iron intake is limited and parasitic diseases are common.

It is vital, especially in developing countries, that the contraceptive method does not interfere with milk production or that the hormone is not transmitted directly via the milk to the infant. Unfortunately, the combined (estrogen and progestrone) oral contraceptive does reduce milk production. Milk production is not, however, affected by the progestogen-only pill.

An important aspect of contraceptive evaluation is postmarketing surveillance. Regardless of the size of the initial study, there are almost invariably too few subjects to uncover rare side-effects. When a new contraceptive is introduced, a program for its continued evaluation should be in place simultaneously.

Organized postmarketing surveillance has only recently been initiated even in developed countries. Postmarketing surveillance of Norplant is being sponsored by the Population Council and Family Health International. This project has been instituted in eight countries and involves follow-up of 8000 Norplant users. The control group consists of 8000 women who use the IUD or have been sterilized. A 5 year follow-up is projected. Recruitment of women for the study was completed in 1991; meaningful results will not be available for several years.

Sexually transmitted diseases

Diseases transmitted sexually are an increasingly worrisome problem. The incidence of chlamydial infections and gonorrhea is once again increasing in the USA, and this pattern has been observed in other developed countries. In the less developed world, the incidence of sexually transmitted diseases varies greatly from one country to the next. In China, for example, there is little, if any, gonorrhea or chlamydia. This is largely the result of social constraints with emphasis on monogamy and nearly complete absence of premarital coitus. In contrast, sexually transmitted diseases, particularly gonorrhea and in recent years the acquired immune deficiency syndrome (AIDS), have increased substantially in subSaharan Africa. AIDS has attained epidemic proportions. This tragedy is compounded by the fact that the human immunodeficiency virus (HIV) is transmitted to up to 40 per cent of infants born to mothers with AIDS. Development of a method that would prevent transmission of HIV and at the same time prevent pregnancy is of particular importance from a humane as well as a public health standpoint. The relationship between the transmission of infection and the use of various methods of family planning is under investigation in a number of centers. The efficacy of the condom or diaphragm, or both in preventing viral transmission has not been completely evaluated. There is some evidence that the commonly used contraceptive spermicide nonoxinol-9 has antiviral properties, although its action is certainly not complete or predictable.

Barrier methods do prevent virus transmission to some degree. Thie is a clear advantage, especially in areas where AIDS has become epidemic. WHO has conducted studies in five subSaharan countries—Zambia, Uganda, Nigeria, Kenya, and Benin—of people from both rural and urban areas (WHO Special Program 1992). Overall, there is an awareness that condoms are effective in preventing STDs as well as pregnancy. There is a considerable gap, however, between knowledge and condom use. Most men know about condoms but many fewer actually use them; even fewer use them consistently. Attitudes differ between countries, even on the same continent. In **some West African** countries, most men view the purpose of marriage as procreation and only rarely use condoms, even though they do favor birth spacing. In **other** parts of **Western Africa**, there is even more reluctance to use condoms within marriage as they are perceived as somehow lowering the woman's position to that of a prostitute.

On the positive side, there seems to be a changing attitude among younger men. In Nigeria, for example, more men now marry for love rather than for procreation. Such social factors have a significant impact on contraceptive use. With a lethal disease such as AIDS, however, there is urgent need for education not only in the developing world but also in developed countries and the concept of safe sex cannot be overemphasized.

Since attitudes and social situations vary widely, contraceptive methods should be evaluated in the context of the social circumstances in which they are used. World-wide, attitudes toward contraception are influenced dramatically by the status of women. This area has been explored recently by the WHO Special Programme, which has evaluated the influence of sex roles on marriage and childbearing on patterns of fertility and contraceptive behavior, the status of women and their ability to insist on contraception, and the way in which cultures and traditions influence the effectiveness of a given method. Preliminary studies are critical before introduction of any new method.

It has long been known that the effectiveness of a given method varies among groups. For example, the failure rate of the Pill in women under 18 is much higher than in women over 25. The efficacy of the Pill is substantially greater among well-educated, monogamous couples. The differences are largely the result of failure to remember to take the Pill and/or lack of motivation to use it consistently among some women. It appears that those who are in greatest need of protection and whose unplanned pregnancy has the most serious effect are at highest risk. Although educational programs have improved the effectiveness of contraception among younger users, the pregnancy rate in this group nevertheless remains high. In general, sexual behavior is influenced greatly by social circumstances. Teenagers in Sweden, for example, have a higher rate of sexual activity than do their US counterparts and yet they have a substantially lower rate of unintended pregnancy. In Argentina, 40 per cent of all adolescent births (less than 21 years of age) occur in women under the age of 18, in contrast to other Latin American countries, in which the rate is 25–30 per cent. Not surprisingly, those who have limited education and live in rural areas suffer the highest levels of unintended pregnancy. Of the sexually active teenagers in Argentina only 40 per cent have ever used contraception. Most men believe that contraception is a woman's responsibility. The incidence of teen pregnancy in the USA remains the highest in the developed world and was the subject of a comprehensive study by the National Research Council (Hayes 1987).

Contraception and abortion

Contraception and abortion remain inexorably entwined. In the USA, there are approximately 1.5 million abortions annually. In at least half the women having an abortion, conception was a result of contraceptive failure. By and large, these women were using the less effective methods. It is clear that using any method is more effective than using none. The problem is that, given human frailty, the method selected is not always used consistently. In countries where safe, legal abortion is available, it can be used as a back-up for failed contraception. This allows the safer use of a less effective method.

When abortion is not available or for women who cannot accept pregnancy termination as an alternative, it is all the more imperative to encourage the selection of the most effective methods. Contraceptive counseling should include a thorough discussion of the effectiveness of the available methods. The consequences of an unplanned pregnancy are substantially different for a woman who accepts abortion as an alternative and one who does not. Abortion is a major political and social problem in most countries and although elective pregnancy termination is legal the discussion is particularly strident in the USA.

There are still misunderstandings about the mechanism of action of various contraceptives. Many still believe that the Pill acts to abort an early embryo prior to implantation. The Pill does affect the development of the endometrium, but it clearly exerts its effect prior to fertilization. It prevents ovulation and, by its action on cervical mucus, also interferes with sperm migration. Those with a strongly held belief that contraception is immoral look to scientific information to justify their position. When there is profoundly held belief that the newly fertilized egg represents a meaningful and sacred life, there is great concern over the mechanism of action of any new method. This spills over into political action to discourage the introduction of new methods. Often the opinions of vociferous minorities take precedence over those of a less committed majority.

Natural family planning

Since the discovery that ovulation occurs in the middle of a normal 28 day cycle, 14 (± 2) days before the onset of the next menstrual period, efforts have been made to time intercourse so as to avoid the so-called fertile phase. Observations on bodily changes are used to supplement the temperature chart as an indicator of ovulation. This approach is referred to as natural family planning. As with other methods, the success rate varies, depending on the level of motivation and ability to follow through. Natural family planning requires a high degree of cooperation between partners and a mutual commitment to tolerating long periods of abstinence.

Any intercourse in the preovulatory phase of the menstrual cycle is associated with some risk of pregnancy because spermatozoa migrate into the mucus almost immediately on ejaculation and can survive in the reproductive tract for many days. A reliable indicator that would signal that ovulation has already occurred two or more days previously would represent an ideal refinement of natural family planning and would allow virtually risk-free postovulatory intercourse (Djerassi 1991). A method to detect the presence of postovulatory progesterone in urine by color indicator is in development. Such a method, which would allow a couple to be contraception-free for 10 or more days between ovulation and the onset of menses, would be most welcome. Those using barrier methods could safely discard them during that interval. As presently constituted, natural family planning is associated with a variable failure rate, of up to 20 per cent. Among highly motivated and carefully instructed couples, success is considerably greater, however.

Male methods of fertility regulation

There are vast differences in the function of the reproductive tracts of men and women which make development of male-oriented contraception a more difficult task (Segal 1972). At the same time, there is an acknowledged need to increase awareness in men of their responsibility in procreation. The woman typically discharges only one egg during each ovarian cycle, and this results in the release of perhaps of 400 eggs in a whole lifetime. Compare this with the thousands of eggs released by amphibians and fish. The human male has escaped this evolutionary modification and has retained the capacity to release millions of spermatozoa in each ejaculate. In contrast to the cyclic function of the female reproductive tract, spermatogenesis is a continuous process, initiated at puberty and proceeding into senescence. Thus, there are fewer areas of attack and a higher possibility of failure. It is much easier to suppress the release of one egg per month than it is to suppress the continuous release of billions of spermatozoa.

In men, the four reproductive mechanisms that might be targeted are sperm production in the testis, sperm storage and maturation in the epididymis, sperm transport in the vas, and the chemical constitution of the seminal fluid. A man does present the advantage of having his reproductive organs located in a more accessible place. Vas ligation has proved to be the most effective method of male-oriented contraception. The procedure can be done under local anesthesia and is a less complicated procedure than is tubal sterilization. If the man in a couple has been sterilized, the woman remains fertile and could still become pregnant in an extramarital relationship. Thus, vasectomy is looked upon by some as a modern chastity belt, as the control of reproduction is delegated entirely to the male.

The increasing prevalence of vasectomy certainly is evidence that in many societies men have a sincere interest in fertility control, although, world-wide, twice as many female sterilizations are performed as vasectomies. Yet in some parts of the world—particularly in developed countries—vasectomy is substantially more popular than tubal sterilization. In some provinces of China, four to five times as many vasectomies are performed as are tubal ligations. The Chinese have developed a method of vas occlusion, which involves injection through the skin of polyurethane plugs which occlude the vas. This approach is presumably reversible. Initial studies reveal a return of sperm in the ejaculate when they are removed after 1–2 years. This method is now under investigation in the WHO Special Programme.

It has long been known that the male hormone testosterone, when given in sufficient dose, will suppress spermatogenesis. If it is given for a long enough time, sperm production can usually be halted entirely. The method is not foolproof and in some cases there is an unpredictable release of the effect in spite of continued treatment. For this reason it is difficult to be sure that this or other methods of arresting spermatogenesis will offer a completely effective method. Pharmacologic suppression of spermatogenesis is now under evaluation in the WHO Special Programme.

Other hormonal approaches to inhibiting sperm formation are also under investigation. These require at least a weekly injection, although a long-acting form of testosterone has now been developed with a duration of action of 3–4 months. Unfortunately, testosterone stimulates the growth of the prostate gland and there are also psychosexual effects that remain to be evaluated. Another issue that must be settled is: is testosterone in fact effective as a contraceptive even when sperm production is not completely suppressed? Suppression of spermatogenesis remains a difficult but hopefully not an insurmountable task.

Contraception research

In 1990, the National Research Council and the Institute of Medicine of the National Academy of Sciences in the United States released their report on contraceptive development (Mastroianni *et al*. 1990). In a study spanning 2 years, the committee found that there was clearly a need for newer and better methods of family planning. By and large, contraceptive development has been neglected in the USA, especially when one considers its importance to individuals and to society. There has not been a genuine national commitment to contraceptive development. Political factors play a major role, and the climate of litigation has discouraged many of the major pharmaceutical companies from continuing their efforts to develop contraceptives. Most contraceptive development is carried out in the public sector and by a few small venture capital companies. Support for these endeavours has not kept pace with the complexity of the field, and, until very recently, research support has been declining. The number of trainees in reproductive biology—the basic research underpinning contraceptive development—is considerably smaller than needed, and is minuscule compared with those working on such important diseases as cancer and cardiovascular disease. The lack of long-term commitment discourages bright and able investigators from entering a field which clearly could have a major impact on the health and well-being of women.

Factors behind this seeming neglect of women's health issues have recently been addressed in the USA, and there is now an effort to take remedial action. This initiative is still in its early stages and is influenced greatly by the political climate. The Special Programme of WHO has continued to foster research and development of family planning methods, with worldwide support except in the USA. Again, the political issues supervene, and the abortion issue surfaces as a reason for the failure of the US government to support the Special Programme, which includes abortion research on its agenda. This policy has been maintained despite assurances from WHO that the monies received from the USA would not be used for abortion research.

Planned Parenthood Federation of America (1991) has sponsored a series of conferences on new birth control methods, both to foster the development of contraceptive methods and to encourage family planning programs. The impediments to contraceptive development which were identified included insufficient funding to substitute for the withdrawal of the pharmaceutical industry from research and development, a lack of interest among scientists to enter the field of reproductive biology, lengthy and expensive FDA regulation and approval processes for new methods, fears of product liability lawsuits and high costs of product liability insurance, and the negative impact of abortion politics on biomedical science and on the pharmaceutical industry. One of the speakers, C. Ardin Miller, made the point that 'if only half of all unwanted pregnancies in North Carolina were averted by contraception, the state would save $10 million in neonatal intensive care unit costs. This saving alone would restore family planning services to 50 000 women in North Carolina.' Evaluations of the cost–benefit equation consistently come down in favor of contraceptive programs.

World wide, pregnancy causes vastly more deaths in women than does the use of any birth control method. The effects of a lack of methods for pregnancy prevention and child spacing are clear. Sheldon Segal, distinguished scientist of the Population Council and developer of Norplant, has stated, 'contraceptive research should be viewed as abortion prevention research, teen pregnancy reduction research, or as infant mortality rate reduction research—because that is *exactly* what it is' (Committee on Population 1989). The impact of lack of availability of effective contraception is, of course, more pronounced in developing countries than in the developed world. Many parts of the world suffer staggering maternal mortality, and the rate is accentuated with each unplanned pregnancy. Given the vital importance of this area, should we not look again at the priority it receives, with proper attention to education, but a studied avoidance of any coercion?

References

Alvarez, F., Brache, U., Fernandez, E., Guerrero, B., Guiloff, E., Hess., R., *et al.* (1988). New insights on the mode of action of intrauterine contraceptive devices. *Fertility and sterility*, **49**, 768–73.

American College of Obstetricians and Gynecologists (1969). *Standards for Obstetric-Gynecologic Hospital Services: Surgical Sterilization*, ACOG, Washington.

Cancer and Steroid Hormone Study of the Centers for Disease Control and the National Institute of Child Health and Human Development (1987). Combination oral contraceptive use and the risk of endometrial cancer. *Journal of the American Medical Association*, **257**, 796–800.

Committee on Population, National Research Council (1989). *Contraception and reproduction: health consequences of contraceptive use and controlled fertility*. National Academy Press, Washington DC.

Croxatto, H. (1992). IUD mechanisms of action. In *Proceedings of Conference on a New Look at IUDS—advancing contraceptive choices*. Population Council, New York.

Djerassi, C. (1990). Fertility awareness—jet age rhythm method. *Science*, **248**, 1061–2.

Dunson, T. R., McLaurin, V. L., Aguayo, E. L., de Silva, P., Calventi, V., Genais, A. S., and Serani, R. G. (1993). A multicenter comparative trial of triphasic and monophasic, low-dose combined oral contraceptives. *Contraception*, **47(6)**: 515–25.

Farley, T. M. M., Rosenberg, M. J., Rowe, P. J., Chen, J. H., and Meirik, O. (1992). Intrauterine devices and pelvic inflammatory disease: an international perspective. *Lancet* **339**, 785–8.

Faundes, A. (1992). Factors limiting IUD use in Latin America. In *Proceedings of Conference on a New Look at IUDs—advancing contraceptive choices*. Population Council, New York.

Forrest, J. D. (1992). Acceptability of IUDs in the United States. In *Proceedings of Conference on a New Look at IUDs—advancing contraceptive choices*. Population Council, New York.

Grimes, D. A. (1989). Breast cancer, the pill and the press. In *Oral contraceptives and breast cancer* (ed. R. D. Mann), pp. 309–22. Parthenon Publishing, Carnforth.

Griswold v. Connecticut. (1965). *431 US 687*.

Hartman, C. G. (1962). *Science and the safe period: a compendium of human reproduction*. Williams and Wilkins, Baltimore/London.

Hayes, C. D. (ed.) (1987). *Risking the future: adolescent sexuality*, pregnancy and child bearing. National Academy Press, Washington DC.

Mastroianni, L., Donaldson, P. J., and Kane, T. T. (ed.) (1990). *Developing new contraceptives: obstacles and opportunities. New England Journal of Medicine*, **322**, 482–4.

Mastroianni, L., Jr, Donaldson, P. J., and Kane, T. T. (1990). Development of contraceptives–obstacles and opportunities. *New England Journal of Medicine*, **322**, 482–4.

McLaughlin, L. (1982). *The Pill, John Rock and the Church: the biography of a revolution*. Little, Brown, Boston.

Peterson, H. B. and Lee, N. C. (1989). The health effects of oral contraceptives: misperceptions, controversies and continuing good news. *Clinical Obstetrics and Gynecology*, **32**, 339–55.

Planned Parenthood Federation of America (1991). *New Birth Control Conferences Report* planned Parenthood Federation of America, Washington, DC.

Polaneczky, M., Slap, G., Sondheimer, S., Forke, C., and Rappaport, A. (1994). Levonorgestrel Implant (NORPLANT®) Use in Adolescent Mothers. *New England Journal of Medicine*, in press.

Robertson, W. H. (1989). *History of contraception*. Parthenon Press, Park Ridge, NJ.

Rory, H. W. (1982). The non-contraceptive health benefits from oral contraceptive use. *Family Planning Perspectives*, **14**, 182–4.

Ryder, N. B. and Westoff, C. F. (1971). *Reproduction in the United States, 1965*. Princeton University Press.

Segal, S. J. (1972). Contraceptive research: a male chauvinist plot? *Family Planning Perspectives*, **4**, 21–5.

Segal, S. J. (1987). A new delivery system for contraceptive steroids. *American Journal of Obstetrics and Gynecology*, **157**, 1097.

Segal, S. J., Alvarez-Sanchez, F., Brache, V., Faundes, A., Vilja, P., and Tuohimaa, P. (1991). Norplant implants: the mechanism of contraceptive action. *Fertility and Sterility*, **56**, 273–7.

Shaaban, M. M. (1992). Factors limiting IUD use: North Africa. In *Proceedings of Conference on a New Look at IUDs—advancing contraceptive choices*. Population Council, New York.

Thomas, D. B. (1991). Oral contraceptives and breast cancer: review of the epidemiologic literature. *Oral Contraceptives and Breast Cancer*, (ed. Committee on Relationship between Oral Contraceptives and Breast Cancer, Institute of Medicine, Division of Health Promotion and Disease Prevention). National Academy Press, Washington DC.

Trussel, J. and Kost, K. (1987). Contraceptive failures in the United States: a critical review of the literature. *Studies in Family Planning*, **18**, 237–83.

WHO Collaborative Study of Neoplasia and Steroid Contraception (1991). Breast cancer and depot-medroxyprogesterone acetate: a multinational study. *Lancet*, **338**, 833–8.

WHO Special Programme of Research Development and Research Training in Human Reproduction (1992). *Reproductive health: a key to a brighter future*, biennial report. WHO, Geneva.

9 Female sterilization

Herbert B. Peterson and Lynne S. Wilcox

Introduction

The health of women and infants the world over is affected by the ability of women to control the number and timing of their pregnancies. Although maternal mortality has decreased dramatically in recent decades in developed countries, the risk of death and serious morbidity from pregnancy remains high in much of the developing world. Even in developed countries, maternal morbidity and mortality are important considerations for women's health. It is estimated that, somewhere in the world, a woman dies every minute from pregnancy-related causes. Infant health is inextricably related to maternal health. Further, the health of infants has been conclusively linked to child spacing (Park 1986; Klebanoff 1988).

Except in China, where use of the intrauterine device is common, the two most widely used means for pregnancy prevention are oral contraceptives (see Chapter 8) and surgical sterilization. Although vasectomy is common in some countries, including India, Bangladesh, China, the USA, and the UK, the overwhelming majority of sterilizations globally are performed on women (Ross *et al*. 1985). This chapter will focus on female sterilization and its impact on women's health. However, it should be noted that male sterilization can have the same beneficial impact on women's and infants' health as female sterilization. Further, vasectomy appears at least as effective as female sterilization and is a safer surgical procedure (Liskin *et al*. 1983; Peterson *et al*. 1990).

Prevalence and use

World-wide, based on a review of surveys reported in 1985, more than 95 million women have undergone surgical sterilization (Ross 1985). Data regarding the prevalence of surgical sterilization comes predominantly from surveys conducted in the 1970s and the 1980s and may, therefore, underestimate the prevalence of sterilization today as its use is high or rising in many countries and declining in few or none (Ross 1985). The prevalence is low in Africa and in some countries in Latin American and Asia (although it is very high in a number of other Latin American and Asian countries).

A closer look at the pattern of female sterilizations in the USA is worthwhile in assessing the popularity of sterilization over the last several decades. It was uncommon through the 1960s, but the number of procedures performed increased markedly in the 1970s, rising from approximately 200 000 in 1970 to approximately 702 000 in 1977 (DeStefano *et al.* 1982*a*). Although the number of sterilizations performed in hospitals began to decline after 1977 (Centers for Disease Control 1984), this was largely due to the fact that sterilizations were more often being done outside hospitals. By 1987, one third of all female sterilizations in the USA took place in out-patient facilities (Schwartz *et al.* 1989). The prevalence of female sterilization in the USA continued to increase throughout the 1980s. According to the 1988 National Survey of Family Growth, one-third of women in the USA aged 30–34 who were using contraception had undergone sterilization (excluding hysterectomy). About half of women in that age group were relying on sterilization of themselves or their spouse for fertility control (Mosher and Pratt 1990).

Although there are many likely determinants of the widespread and rapidly increasing popularity of female sterilization, one is clearly the availability of sterilization outside hospitals. New surgical techniques, including the use of the laparoscope for sterilization, have helped to make this possible. The laparoscope is, in essence, a telescope with a light source. When inserted into the abdominal cavity, usually through an incision just below the navel, it can be used to view the pelvic organs. Sterilization is then performed using instruments inserted through the laparoscope or through a second incision. In 1970, less than 1 per cent of female sterilizations in the USA were performed with the laparoscope. By 1975, however, more than one-third were performed using the technique (Peterson *et al.* 1981). Concurrently, the average length of hospital stay for sterilization declined from 6.5 nights in 1970 to 4.0 nights in 1975–1978. As noted earlier, by 1987, one-third of female sterilizations in the USA required no overnight hospital stay. Of these, 79 per cent were performed with the laparoscope (Schwartz *et al.* 1989).

Globally, minilaparotomy is more accessible and more widely used than laparoscopy for sterilization (Liskin *et al.* 1985). Like laparoscopy, however, it can also be used to perform sterilizations on an out-patient basis, and so has contributed to the widespread availability of sterilization services. Minilaparotomy requires a somewhat larger surgical incision than laparoscopy (2–5 cm versus 1 cm) but requires simpler, less expensive, and more widely available equipment. The technique, which involves a transverse incision just above the pubic bone in non-pregnant women and just below the navel after vaginal delivery, requires less specialized training and less sophisticated maintenance of equipment.

Complications

Because millions of women undergo this procedure and because the intent of sterilization is to promote well-being, it is imperative that the risks of the procedure be small and well understood. The risks can be broadly categorized into operative risks and potential late sequelae. The former have been better described than the latter, but large national and multinational studies have been conducted to assess both.

Operative risks

The discussion of mortality risk can be facilitated by briefly reviewing the methods of female sterilization and associated anesthetic techniques. The general surgical approaches for entry into the abdominal cavity (laparoscopy and minilaparotomy) have already been described. Vaginal and transcervical approaches are available but are infrequently used today. Tubal occlusion during sterilization by minilaparotomy is generally accomplished by suture ligation of the fallopian tube with resection of a portion of the tube or, less often, by mechanical occlusion of the tube with devices (clips or rings). Tubal occlusion during laparoscopy usually involves electrocoagulation (bipolar or unipolar) of the fallopian tubes or application of mechanical devices (clips or rings). Both minilaparotomy and laparoscopic sterilization can be performed using either local or general anesthesia (Ross *et al.* 1985), although most laparoscopic sterilizations are done under general anesthesia.

Mortality

The risk of dying from female sterilization in the USA is extremely low; it has been estimated at one or two deaths per 100 000 procedures (Escobedo *et al.* 1989). Estimates from developing countries have been higher (Ross *et al.* 1985). In countries with high maternal mortality rates, however, the net effect of sterilization on women's health can be strongly beneficial. For example, a report from India in 1982 estimated a case-fatality rate for postpartum sterilization of seven deaths per 100 000 procedures, as compared with a maternal mortality rate of 420 deaths per 100 000 live births (Ross 1982). Similarly, a 1979 report from Bangladesh identified 19 deaths per 100 000 female sterilizations. Based on an estimate of maternal risk in Bangladesh, it was estimated that 100 000 female sterilizations would prevent 1015 maternal deaths (Grimes *et al.* 1982).

Studies in both developed (Escobedo *et al.* 1989) and developing (Grimes *et al.* 1982) countries have identified complications of anesthesia as an important cause of death attributable to sterilization. In the USA (Escobedo *et al.* 1989), complications of general anesthesia caused more sterilization-attributable deaths than any other single cause. In Bangladesh (Grimes *et al.* 1982), over-sedation with narcotic analgesics during local anesthesia was the leading cause of death. Careful use of local anesthesia, where feasible and otherwise appropriate, should reduce the risk of death. Other causes of death from sterilization include hemorrhage (particularly from abdominal penetration for laparoscopy) and infection. Thermal bowel injuries with unipolar coagulating instruments have been identified as one preventable cause of death attributable to postoperative infection (Peterson *et al.* 1983).

Morbidity

Major morbidity from female sterilization is uncommon but not rare. A multinational study compared the experiences of approximately 1600 women randomized to sterilization by either minilaparotomy or by laparoscopy using electrocoagulation (WHO Task Force on Female Sterilization 1982). Major complications occurred among 1.5 per cent of the former group and 0.9 per cent of the latter. A multicenter study of laparoscopic sterilizations in the USA found that 1.7 per cent of women experienced an intraoperative or postoperative complication (DeStefano *et al.* 1983). The most frequent complication, however, was unintended major surgery which sometimes occurred because of technical limitations of laparoscopy or incidental pathology identified during laparoscopy, rather than complications caused by the procedure *per se* (Franks *et al.* 1987).

The likelihood that complications of sterilization will be serious appears to vary depending on surgical approach. Complications of minilaparotomy procedures are most often minor and usually related to the surgical incision. Minor wound infections and small amounts of bleeding are the most common complications (Liskin *et al.* 1985). By contrast, when complications occur with the laparoscopic approach, they can be more serious. In particular, rare but life-threatening hemorrhages have occurred after blood vessel laceration during abdominal penetration before insertion of the laparoscope and serious infections have occurred after bowel perforation during abdominal penetration and after bowel injury during tubal coagulation. These serious complications are often preventable; when they occur, early diagnosis and treatment can be critical.

Long-term safety and acceptability

The long-term safety and acceptability of female sterilization is somewhat less well characterized than its short-term safety, but nevertheless substantial information is now available to address these issues. Although longer follow-up of sterilized women will be needed, available information about potential long-term consequences of the procedure is broadly reassuring. Questions about late sequelae of female sterilization have been raised in four areas: menstrual function, increased risk of hysterectomy, regret, and sterilization failure.

Menstrual function

As early as the 1950s, investigators questioned whether female sterilization caused subsequent menstrual disturbances including heavy bleeding, intermenstrual spotting, irregular cycles, and dysmenorrhea (Williams *et al.* 1951). Although numerous studies have been reported since the 1950s, questions remain about the existence of a post-tubal ligation syndrome. Most recent studies of women 1–2 years after sterilization provide little support for the existence of such a syndrome and suggest that most menstrual abnormalities after sterilization are attributable to factors other than sterilization. One explanation for menstrual changes in some women is that, when they stop taking oral contraceptives after sterilization, menstrual abnormalities that had been controlled by the contraceptives resurface. Approximately one-third of women in the USA who undergo sterilization were previously taking oral contraceptives and therefore return to their natural menstrual cycles when they stop.

Despite these generally reassuring findings of short-term follow-up after sterilization, several investigations in which the follow-up periods were 5 or more years are somewhat less reassuring (Vessey *et al.* 1983; DeStefano *et al.* 1985; (Wilcox, in press). They suggest that any poststerilization menstrual changes attributable to the procedure may take at least several years to develop. However, it is still unclear whether such late menstrual abnormalities are attributable to sterilization *per se* or to other factors such as age.

Hysterectomy after tubal sterilization

Hysterectomy is common in many countries in which female sterilization is popular. Whether important relationships exist between these surgical procedures is uncertain. There are, however, at least three means by which female sterilization could potentially increase the risk of subsequent hysterectomy. First, sterilization could cause menstrual changes (the 'post-tubal ligation syndrome') which are then managed by hysterectomy. Second, the perception that a post-tubal ligation syndrome exists, even if it does not, might increase the use of hysterectomy to manage menstrual complaints after sterilization. Third, after sterilization, a woman and her physician may be more likely to choose surgical management of a gynecologic problem.

Data to address these possibilities are limited but, for the most part, reassuring. A large cohort study in the UK found no increase in the likelihood of hospital referral for hysterectomy among sterilized women 3 and 6 years after sterilization compared with women whose husbands had undergone vasectomy (Vessey *et al.* 1983). Two other studies, one in the USA (Stergachis *et al.* 1990) and one in Canada (Cohen 1987), found increased risks of hysterectomy only for women in certain age categories at the time of sterilization. In the US study, women 20–29 years old at the time of sterilization were 3.4 times more likely to have a subsequent hysterectomy than a population-based cohort of non-sterilized women. In the Canadian study, women 25–29 years old at sterilization were 60 per cent more likely than a population-based comparison group to have a subsequent hysterectomy. No increased risk of hysterectomy was found in either study among women who underwent sterilization at age 30 or older. All these findings suggest that any relationship between sterilization and subsequent hysterectomy is probably attributable to factors other than menstrual changes.

Regret

Although sterilization is intended for women who are certain that they have completed childbearing, some women will ultimately regret having undergone the procedure. Estimates of the likelihood of such regret vary widely, in part, depending on the definition of regret used for study purposes. For example, in a national survey of women in the USA, 26 per cent responded affirmatively to the question, 'If it were possible for you to have another baby, would you, yourself like to have one?' (Henshaw and Singh 1986.) In one US follow-up study, 6 per cent of women at 5 years after sterilization reported that they had sought information regarding surgical reversal of sterilization, and 0.2 per cent had actually undergone a reversal procedure (Wilcox *et al.* 1990). The likelihood of regret in that follow-up study increased over time, a phenomenon reported also in Panama and Puerto Rico (Wilcox *et al.* 1991). This is understandable, particularly in countries where divorce and subsequent remarriage are common.

Young age at sterilization is an important predictor of later regret and should be considered during presterilization counseling. Life changes such as changes in marital status are the likely reason for the importance of age as a risk factor. The follow-up study by Wilcox *et al.* (1991) found that age at sterilization was the strongest risk factor for later regret. In that study, women who were less than 20 years old at the time of sterilization had 2.9 times the risk of regret as women 30–34 years old, who in turn had twice the risk of women more than 34 years old. This age effect was independent of the number of living children a woman had or her marital status at the time of sterilization.

Although fertility can sometimes be surgically restored after sterilization, reversal surgery is expensive and not always available. Further, the likelihood of success is dependent on a variety of factors including the method of sterilization performed. Although pregnancy rates after reversal surgery are often reported to be in the 50–70 per cent range, such rates are usually based on selected patients operated on by highly skilled surgeons using special techniques. These rates should not, therefore, offer false expectations to women considering sterilization. The decision to undergo sterilization should be made with the intended permanence of the procedure in mind.

Sterilization failure

Although female sterilization is undoubtedly highly effective, sterilization failures can and do occur. Because few studies are available with long-term follow-up to estimate failure rates according to sterilization method, precise effectiveness rates are not available. On the basis of the known methodologic limitations of available studies, the often quoted estimate of four failures per 1000 procedures is probably an underestimate for most procedures under most circumstances. The likelihood of failure appears to be influenced by a variety of considerations including the method of sterilization and certain physician and patient characteristics. The precise impact of these factors on sterilization effectiveness remains incompletely understood. It is clear, however, that failure can occur even under ideal circumstances.

Further, when sterilization failure occurs, the likelihood of ectopic (tubal) pregnancy is increased. The degree of increase in risk of ectopic pregnancy is influenced by the method of sterilization. Methods which involve coagulation of the fallopian tubes are more likely than other techniques to result in tubal pregnancy when sterilization fails (Chi *et al.* 1980). The absolute risk of ectopic pregnancy after sterilization is reduced, however, for many women because sterilization is highly effective in preventing pregnancies, including ectopic gestations (DeStefano *et al.* 1982*b*). The extent to which sterilization protects against ectopic pregnancy depends on the effectiveness of the methods of temporary contraception a woman was using before sterilization (DeStefano *et al.* 1982; Holt *et al.* 1991). Women using highly effective methods (such as oral contraceptives) have an increased risk of ectopic pregnancy after sterilization and cessation of temporary contraception, particularly after sterilization by tubal coagulation (Holt *et al.* 1991). By contrast, women using less effective temporary methods (such as spermicides) have a reduced risk of ectopic pregnancy after sterilization (Holt *et al.* 1991).

Some apparent sterilization failures or so-called 'luteal phase pregnancies' are the result of conceptions which occurred before the sterilization but were diagnosed after the sterilization (Grubb and Peterson 1985). The likelihood of luteal phase pregnancy can be greatly reduced by either timing the sterilization surgery for before the estimated date of ovulation, protection by sexual abstinence, or use of highly effective contraceptives in the month before sterilization. Use of pregnancy tests at the time of sterilization and performance of dilation and curettage at the time of sterilization are less effective in reducing the risk (Grubb and Peterson 1985).

Summary

The global prevalence of female sterilization is high and rising. In general, operative risks of the procedure are low—major morbidity and death are uncommon. Serious complications are often preventable; when they occur, early diagnosis and treatment may be critical. The long-term health effects of female sterilization are currently being studied. Most findings to date are reassuring about potential adverse effects on menstrual function and risk of hysterectomy, but indicate that young age at sterilization is an important risk factor for later regret. Although female sterilization is highly effective, the often quoted estimate of four failures per 1000 procedures is probably an underestimate for most procedures. When failure does occur, the likelihood of ectopic pregnancy is increased, particularly after coagulation procedures. Timing of sterilization before the estimated date of ovulation and sexual abstinence or use of effective contraceptives before sterilization will reduce the risk of luteal phase pregnancy.

References

Centers for Disease Control (1984). Tubal sterilization among women of reproductive age, United States, update for 1979–1980. *Morbidity and Mortality Weekly Report*, **32** (Surveillance Summary 3), 9–14ss.

Chi, I. C., Laufe, L. E., Gardner, S. D., and Tolbert, M. A. (1980). An epidemiologic study of risk factors associated with pregnancy following female sterilization. *American Journal of Obstetrics and Gynecology*, **136**, 768–73.

Cohen, M. M. (1987). Long-term risk of hysterectomy after tubal sterilization. *American Journal of Epidemiology*, **125**, 410–19.

DeStefano, F., Greenspan, J. R., Ory, H. W., and Peterson, H. B. (1982*a*). Demographic trends in tubal sterilization: United States, 1970–1978. *American Journal of Public Health*, **72**, 480–4.

DeStefano, F., Peterson H. B., Layde, P. M., and Rubin, G. L. (1982*b*). Risk of ectopic pregnancy following tubal sterilization. *Obstetrics and Gynecology*, **60**, 326–30.

DeStefano, F., Greenspan, J. R., Dicker, R. C., Peterson, H. B., Strauss, L., and Rubin, G. L. (1983). Complications of interval laparoscopic tubal sterilization. *Obstetrics and Gynecology*, **61**, 153–8.

DeStefano, F., Perlman, J. A., Peterson, H. B., and Diamond, E. L. (1985). Long-term risk of menstrual disturbances after tubal sterilization. *American Journal of Obstetrics and Gynecology*, **152**, 835–41.

Escobedo, L., Peterson, H. B., Grubb, G. S., and Franks, A. L. (1989). Case-fatality rates for tubal sterilization in U.S. hospitals, 1979 to 1980. *American Journal of Obstetrics and Gynecology*, **160**, 147–50.

Franks, A. L., Kendrick, J. S., and Peterson, H. B. (1987). Unintended laparotomy associated with laparoscopic tubal sterilization. *American Journal of Obstetrics and Gynecology*, **157**, 1102–5.

Grimes, D. A., Peterson, H. B., Rosenberg, M. J., Fishburne, J. I., Rochat, R. W., Khan, A. R., *et al*. (1982). Sterilization-attributable deaths in Bangladesh. *International Journal of Obstetrics and Gynecology*, **20**, 149–54.

Grubb, G. S. and Peterson, H. B. (1985). Luteal phase pregnancy and tubal sterilization. *Obstetrics and Gynecology*, 66, 784–8.

Henshaw, S. K. and Singh, S. (1986). Sterilization regret among U. S. couples. *Family Planning Perspectives*, **18**, 238–40.

Holt, V. L., Chu, J., Daling, J. R., Stergachis, A. S., and Weiss, N. S. (1991). Tubal sterilization and subsequent ectopic pregnancy. A case-control study. *Journal of the American Medical Association*, **266**, 242–6.

Klebanoff, M. A., (1988). Short interpregnancy interval and the risk of low birthweight. *American Journal of Public Health*, **78(6)**, 667–70.

Liskin, L., Pile, J. M., and Quillen, W. F. (1983). Vasectomy—safe and simple. In *Population Reports*, (Series D), No. 4, (ed. W. Reinhart), pp. 63–100. Johns Hopkins University, Baltimore.

Liskin, L., Rinehart, E. W., Blackburn, R., and Rutledge, A. H. (1985). Minilaparotomy and laparoscopy: safe, effective, and widely used. In *Population Reports*, (Series C), No. 9, (ed. W. Rinchart), pp. 127–67. Johns Hopkins University, Baltimore.

Mosher, W. D. and Pratt, W. F. (1990). Contraceptive use in the United States, 1973–1988. Advance data from *Vital and Health Statistics*, 20 March. National Center for Health Statistics.

Park, C. B. (1986). The place of child-spacing as a factor in infant mortality: a recursive model. *American Journal of Public Health*, **76(8)**, 995–9.

Peterson, H. B., Greenspan, J. R., DeStefano, F., Ory, H. W., and Layde, P. M. (1981). The impact of laparoscopy on tubal sterilization in United States hospitals, 1970 and 1975–1978. *American Journal of Obstetrics and Gynecology*, **140**, 811–4.

Peterson, H. B., DeStefano, F., Rubin, G. L., Greenspan, J. R., Lee, N. C., and Ory, H. W. (1983). Deaths attributable to tubal sterilization in the United States, 1977–81. *American Journal of Obstetrics and Gynecology*, **146**, 131–6.

Peterson, H. B., Huber, D. H., and Belker, A. M. (1990). Vasectomy: an appraisal for the obstetrician–gynecologist. *Obstetrics and Gynecology*, **76**, 568–72.

Ross, J. A., Hong, S., and Huber, D. H. (1985). *Voluntary sterilization: an international fact book*. Association for Voluntary Sterilization, New York.

Schwartz, D., Wingo, P. A., Antarsh, L., and Smith, J. C. (1989). Female sterilization in the United States, 1987. *Family Planning Perspectives*, **21**, 209–12.

Stergachis, A., Shy, K. K., Grothaus, L. C., Wagner, E. H., Hecht, J. A., Anderson, G., *et al.* (1990). Tubal sterilization and the long-term risk of hysterectomy. *Journal of the American Medical Association*, **264**, 2893–8.

Vessey, M., Huggins, G., Lawless, M., McPherson, K., and Yeates, D. (1983). Tubal sterilization: Findings in a large prospective study. *British Journal of Obstetrics and Gynecology*, **90**, 203–9.

WHO Task Force on Female Sterilization. (1982). Minilaparotomy or laparoscopy for sterilization: a multicenter, multinational, randomized study. *American Journal of Obstetrics and Gynecology*, **143**, 645–52.

Wilcox, L. S., Chu, S. Y., and Peterson, H. B. (1990). Characteristics of women who considered or obtained tubal reanastomosis: results from a prospective study of tubal sterilization. *Obstetrics and Gynecology*, **75**, 661–5.

Wilcox, L. S., Chu, S. Y., Eaker, E. D., Leger, S. L., and Peterson, H. B. (1991). Risk factors for regret after tubal sterilization: 5 years of follow-up in a prospective study. *Fertility and Sterility*, **55**, 927–33.

Wilcox, L. S., Martinez-Schnell, B., Peterson, H. B., Ware, J. H., and Hughes, J. M. (1992). Menstrual function after tubal sterilization. *American Journal of Epidemiology*, **135(12)**, 1368–81.

Williams, E. D., Jones, H. E., and Merril, R. E. (1951). The subsequent course of patients sterilized by tubal ligation. *American Journal of Obstetrics and Gynecology*, **61**, 423–6.

10 Induced abortion

Stanley K. Henshaw and Rachel Benson Gold

Attitudes to abortion

Induced abortion has been practiced for thousands of years. Descriptions of methods of inducing abortion have been found in writings from ancient Egypt, China in the twenty-eighth century BC, and Rome (David 1981). Abortion was common in nineteenth century Europe and North America and is usually considered to have been an important factor in the sharp reduction in birth rates that began in that century in France and other countries. In the twentieth century, abortion has become one of the most common surgical procedures in industrialized countries.

Ethical and moral views of abortion vary widely from culture to culture and over time within the same culture, as do views of other aspects of sexuality. At one end of the spectrum are cultures where abortion is generally viewed as a normal way to regulate fertility. This is the case in some East Asian countries such as China, Japan, Korea, and Taiwan. Abortion is also used as a major method of fertility control in Eastern Europe and the former Soviet republics, and there are reports of women in those areas who regard abortion as a healthy 'cleaning out' that should be done periodically. In some cultures, there is little awareness that abortion could be viewed as murder or as an immoral act.

At the other end of the spectrum are cultures where abortion is viewed as the taking of human life, morally wrong, and/or a violation of religious precepts, although there are no cultures where an early spontaneous miscarriage is treated with the same gravity as the death of an infant, with funeral and burial. In most Western industrialized countries, varying views co-exist, the predominant one being that abortion is a matter of moral concern but must be legally available in many circumstances.

Religious views of abortion have evolved over time and may continue to change in the future. The Catholic Church did not consider abortion before quickening (which occurs at about the sixteenth week), to be a mortal sin until 1869, when Pope Pius IX eliminated the distinction between a formed and unformed fetus, making abortion a mortal sin even to save the life of the woman (Callahan 1970). Today, in addition to Catholics, some fundamentalist Christian groups are among the strongest opponents of abortion, while most of the major Protestant and Jewish denominations believe that abortion is morally justified or even required under some circumstances. In Islam (Musallam 1983) and many Christian groups, the religious authorities are not in agreement as to the moral status of abortion, in part because the Koran and Bible say little on the subject.

The legal status of abortion has also varied over time. Abortion before quickening was not a crime under English common law, but during the nineteenth century heavily restrictive laws were passed in most of the world, including Europe and America. There were several reasons for the change: concern about the harm to women's health caused by abortion, which was relatively unsafe at the time, whether attempted by medical or surgical means, new understanding that fetal development is continuous and that quickening does not represent an important change in the character of the fetus, and changing sexual attitudes, which also led to the outlawing of contraception. In the USA, other conditions contributed to the increased restrictions: the attempt of physicians to undermine the economic base of midwives, who were competing for women's health care and who provided many of the abortions and concern about the low birth rate among Americans of European ancestry, who were threatened by the large numbers of recent immigrants who had many children (Mohr 1978).

The twentieth century has seen a large-scale reversal in industrialized countries of the restrictive nineteenth century laws. Today, induced abortion is legal during the first trimester on request, for social reasons, or to preserve the health of the pregnant women in all industrialized countries except the Republic of Ireland (Tietze and Henshaw 1986; Henshaw 1990). Induced abortion is also legal on request or for social indications in many developing countries, including China and India, but is not legal in most countries of Africa and Latin America, and in parts of Asia. Further liberalization of laws is likely in developing countries, but powerful efforts to restrict abortion again are occurring in some of the former socialist bloc countries and former Soviet republics.

Public opinion in the Western developed countries generally favors the legal availability of abortion services, although many people have ambivalent feelings and believe that some restrictions may be appropriate. Opinion polls show surprisingly similar views in most countries, with only about 5–20 per cent of the public believing that abortion should be prohibited in almost all circumstances (Sachdev 1988). In the USA, a 1992 poll showed that 14 per cent believed that abortion should be illegal in all circumstances, while 31 per cent favored abortion on request. Approval of legal abortion increased rapidly during the 1960s and has continued to increase gradually since abortion was legalized nationally in 1973 (Hugick and Saad 1992).

Rates of legal abortion vary widely from country to country (Table 10.1). Among the Western industrialized countries, these rates are largely a function of the rate of unintended pregnancy, which in turn depends on the prevalence of the use of the most effective contraceptive methods, the Pill, IUD, and sterilization (Jones *et al.* 1989). Public opinion has less effect on the abortion rate; for example, the Netherlands, which has the lowest abortion rate of any industrialized country (five abortions per 1000 women aged 15–44), has very liberal attitudes toward sexuality and abortion as well as a law permitting abortion on request up to viability of the fetus. Rates in Western industrialized countries except the USA are generally in the range 10–20 per 1000, while those in the former Soviet bloc countries and the USA are higher. Developing countries tend also to have higher rates because of lower contraceptive prevalence and less effective contraceptive use.

For most countries, abortion rates were relatively stable during the 1980s. Of the countries shown in Table 10.1 for which trend data are available, the abortion rate increased 10 per cent or more since 1985 in Canada, Czechoslovakia, England and Wales, Hungary, and Sweden, and decreased by that amount in Italy, Singapore, and the USSR. Official statistics suggest that the abortion rate is also declining in France.

Table 10.1 Number of abortions and abortion rate per 1000 women aged 15–44, selected countries

Country	Year	Number of abortions	Rate
Australia	1988	63 200	16.6
Bulgaria	1987	119 900	64.7
Canada[a]	1990	94 100	14.8
China	1989	10 600 000	37.6
Cuba	1988	155 300	58.0
Czechoslovakia	1990	157 300	45.7
Denmark	1990	20 600	18.2
England and Wales[b]	1990	173 900	15.8
Finland	1990	12 700	11.5
France[c]	1988	163 000	13.3
Hungary	1990	90 400	41.2
Italy[c]	1989	166 300	13.1
Japan[c]	1987	497 800	18.6
Netherlands[b]	1988	18 000	5.1
Norway	1990	15 600	16.7
Singapore	1987	21 200	30.1
Soviet Union[c]	1990	6 426 500	101.0
Sweden	1990	37 500	21.3
Tunisia	1988	23 300	13.6
United States	1988	1 590 800	27.3
Yugoslavia	1988	343 300	66.7

[a] Including abortions obtained by Canadian residents in the United States.

[b] Residents only.

[c] Abortions are underreported.

Sources: official statistics for all countries except the USA, for which the number of abortions was taken from a survey of providers conducted by the Alan Guttmacher Institute.

Induced abortion has a number of social and health benefits when provided under modern medical conditions. The procedure is relatively safe; mortality associated with first-trimester abortion is about one-tenth that of mortality from pregnancy and childbearing and although the risk of complications and death increases sharply with the length of the pregnancy, at no time in pregnancy is abortion mortality higher than that of pregnancy and delivery (Gold 1990). Serious complications accompany less than 1 per cent of abortions and are much less common than cesarean section and other complications of delivery. Although infection after induced abortion can undoubtedly impair fecundity in some women, adverse effects of vacuum aspiration on reproductive capacity are so rare as to be undetectable in epidemiologic studies (Hogue *et al.* 1982; Hogue 1986). The effects of multiple abortions and second-trimester procedures have been less extensively studied but are probably also small.

Thus, as a backup for contraception, induced abortion has few risks and offers the benefits that accrue from the ability to control fertility: it allows couples to postpone childbearing to the time when they are best able to assume the responsibilities of child rearing, it permits women to participate more fully in economic activities, and it prevents the life-changing stigma of childbearing in socially disapproved circumstances (for example, when women are pregnant outside marriage in some cultures, or because of rape or incest). Abortion has health benefits for women who are at high risk of complications of pregnancy because of medical or nutritional conditions or too recent delivery. Because many legal abortions are obtained by women with high-risk pregnancies and many replace unsafe illegal abortions, an estimated 1500 women's lives were saved in the USA by the availability of legal abortion during the first 10 years after the Roe v. Wade decision legalized abortion nationally (Tietze 1984). Similarly, the ability of women to terminate unwanted pregnancies safely has contributed to the lowering of infant mortality in the USA (Joyce 1987).

Among the other benefits of safe induced abortion has been the reduction in the number of infants born with serious congenital abnormalities. Amniocentesis, chorionic villus sampling, and other diagnostic procedures allow many fetal anomalies to be detected in time for the pregnancy to be terminated by abortion. While the absolute number of abnormalities found by screening is small, each one prevents a major tragedy for a family. Prenatal screening backed up by abortion when indicated makes procreation possible for couples who would otherwise avoid childbearing because of their high risk of having abnormal children. Selective fetal reduction of multiple pregnancies increases the probability of a healthy outcome for the remaining fetuses (Lynch *et al.* 1990)

Many of the above effects of induced abortion are reduced or non-existent when the procedure is performed in unsafe conditions because of legal restrictions or because of inadequate medical services. On the contrary, complications from unsafe abortions are a major medical problem for women in developing countries. The WHO has estimated that unsafe abortions cause between 50 000 and 100 000 deaths in developing countries each year; these amount to approximately 13 per cent of all maternal deaths (WHO 1994).

Legal issues

The controversy surrounding abortion stems from conflicting religious, moral, and legal viewpoints. The fundamental issues are the moral and religious value of the fetus and when personhood begins and whether a particular viewpoint should be embodied in the law.

Those opposed to legal restrictions on abortion argue that where the law treats abortion in the same way as any other medical procedure, no one is forced to act against her or his beliefs, while restrictions would prevent the exercise of conscience for pregnant women who believe that ending the pregnancy is the morally responsible thing to do. Many of those who believe that abortion is murder or perhaps a lesser moral offense, on the other hand, believe society should use the law to make a forceful statement that abortion is wrong and to prevent its being performed. In practice, the political and legal processes in most countries have produced a compromise position that recognizes the moral reservations that many people feel but allows the procedure to be performed legally for most women who seek it. Since no compromise can satisfy all viewpoints, attempts to change the law are likely to recur from time to time.

Grounds for abortion

One common type of limitation on legal abortion is to allow the procedure only for certain indications. Laws based on this principle range from extremely restrictive to not restrictive. The most restrictive laws allow abortion only if continuing the pregnancy would seriously threaten the life of the pregnant woman. Such laws are found in the Republic of Ireland and in some countries of Africa, the Middle East, and Latin America. Brazil, Ecuador, and Mexico have slightly more permissive laws that permit abortion in cases where the pregnancy resulted from an illegal act (rape or incest) as well as where it endangers life.

More liberal laws allow abortion to protect the health of the pregnant woman. These are sometimes worded restrictively to apply only when there is a risk of serious and lasting damage to the woman's health, as in Portugal and Spain. The laws of some countries, including Great Britain, Japan, and West Germany (before reunification) specify that the social conditions of the pregnant woman as well as her physical state can be taken into account in assessing the risk to her health. Not all such laws specify that the risk to health must be grave or serious; in Great Britain, for example, abortion is permitted for the protection of the health of the pregnant woman if the danger of continuing pregnancy is greater than the danger of having the abortion. Since abortion up to about 16 weeks of pregnancy is almost always safer than carrying a pregnancy to term, abortion before that point in gestation is generally permissible under the Great Britain law.

Some countries allow abortion under certain social or economic conditions as well as for health risks. For example, in Romania before 1986, abortion was allowed on request to women over the age of 40 and to women with four or more living children (Tietze and Henshaw 1986). Besides age and number of children, other conditions specified in laws include having inadequate housing (Hungary before 1992), being unmarried (Bulgaria before 1990), and contraceptive failure (India).

Laws incorporating the principle that abortion is permissible under some conditions but not others must contain a mechanism for determining whether the requirements are met in each specific case. In Great Britain, this is accomplished by the certification of two physicians. In Eastern European countries when such laws were in effect, committees were established by governmental authorities. Another approach is to leave to the physician performing the abortion the responsibility for interpreting and applying the terms of the law. This approach has the disadvantage that a physician could be subject to sanctions and possibly criminal penalties after the abortion if his or her judgment or interpretation of the law were later found to be incorrect. A proposed law of this type was widely opposed by physicians in Canada because they feared they could be the target of unpredictable legal action.

Laws allowing abortion only for certain indications are subject to widely varying interpretations, especially when the indications involve risk to the woman's health. An extreme example is Switzerland, where the law permits abortion only to prevent an otherwise unavoidable danger of serious and lasting injury to the woman's health. The law is interpreted so liberally in some cantons that abortion is available virtually on request and so restrictively in other cantons that no abortions are performed (Dondenaz *et al.* 1992). Such variations in implementation of the law result in inequities based on the place of residence of a woman.

Other inequities may be introduced when it is possible for some women but not others to find physicians who will certify that they meet the requirements for an abortion. For example, in New York before 1970, abortions were difficult to obtain for women who could not afford a private consultation with a psychiatrist who would certify that they were suicide risks (Belsky 1992).

Gestation limits

Many countries, including Canada, China, France, Scandinavia (except Finland), the republics of the former Soviet Union, and the USA, permit abortion on the request of the woman without regard to her reasons. Most countries, however, specify a point in gestation beyond which the procedure is no longer permitted or is permitted only for specified indications such as danger to a woman's life. The limit is usually set between 12 and 24 weeks after the last menstrual period (LMP). France, for example, allows abortions past 12 weeks only if the pregnancy poses a grave danger to the woman's health or if there is strong risk of serious incurable fetal abnormality. Some countries, including France and Great Britain, allow abortions at any point in gestation under these circumstances.

Even where no limit is specified by law, few abortions take place after around 24 weeks, because few women seek abortions at that point and most physicians are unwilling to provide them. In the USA, for example, although many states have no law specifying a gestation limit, only about 100–400 abortions per year or about 0.01–0.03 per cent of all abortions, are performed past 24 weeks.

The question of whether there should be a legally defined upper gestational limit for abortion and if so where it should be set, is a continuing issue with no clear answer. Some states in the USA, using the language of the Supreme Court in the Roe v. Wade decision, have set fetal viability as the legal limit. This limit, however, is not clearly defined, since it could be the point at which 1 per cent of fetuses survive, or 50 per cent, or 90 per cent; the probability of mental and physical handicap could also be considered in determining when viability occurs. Viability has generally been interpreted as viability with intensive medical intervention, so the gestation limit moves lower as medical technology improves. If technology were to improve to the point where an early embryo could be grown in an artificial environment, abortion would become illegal at all points in gestation.

England and Wales set the maximum at a fixed number of weeks, which was recently reduced to 24 weeks, in part because viability occurs earlier now than when the original standard of 28 weeks was set. Although this reduction affected relatively few women, those affected were among those most in need of abortions and least able to care for a child. According to one study in England, women who request late abortions tend to have severe social or psychological problems or both (Savage 1985).

Other restrictions

A number of other conditions may apply to abortion that are not applied to most other surgical or medical procedures. In France, for example, all women having abortions must consult with a social welfare or family counselor. In some states in the USA, regulations detail that women must be informed about such matters as all possible complications of abortion, the characteristics of the fetus or embryo at the woman's stage of gestation, the medical and social services available to mothers and to women who wish to place a baby for adoption, and methods of contraception. In 1991, Poland began to require that women seeking abortions be counseled by approved psychologists who are to try to dissuade the women from having abortions.

Sometimes associated with counseling requirements are mandatory delay periods ranging from 24 h to 1 week, the purpose being to assure that women have time to carefully consider their decision. Both the delay and the counseling may force women to make two or more trips to the abortion facility; this may be a serious barrier to services for women who live a long distance from them or who lack transportation.

In many jurisdictions, notification or consent of one or both parents is required for minors, usually defined as unmarried women under the age of 18. In some cases, a minor can seek a court order allowing the abortion as an alternative to involving her parents. In the USA, at least, the purpose of these laws appears to be to discourage abortion, since no such consent or notification requirements are applied to minors seeking prenatal care, although pregnancy and childbirth are more dangerous than abortion and have more long-lasting effects on the woman's future life (Donovan 1992). Consent or notification of husbands is not currently required in any industrialized country but is common in developing areas.

A final restriction is that the provision of abortion services is sometimes organized in ways different from other medical care. Some countries charge fees for abortion that are not charged for other procedures, although the fees are usually only a fraction of the actual cost of the service. In the USA, public health insurance for low-income women does not cover abortion in most states and private health insurance often excludes elective abortion. The types of facility in which abortion may be provided are sometimes regulated, for example a number of countries require that abortions be performed only in hospitals or other approved facilities.

Public health effects of restrictions

A number of undesirable health and social effects can result from many of the common restrictions on abortion. Restrictions can cause women to resort to unsafe illegal abortion methods or practitioners, with higher risks of maternal mortality and morbidity. In the USA during the 1950s and 1960s before state laws began to be liberalized in 1968, at least 200–300 deaths a year were caused by illegal abortions (Council on Scientific Affairs, American Medical Association 1992). Romania, which outlawed abortion under most circumstances (as well as contraception) in 1966, provides a striking example of the consequences of severe restrictions. The government reported that 421 000 women were treated for abortion complications in 1983, a rate of 91 per 1000 women aged 15–44, and 449 abortion deaths were reported for 1984 (Henshaw 1990). These figures illustrate two points: that the motivation of women to control their fertility can be high enough to cause large numbers to seek abortions despite serious risks to their health and that when abortion is restricted, there may not be enough trained medical personnel willing to provide abortion services outside the law to meet the demand.

Unsafe illegal abortions can occur in response to restrictions much less severe than complete prohibition. In the USA, deaths from illegal abortions still occur at the rate of about one a year and several deaths have resulted because insurance for low-income women did not cover the procedure (Binkin *et al.* 1982). In the Soviet Union, although abortions were provided without charge through the various health systems, many women sought abortions from illegal lay practitioners or by self-induction because of the lack of confidentiality in the governmental health system or because of distance from a service provider. These abortions resulted in 536 deaths or 23 per cent of all maternal deaths in 1988 (Popov 1991).

A second consequence of most restrictions is that they delay abortions, thereby exposing many women to increased risk of complications and prolonged psychological stress. Where committee approval is required, time is needed for the woman or her physician to prepare the application and for the committee to make its decision; additional delay occurs if an appeal is necessary. For example, when approval was required in Canada before 1988, the application and committee approval process usually involved significant delay, although some large urban hospitals had committees that provided almost immediate approval. In 1987, only 33 per cent of abortions were performed before 9 weeks after the last menstrual period (Statistics Canada 1989), compared with 51 per cent in the USA (Henshaw *et al.* 1991).

A requirement for counseling may not in itself cause delay if the services are readily available, but waiting periods of 1–7 days—which often accompany counseling requirements—almost inevitably cause delay for some women. In the USA, such requirements usually increase the number of visits a woman must make to the abortion facility; where women live long distances away, the extra trip can cause hardship and delay.

A requirement that minors' parents be notified of the abortion in advance or that they provide consent can cause minors to postpone seeking abortion services. Even where no requirements exist, adolescents usually are later than older women in obtaining abortions, in part because they want to avoid involving their parents. The experience of US states that have imposed parental involvement requirements shows that minors who obtain abortions tend to have them at later gestations (Cartoof and Klerman 1986; Rogers *et al.* 1991). Even where minors can obtain a court order allowing abortion without parental involvement, obtaining it can itself cause delay.

Although few countries expect patients to pay a significant proportion of the cost of an abortion, low-income women may experience delay because of the time they need to accumulate any payment which is required. Studies in the USA have shown that this is a significant cause of delay in the absence of insurance coverage for low-income women (Henshaw and Wallisch 1984; Torres and Forrest 1988). On the other hand, financial incentives to present early for abortion services may reduce average gestational age. In the USA, women must pay higher fees if their abortions are past 12 weeks and in Czechoslovakia, the proportion of abortions performed before 9 weeks increased from 65 per cent in 1986 to 85 per cent in 1987 because of new regulations that provide free 'miniabortions' before 8 weeks (46 days for nulliparous women) but require a fee to be paid at later gestations (Henshaw and Morrow 1990).

Gestational age limits may also encourage women to seek services before they become difficult or impossible to obtain. For a woman who becomes aware of her pregnancy only after the limits have been passed, however, the restrictions may cause hardship or may actually cause delay while she applies for approval for a second-trimester procedure.

Yet another effect of abortion restrictions is to force women to travel to other countries or jurisdictions where services are more available. For example, in 1983, 22 000 Spanish women had abortions in England because of the restrictive law in Spain. In 1990, 2800 French women went to England for abortions even though abortions are available on request in France up to 10 weeks, presumably because of the need for second-trimester services or parental involvement requirements for minors (Office of Population Censuses and Surveys 1991). In the USA a parental consent law implemented in

Massachusetts in 1981 resulted in 1117 adolescents traveling to neighboring states for abortions during the next year (Cartoof and Klerman 1986). The need to travel causes delay and increases the likelihood that a woman will receive inadequate follow-up care.

Besides delay, another effect of most restrictions is that they differentially affect disadvantaged women and those who live in areas remote from abortion services. Women who have access to information and financial resources can usually find ways to obtain services where abortions are limited to certain indications, if necessary by traveling to other jurisdictions. The women least able to overcome barriers are adolescents and women with low income, low education, inability to speak the dominant language, or other limitations.

From a public health point of view, the best approach to the abortion issue is to reduce the number of unintended pregnancies, thereby reducing the need for abortion. While different measures to reduce unintended pregnancies may be appropriate in different communities, increasing the availability of contraceptive services, developing and making available more contraceptive methods, and promoting attitudes conducive to better contraceptive practice would be helpful in most contexts (Jones *et al.* 1989).

Since unwanted pregnancies can never be completely prevented, abortion services should be made readily available without barriers that cause delay or result in preferential treatment for some women over others. Public education efforts should assure that women are aware that safe abortion services are available and that early action is needed when pregnancy is suspected, to obtain termination or prenatal care as early as possible.

RU-486

The controversy surrounding abortion has affected not only laws but also the development and introduction of new abortion technologies, specifically the use of antiprogestins. The combination of the antiprogestin mifepristone, popularly known as RU-486, and a prostaglandin has been approved for use in China, France, the UK, and Sweden for the termination of pregnancies up to 8 or 9 weeks after the LMP. By 1991, 80 000 women in France had had induced abortions by taking 600 mg of RU-486, followed 36–48 later by an injection of sulprostone or a vaginal suppository of gemeprost (Klitsch 1991). Several studies have found the regimen to be 95–96 per cent effective in terminating the pregnancy, including one based on 10 000 patients (Goldsmith 1991). Research is continuing on the dosage, the use of different prostaglandins, and the length of gestation at which the method is effective. Recent studies have found that pregnancies up to 9 weeks can be equally effectively terminated (UK Multicentre Trial 1990) and that a different prostaglandin, misoprostol is (trade name Cytotec), is effective. Misoprostol is less expensive than sulprostone or gemeprost, more convenient because it can be taken by mouth, easier to store, available in more countries, and may have fewer side-effects.

The disadvantages of RU-486 with prostaglandin are nausea and diarrhea caused by the prostaglandin, bleeding that can last for weeks and on rare occasions require transfusion, and cardiac complications caused by the prostaglandin. Advantages are that the risks associated with anaesthesia and surgery—including damage to the uterus or cervix, and infection—are avoided and women may feel more in control.

RU-486 has attracted the opposition of antiabortion groups because they believe that a safe medical abortifacient will make abortion simpler to provide, less easily subject to legal controls, more accepted by the public, and therefore more frequent. Because of the opposition of these groups and their threats to boycott the products of companies that manufacture abortifacients, Roussel-UCLAF, RU-486's manufacturer, has made no attempt to introduce it into the USA and other countries where opposition is strong. Similarly, antiabortion opposition may have been a factor in causing other companies to stop research on other antiprogestins.

Opposition to RU-486 is particularly unfortunate because of other possible uses of the drug. Among these are speeding up delivery by causing contractions, and treatment of breast cancer, certain brain tumors, glaucoma, and Cushing's syndrome. Most recently, a British study found RU-486 to be effective as a postcoital contraceptive and possibly more effective than the contraceptive pills, especially Ovral (0.5 mg norgestrel and 0.05 mg ethinyl estradiol; Wyeth-Ayerst Laboratories) that are currently used (Glasier *et al.* 1992).

While it is not clear exactly what proportion of women would choose RU-486 over surgical abortion, the drug is an important innovation that will make abortion safer and will meet the needs of many women, and its availability should not be restricted as a means of limiting access to abortion. If it proves to be uniquely effective as a postcoital contraceptive, its availability will be even more important, especially in countries like the USA, where unintended pregnancies are common and postcoital contraception is not widely used.

Summary

The most pressing issues relating to abortion are legal and political, not medical. The question of whether induced abortion should be legally permitted even when a woman's health is threatened is being actively debated in many developing countries and in some of the former Soviet bloc countries, especially Croatia, Hungary, Lithuania, Poland, and Slovakia, although it has been answered in the affirmative in all Western developed countries except The Republic of Ireland.

Even in many Western countries, moral reservations about abortion have led to political compromises that have resulted in various types of restrictions on abortion, including limitation to women with health or other indications for abortion, gestation limits, required counseling and waiting periods, and mandatory parental consent or notification for minors. While in some cases these restrictions are ostensibly intended to benefit pregnant women—for example, by ensuring that they have time to give careful consideration to the abortion decision—such benefits have not been demonstrated, and the most ardent supporters of the restrictions are those who would prohibit abortion completely. Virtually all the restrictions exact a price from women seeking abortions: health risk resulting from delay, psychological stress, expense, or inability to obtain abortion services at all. The challenges for those concerned for the welfare of women are to reduce the rate of unintended pregnancy, to eliminate restrictions on abortion, to agree to the least intrusive restrictions where compromise is necessary, and to minimize the detrimental effects of unavoidable restrictions.

A related issue is the extent to which opponents of abortion have succeeded in blocking research and innovation in pregnancy prevention and termination. In particular, abortion opponents have delayed the introduction of RU-486 into the USA, Germany, and other countries, and their threats have discouraged pharmaceutical companies from developing other antiprogestins and prostaglandins. Here the challenge is to reassure companies that the goodwill and economic benefits of developing abortion-related products outweigh any possible harm from abortion opponents.

References

Belsky, J. (1992). Medically indigent women seeking abortion prior to legalization: New York City, 1969–1970. *Family Planning Perspectives*, **24**, 129–34.

Binkin, N., Gold, J., and Cates, W. (1982). Illegal-abortion deaths in the United States: why are they still occurring? *Family Planning Perspectives*, **14**, 163–7.

Callahan, D. (1970). *Abortion: Law, Choice, and Morality*. Macmillan, New York.

Cartoof, V. and Klerman, L. (1986). Parental consent for abortion: impact of the Massachusetts law. *American Journal of Public Health*, **76**, 397–400.

Council on Scientific Affairs, American Medical Association (1992). Induced termination of pregnancy before and after Roe v. Wade. *Journal of the American Medical Association*, **268**, 3231–9.

David, H. P. (1981). Abortion policies. In *Abortion and sterilization: Medical and Social Aspects* (ed. J. E. Hodgson), pp. 1–40. Academic Press, London.

Dondénaz, M., Gloor, P.-A., Hagmann, H.-M., Hurni, M., Rey, A.-M., Stamm, H., *et al*. (1992). L'interruption de grossesse en Suisse: période 1987–1990. *Medicine Hygiene*, **50**, 926–34.

Donovan, P. (1992). *Our daughters' decisions: The conflict in state law on abortion and other issues*. The Alan Guttmacher Institute, New York.

Glasier, A., Thong, K. J., Dewar, M., Mackie, M., and Baird, D. T. (1992). Mifepristone (RU 486) compared with high-dose estrogen and progestogen for emergency postcoital contraception. *New England Journal of Medicine*, **327**, 1041–4.

Gold, R. (1990). *Abortion and women's health*. The Alan Guttmacher Institute, New York.

Goldsmith, M. (1991). As data on antiprogesterone compounds grow, societal and scientific aspects are scrutinized. *Journal of the American Medical Association*, **265**, 1628–9.

Henshaw, S. K. (1990). Induced abortion: a world review, 1990. *Family Planning Perspectives*, **22**, 76–89.

Henshaw, S. K. and Morrow, E. (1990). *Induced abortion: a world review, 1990 supplement*. The Alan Guttmacher Institute, New York.

Henshaw, S. K. and Wallisch, L. (1984). The Medicaid cutoff and abortion services for the poor. *Family Planning Perspectives*, **16**, 170–80.

Henshaw, S. K., Koonin, L., and Smith, J. (1991). Characteristics of U.S. women having abortions, 1987. *Family Planning Perspectives*, **23**, 75–81.

Hogue, C. J. R. (1986). Impact of abortion on subsequent fecundity. *Clinics in Obstetrics and Gynecology*, **13**, 95–103.

Hogue, C. J. R., Cates, W., Jr, and Tietze, C. (1982). The effects of induced abortion on subsequent reproduction. *Epidemiologic Reviews*, **4**, 66–94.

Hugick, L. and Saad, L, (1992). But public seeks middle ground on abortion, supports Pennsylvania law. *The Gallup Poll Monthly* No. 316, January, pp. 6–8.

Jones, E., Forrest, J. D., Henshaw, S. K., Silverman, J., and Torres, A. (1989). *Pregnancy, conception and family planning services in industrialized countries*. Yale University Press, New Haven.

Joyce, T. (1987). The impact of induced abortion on black and white birth outcomes in the United States. *Demography*, **24**, 229–44.

Klitsch, M. (1991). Antiprogestins and the abortion controversy: a progress report. *Family Planning Perspectives*, **23**, 275–82.

Lynch, L., Berkowitz, R. L., Chitkara, U., and Alvarez, M. (1990). First-trimester transabdominal multifetal pregnancy reduction: a report of 85 cases. *Obstetrics and Gynecology*, 75, 735–8.

Mohr, J. C. (1978). *Abortion in America*. Oxford University Press, New York.

Musallam, B. F. (1983). *Sex and society in Islam*. Cambridge University Press, London.

Office of Population Censuses and Surveys (1991). *Abortion statistics, 1990*. HMSO, London.

Popov, A. (1991). Family planning and induced abortion in the USSR: basic health and demographic chasracteristics. *Studies in Family Planning*, **22**, 268–77.

Rogers, J. L., Boruch, R. F., Stoms, G. B., and DeMoya, D. (1991). Impact of the Minnesota parental notification law on abortion and birth. *American Journal of Public Health*, **81**, 294–8.

Sachdev, P. (1988). *International handbook on abortion*. Greenwood Press, New York.

Savage, W. (1985). Requests for late termination of pregnancy: Tower Hamlets, 1983. *British Medical Journal*, **290**, 621–3.

Statistics Canada (1989). *Therapeutic abortions 1987*. Government of Canada, Ottawa.

Tietze, C. (1984). The public health effects of legal abortion in the United States. *Family Planning Perspectives*, **16**, 26–8.

Tietze, C. and Henshaw, S. K. (1986). *Induced abortion: a world review, 1986*. The Alan Guttmacher Institute, New York.

Torres, A. and Forrest, J. (1988). Why do women have abortions? *Family Planning Perspectives*, **20**, 169–76.

UK Multicentre Trial (1990). The efficacy and tolerance of mifepristone and prostaglandin in first trimester termination of pregnancy. *British Journal of Obstetrics and Gynaecology*, **97**, 480–6.

World Health Organization (1994). *Abortion: a tabulation of available data on the frequency and mortality of unsafe abortion*, 2nd edition. WHO, Geneva.

11 Assisted fertilization

Carl Wood and Karen Dawson

By 1989, a total of more than 45 000 children had been born from the use of assisted fertilization techniques, according to the World Collaborative Report released at the Seventh World Congress on *In Vitro* Fertilization and Assisted Procreations in 1989 (Seventh World Congress on *in vitro* fertilization and assisted procreation 1991). Since the birth in England in 1978 of Louise Brown, the world's first baby to be born from the use of *in vitro* fertilization (IVF) (Steptoe and Edwards 1978), the use of assisted fertilization techniques has grown rapidly. The development of this technology has, however, not been without controversy; many social, legal, ethical, and religious concerns about its use have been raised and debated.

The development of assisted reproduction techniques, their present status and possible future, and some of the issues raised by the use of these technologies will be considered in this chapter.

The history of assisted fertilization

Despite the long history of IVF and embryo transfer (ET) in animals (Westmore 1984), the modern approach to human fertility problems—which involves exposing the human ovum to spermatozoa outside the mother and transferring the resulting embryo to her uterus—has been in use for a relatively short time. The first reports of pregnancies following the use of this technique in humans were published during the 1970s (de Kretser *et al.* 1973; Steptoe and Edwards 1976, 1978), and the use of IVF, ET, and gamete intrafallopian transfer (GIFT) have since resulted in many live births for couples with infertility problems. The recent rapid growth of these techniques has demonstrated their potential for treating a range of infertility conditions and has required considerable back-up support. Perhaps more than most therapies, assisted fertilization has relied for its development and growth on a favorable social and scientific climate.

Embryo culture

Since the work of Heape (1891) in the late nineteenth century, scientists have been interested in the possibility of culturing embryos in the laboratory to study their early development. For many years, however, progress was frustratingly slow. The scientists usually tried to grow the embryos in a culture medium based on blood plasma, serum, or undefined biological fluids. In 1949, John Hammond Jr devised a complex medium that allowed eight-cell mouse embryos to develop into blastocysts. Whitten (1956) later showed that a simpler chemically defined medium could sustain *in vitro* mouse embryo development. Soon afterwards, McLaren and Biggers (1958), combining the culture fluid of Whitten with the transfer techniques of Heape, cultured mouse embryos to the blastocyst stage and then transferred them to foster mothers, where they developed normally.

Events in the development of IVF and ET

Following the discovery of sperm capacitation (the process which results in the sperm being capable of fertilizing an oocyte), investigators became conscious of the difficulty of selecting suitable criteria for IVF and of discriminating it from parthenogenic activation. In 1959, Chang overcame this difficulty and, in work with rabbits, achieved the first live births following IVF.

In 1970, Patrick Steptoe and Bob Edwards referred to unpublished work on rabbits in which oocytes stimulated by the hormone human chorionic gonadotropin (hCG) were extracted shortly before the expected time of ovulation, and allowed to mature *in vitro* and fertilized *in vivo*. These manipulations resulted in normal term fetuses. Within a few years, Steptoe and Edwards had adopted the procedure of injecting hCG and recovering oocytes before the expected time of ovulation. The technique of laparoscopy, of which Steptoe was a pioneer, proved ideal for the recovery of mature oocytes from the ovaries.

The freezing of human embryos by Trounson and Mohr (1983) in Melbourne resulted in the world's first frozen embryo baby. This technique is useful for storing excess embryos that cannot be safely transferred in one cycle or for storing embryos when the patient is not fit for embryo transfer.

The world's first donor egg baby was born in 1984 in Melbourne, to a woman who had no ovaries. By using donor oocytes and the husband's sperm, an artificial menstrual cycle, IVF, and embryo transfer, a normal pregnancy resulted. Some women who had no eggs or whose eggs were unsuitable because of the risk of chromosomal or genetic diseases were also treated.

As well as a possible treatment for a significant proportion of couples with fertility problems, the potential of IVF and ET is increasingly recognized in other areas, including contraceptive research, cancer studies, and the exploration of our evolutionary origins (Short 1979). The techniques have also stimulated interest in defining the causes and incidence of spontaneous human embryonic wastage and in exploring the factors regulating oocyte maturation. Whilst scientific research and clinical developments have proceeded, debate within communities has escalated, centered largely on the moral and legal aspects of the IVF and ET procedures. However, clinics have been established, as fears that the procedure would result in malformation have diminished. There is now evidence that the incidence of genetic and developmental abnormalities in babies born from IVF and other assisted fertilization techniques is no higher than the incidence of birth defects in the general population (Seventh World Congress on *in vitro* fertilization and assisted procreation).

The social impact of infertility

The extent of infertility

Textbooks about human reproduction generally give the rate of involuntary infertility as 10 per cent (Behrman and Kistner 1975). A reassessment of the census from Canada and analysis of data from the World Fertility Survey and other studies, however, do not substantiate this core rate. Instead, there appear to be wide variations in the rates of primary and secondary infertility (Behrman and Kistner 1975). Although there has been little research carried out to document these differences, it is likely that the causes and extent of infertility differ among societies.

About 8–10 per cent of couples in Australia may be infertile, although the prevalence of infertility is not known with any confidence. The only data to support this suspicion is the percentage of couples not pregnant 1 year after stopping the oral contraceptive pill (Vessey *et al.* 1976). At least two-thirds of Australian couples will seek medical advice after 1–2 years of infertility. In half of these couples, the women become pregnant while undergoing infertility treatment and the remainder either become pregnant naturally (and are therefore not sterile), adopt a child, or give up any attempt to conceive. Thus, this estimate of the percentage of infertile couples in the community may actually be too high.

The widely held perception that infertility is becoming more common may not be true. In 1982, a US survey found the prevalence of infertility among married couples to be 8.5 per cent, not significantly increased since 1965 (US Department of Health and Human Services 1988). According to a report published in 1987, a survey of general practice records in the UK found that the incidence of involuntary infertility was the same among women aged 35 at the time of the survey as it was for women who had been 35 years old 15 years earlier. One difference was that modern 35-year-old women were more likely to have sought advice and treatment for infertility or fertility problems (Johnston *et al.* 1987).

The widespread use of contraception to induce voluntary infertility has complicated the definition of infertility and any perception of its incidence. It is likely that the ability to control fertility for long periods has also altered individual and social expectations about the ability to plan conception at will. If the age at which women first attempt conception is increasing, more women will be exposed to diseases that become more common as age increases, such as endometriosis, fibromyomata, and oocyte abnormalities. It might then appear that infertility is becoming more common.

The effect of assisted fertilization on population

The contribution of assisted fertilization procedures to the population is small. It has been estimated that 5 per cent of babies in the USA result from these procedures and that the contribution of these techniques to the population in Australia is about 3 per cent.

The emphasis currently being given to the need for population control has indirectly had an adverse affect on the position of the involuntary childless, who are increasingly being called upon to justify their decision to pursue fertility treatments in their quest to have their own child. In an environment of widespread ignorance about infertility, it is sometimes considered immoral or irresponsible for these couples to be preoccupied with their personal need for a child, when the world is already unable to provide adequately for the majority of existing children.

The number of children likely to be born from assisted fertilization treatments will not have a significant effect on global population. It takes at least 2.3 children per family for a population to be maintained and many childless couples would be satisfied with only one child.

Advantages and disadvantages of assisted fertilization

The most evident advantages and disadvantages of assisted fertilization relate to outcome. Couples with a healthy infant after one or more treatment cycles benefit by achieving their important goal of commencing a family. Couples with outcomes other than a healthy infant after one or more treatment cycles may suffer psychological, physical, social, and economic costs.

In addition, the emotional costs may be high for individuals or couples seeking access to the technology who are excluded by discretionary criteria (such as age or marital status). Conversely, individuals or couples seeking access to treatment may decide to withdraw after receiving counseling and information about the program. In this case the benefits to the individual or couple may be great.

To consider the costs and benefits of assisted fertilization only in terms of the outcome of the treatment, however, is an oversimplification. Despite eventual failure, many couples find it easier to accept their childlessness after having learned about the cause of their infertility or having attempted a novel method of conception and producing embryos. Whether assisted fertilization is advantageous or disadvantageous for an individual or couple is a personal matter that cannot be measured solely in terms of the outcome of treatment.

There are several benefits of assisted reproduction to society:

(1) infertility may be resolved for thousands of women with tubal disease;

(2) new causes of infertility have been discovered;

(3) and the increased knowledge about human fertilization may lead to the development of new contraceptives and new insights into the occurrence of congenital malformations.

The provision of this basic information concerning fertilization and embryo growth also increases respect for the creative process.

Emotional effects on parents

The emotional effects of assisted fertilization procedures have been well documented (Newman and Zoures 1991). It is difficult, however, to compare these experiences with other emotional life experiences, such as the failure to conceive naturally.

Newman and Zoures (1991) studied the emotional profile of infertile couples during a treatment cycle and found that their feelings changed during the various stages of therapy. Both women and men became more anxious waiting for the result of treatment. The failure of a cycle understandably exacerbated depression for the couple and in a majority of women resulted in a feeling of loss of control. Between cycles feelings were similar to those during the stimulation stage of a cycle, except that anxiety was less common for women. With the exception of anxiety, many of the feelings associated with the treatment may be related to infertility rather than to the treatment itself. The need for emotional support and counseling during infertility treatment is obvious if this pattern of anxiety peaks and letdowns is considered. The stress of these treatments is hard to compare with that of other therapies. The physical risk is small, but there is great social and emotional strain for the couple over a long period.

Effects on children

The effects of reproductive technology on the offspring are largely unknown. Ill effects might possibly include emotional disturbance when the child becomes aware of how he or she was conceived, discrimination by other children and late onset of minor physical or mental handicaps as a result of the technology. Most parents tell their children of their mode of conception without ill effect. The children are often pleased with their 'special status' since the social parents are usually the biological parents and they have prepared themselves for parenthood more carefully than many fertile couples.

For children conceived by assisted reproduction the passage from puberty to adulthood will be important for determining whether their special conception influences their eventual attitude to reproduction and childbearing. There is also the possibility that the careful parenting of these children may be very favorable to their later development.

Small studies of children of up to 3 years old have shown nothing remarkable about their intellectual, social, or physical status. Long-term studies of older children with a matched control group have started in Australia.

Funding of assisted fertilization treatments

A global fee has been established recently in Australia to cover services used in assisted reproduction. To this extent, the government has accepted that the new reproductive technologies form part of an adequate level of care which must be accessible to all.

Arguments in support of public subsidy reflect judgements about the worth of reproductive technology programs and their essential comparability with other funded treatments for infertility, in terms of cost and efficacy.

Two arguments are used against public subsidy of reproductive technologies. The first is that these technologies should not be publicly funded because they are morally unacceptable to some members of the community. This is the same argument proposed against any public funding of abortion. The problem with this argument is that is overlooks an individual's right to choose in situations where others will not be harmed by that choice. The second argument against any public funding for reproductive technology is proposed by some radical feminists who claim the technology is unnecessary, unsuccessful, unkind, unsafe, or unwise (National Bioethics Consultative Committee 1991). The counter-arguments to these claims are that assisted fertilization is necessary because the desire to grow a baby inside one's body is a female biological imperative, reinforced by society; is successful because the optimum live birth pregnancy rate closely resembles normal reproduction statistics; is kind because the technology offers infertile couples hope for having their own children; is safe because the procedures are constantly being improved and adverse effects have never been clearly demonstrated; is wise because preventative programs have never been demonstrated to be successful, and because there are currently no social alternative available which satisfy the desire of most couples to reproduce.

Costs

Complex medical technology is expensive and may distort health budgets disproportionately relative to the gains by the community. The total cost of assisted reproduction techniques in Australia was 0.1 per cent of the National Health Budget, which may not be excessive for the estimated 1 per cent of Australians requiring the technology.

Australian couples who have used reproductive technology whether with a successful or unsuccessful outcome spent on average $1300. The average number of cycles to achieve a pregnancy was 2.5, with the Government covering about 60 per cent of the treatment costs. About 60 per cent of couples seeking treatment did not achieve pregnancy, but still spent on average $1300 before stopping treatment.

It has been claimed that infertile couples are depriving others of medical care. The childless are only depriving others of treatment if the concept of a fixed health budget is accepted. There are several areas of national spending which are quite controversial; the defense budget, for example, is a source of contention in almost every country in the world. The case must be made that the childless are not attempting to deprive the sick of vital resources but rather to receive adequate consideration from the national budget as a whole.

Political views

Governments have reacted to the new technology in different ways. In the USA no funding was available for this research for some years, while in the UK the government has placed some restrictions on the technology and was in a limited way support the procedure under the National Health Service. The Australian states of Victoria (Parliament of Victoria 1984), South Australia (Parliament of South Australia 1988), and Western Australia (Parliament of Western Australia 1991) have legislation which controls assisted fertilization procedures by allowing them only at designated hospitals, ensuring compulsory counseling of patients, protecting sperm and egg donors from claims by the offspring and making the infertile couple the legal parents, and restricting embryo experimentation. Neither the USA nor the UK has supported the technology for uninsured patients, in effect restricting access to wealthier patients.

Religious and ethical considerations

The moral status of the human embryo

The most vehement opposition to assisted fertilization has come from those who believe that as soon as the egg and sperm unite at fertilization, either a new human being or a new potential human being has come into existence. Those who hold this view of the starting point of human life reject the use of assisted fertilization. They consider *in vitro* fertilization and embryo transfer to be 'playing God', interfering with the procreative aspects of marriage, or experimenting on human beings without their consent. At worst, when assisted fertilization involves the disposal of an embryo which for one reason or another cannot be transferred to a woman, it is considered as the taking of innocent human life (Kuhse and Singer 1982).

This criticism comes mainly from the Roman Catholic Church. The argument overlooks that the aim of assisted fertilization is to help infertile couples to procreate, however. Vatican policy about assisted reproduction contends that the scientist is an unacceptable intruder into the procreative aspects of the marital relationship (Congregation for the Doctrine of the Faith 1987). Supporters of assisted fertilization argue in return that the role of the scientist is a facilitator, rather than an intruder, in the process of procreation within this loving relationship.

Arguments against IVF also often exaggerate the attributes of the early embryo. The early IVF embryo consists of only a few cells and has none of the characteristics that we may normally think of as making human life worthy of respect and preservation. As argued by one Roman Catholic theologian, until 14 days after fertilization, the embryo is not yet an individual (Ford 1988). At this stage of its life, the embryo is not even assured of survival throughout development to birth (Dawson 1987*a*,*b* 1988). For an IVF embryo to have any chance to fulfil its claimed potential it is necessary that it be transferred by the clinicians (another intrusion) (Singer and Dawson, 1988), but the embryo at this stage is not sentient. Thus, there are lines that can be drawn in a non-arbitrary manner between the embryo and the mature human being.

Conclusive arguments against assisted fertilization cannot be based on the moral status of the embryo. In addition, if the prospects of successful fertilization can be improved by the production of more embryos than can be safely transferred back into the woman seeking to become pregnant, this should be regarded as ethically acceptable. It is equally acceptable for excess embryos preserved by freezing to be donated to another couple or for research, or disposed of, in accordance with the preferences of the biological parents.

Medical ethics

The right of every individual to have children was stated in the Declaration of Human Rights in Geneva in 1948. Codes of medical ethics since Hippocrates have emphasized the doctor's duty to relieve suffering, and suffering is certainly experienced by the infertile patient who desires a child. The plight of infertile couples is made even worse by the decreasing numbers of babies available for adoption as a result of contraception, abortion, and the increasingly greater acceptance of children being born to unmarried mothers. In this context, codes of medical ethics support the use of IVF and ET.

Available technologies

A range of assisted fertilization techniques are available for overcoming infertility of different causes. Procedures for the storage and genetic diagnosis of IVF embryos prior to transfer have been developed in association with these techniques.

Artificial insemination

Donor insemination (DI), which has been used for centuries, is implemented when the husband has no sperm or sperm of poor quality. Artificial insemination by husband's sperm (AIH) may be used if the husband has a mild semen defect or a coital ejaculatory defect.

In vitro fertilization

IVF and ET are used when the woman's tubes are severely damaged or when the husband has poor sperm quality and fertilization has to be shown to occur. IVF may be carried out using the gametes of the infertile couple, using donated sperm or oocytes, or using both donated sperm and donated oocytes.

IVF with donor gametes

At present sperm and oocyte donors may be known or unknown to the couple. Known donors are most often relatives, brothers, sisters, fathers, or daughters, or close friends; anonymous donors have usually responded to an advertisement. Sometimes, anonymous oocyte donors are women on IVF programs who have excess oocytes. One disadvantage of this source of oocytes is that a donor who knows the recipient may fail to become pregnant, yet see the recipient of her eggs become pregnant.

Known donors have the advantage that the recipient knows the social, emotional, and biological characteristics of the donor. Much has been made of the risks of using known donors; the major risk is felt to be that the donor may attempt to interfere with the future parenting of the child. However, when both donors and recipients are well counseled, the recipient couple can be cautioned about the source of donation if the potential donor is thought to be potentially manipulative.

Donor oocyte IVF

Donor oocyte IVF is used when the woman carries the risk of a serious genetic disease, or if she was born without normal ovaries, suffered a premature menopause, or had her ovaries removed because of disease. Donor oocytes have also been used in patients who respond poorly to preliminary hormonal preparation for IVF, and in older patients who have few oocytes or who have already reached the menopause. The use of donor oocytes can produce pregnancy rates of at least 30 per cent in women over the age of 40 years.

Donor sperm IVF

Donor sperm IVF is used when the husband has a severe sperm problem.

Donor sperm and donor oocyte IVF

Donor sperm and donor oocyte IVF is used when the husband has a severe sperm problem and the wife has no oocytes or is at risk of transmitting genetic abnormalities to any child born.

Natural cycle IVF

The disadvantages of the stimulated cycle include the high risk of multiple pregnancy and the risk of overstimulation and behavioral changes from the drugs used during the treatment. The use of natural cycle IVF has not been successful in many clinics, although some have reported success rates around 20 per cent treatment (Muasher *et al.* 1990). By restricting treatment to patients under the age of 35 years, repeating treatments on consecutive cycles if desired, using one blood collection, one injection of hCG to time egg pick-up, one or two ultrasound scans, and carrying out the pick-up in the doctor's office, the natural cycle method may be acceptable to many women, and the treatment may intrude less into normal life style. The success rate varies between 6 and

20 per cent, perhaps depending on the selection criteria for patients (Lim *et al.* 1990; Muasher *et al.* 1990).

IVF surrogacy

An IVF surrogate can be used for women who have ovaries but no uterus because of either a congenital disorder or surgical intervention, for women who repeatedly miscarry, or for women for whom pregnancy would be dangerous.

The procedure involves collection of oocytes from the infertile woman and fertilizing them *in vitro* using her husband's sperm. The resultant embryo is either transferred to a surrogate whose menstrual cycle has been coordinated with the infertile woman's, or frozen for transfer to the surrogate at a later date.

The GIFT procedure

The GIFT (gamete intrafallopian transfer) procedure is used for couples with otherwise incurable infertility where the fallopian tubes are normal. The sperm and oocytes are collected artificially and placed into the woman's tubes so that the gametes move to the normal place of fertilization. Women with endometriosis or ovarian cysts and men with less severe semen problems, as well as couples in whom no cause of infertility has been found, are suitable for GIFT. The overall success rates of assisted reproductive technology have been improved markedly by the introduction of the GIFT procedure.

The ZIFT, TEST, and PROST procedures

The ZIFT (zygote intrafallopian transfer), TEST (tubal embryo stage transfer) and PROST (pronuclear ovum stage transfer) procedures involve initial IVF, and then transfer of the embryo to the fallopian tube between 1 and 3 days after fertilization. These techniques are used when the tubes are normal but when the occurrence of fertilization needs to be verified, for example, when the male has a fertility problem.

Sperm microinjection

Microinjection of sperm is used for men with severe infertility who have not been successful on GIFT or IVF programs. This technique involves either the insertion of two or three sperm under the shell of the oocyte or the injection of a single sperm into the cytoplasm of the oocyte to achieve fertilization and embryo development. Research has shown that the technique itself does not prejudice the development of the embryo and that the selection of sperm does not result in an increased risk of producing an abnormal embryo. This is a new technique; only a small number of babies have been born as a result of sperm microinjection.

Embryo biopsy

Embryo biopsy is a technique involving the removal of one or two cells from the four or eight-cell embryo for genetic or chromosomal analysis. Embryo biopsy has been used at the Hammersmith Hospital in The UK (Handyside, *et al.* 1989) to determine the sex of the embryos of couples who are at risk of having a child with a serious sex-linked genetic disorder. The technique has been shown to be harmless to the embryo and not to increase the risk of subsequent miscarriage or abnormality. Embryo biopsy could be used for sex selection for other reasons and in future could become available for detecting genetic and chromosomal abnormalities. The limitations of the technique result from the need for the couple to go through an IVF program to produce an embryo when the success rate for pregnancy is low.

Embryo freezing

Embryo freezing was developed because the use of ovulatory stimulants in IVF often means that more embryos result than can be safely transferred in one cycle. These excess embryos can be frozen, rather than being discarded, so that the couple can use them subsequently to attempt a pregnancy. Embryos can also be frozen if a couple develop an acute illness during their treatment cycle which may prevent or preclude a pregnancy, or when urgent medical treatment involving exposure to radiation is required.

Techniques for tranfer of frozen embryos have contributed to the overall success rate of GIFT and IVF, which continues to increase. The success rate per frozen cycle is 18 per cent, and the average number of embryos transferred is two. This means that for the 25 per cent of women who have embryos frozen, there is a doubling of the overall pregnancy rate from a single stimulated cycle. The results from embryo freezing have gradually improved, and the ultra-rapid freezing method also makes freezing more simple and easily carried out by clinics (Wood 1992).

The current state of the technology

Although the use of assisted fertilization has enabled thousands of otherwise infertile couples around the world to bear children, these pregnancies and deliveries seem to be more problematic than those in the general population.

Pregnancy rates

The chance of becoming pregnant by means of assisted fertilization depends on the treatment carried out. For the IVF procedure, the pregnancy rate varies from 7 to 25 per cent for each cycle of treatment. The most common result is about 15 per cent. Patients who are older, have active endometeriosis, have only one ovary, or have more than one factor causing infertility may have a lower success rate. The remaining patients who are under 35 and have tubal disease would have a success rate of at least 20 per cent. Women over 40 have the lowest chance—only 7 per cent per treatment cycle.

The GIFT procedure has about twice the success rate of IVF, because the sperm and oocytes are fertilized and grow in the woman's fallopian tube, an environment which it is not yet possible to duplicate in the laboratory. Figures for the Australian clinics for GIFT pregnancies range from 20 to 40 per cent, the average being 30 per cent. Again, age affects the success rate, with women over 40 having a success rate of 15 per cent.

Factors influencing pregnancy rates

In a very small number of patients, physicians are unable to extract any oocytes, either because there are very few ripe follicles, or because the follicles have not properly ripened. Also, in a small group of patients collected oocytes will not fertilize, either there is something wrong with the sperm quantity or quality, or because the oocyte is unripe or is structurally defective. These problems may be overcome by changing the method of stimulation of egg development or changing the method of preparation of the sperm. Since the same result will not necessarily occur in a subsequent treatment cycle, it is often worth repeating the treatment at least once.

Couples often wonder how many treatments they should have. The factors most likely to determine how many treatments a woman has are the costs, the stress, the social dislocation, and the emotional reaction to failure. Patients are advised to have at least five IVF attempts in order to have at least a 50 per cent chance of having a baby and four attempts at GIFT to have a 65 per cent chance of having a baby. Some women pursue up to 12 or more treatments.

The major factor determining the success rate of these treatments is the number of oocytes collected and the consequent number of embryos that develop. Women who have only one embryo transferred in IVF have a success rate of around 7–8 per cent, whereas the success rate is about 15 per cent when two embryos are transferred, and 25 per cent with three or more (Trounson *et al.* 1981). The success rate for GIFT is around 20 per cent with only one oocyte, rising to at least 30 per cent when three or more oocytes are transferred.

Early pregnancy monitoring

Pregnancy can be confirmed by a blood test around the expected time of the patient's period and the levels of estrogen and progesterone will also give some indication of whether the pregnancy is likely to be successful. Ultrasound scans are performed at about 8 weeks of pregnancy.

Miscarriage rates

Miscarriage is more common with reproductive technology, occurring in about 20 per cent of IVF and GIFT pregnancies, the Australian figure being 13 per cent. One reason for this is that women are older than most pregnant women: miscarriage is twice as common in women at 40 (26 per cent) as in women aged 25 (12 per cent). Other factors such as embryo quality, failure of implantation, and the effects of infertility could also contribute to this rate of miscarriage (AIH National Perinatal Statistics Unit 1991). Women of 40 or more who undergo IVF have a miscarriage rate of 40 per cent. Chances for a successful outcome in these women are improved when donated oocytes from younger women are used (Leeton *et al.* 1991). The most likely explanation for this is a poorer quality of oocytes in older women.

A patient who is likely to have a miscarriage will be counseled about this possibility. When early pregnancy loss does occur, most women find it helpful to know as soon as possible; a termination can be performed to save several weeks of carrying a dead fetus.

Ectopic pregnancy

Ectopic pregnancy (pregnancy outside the uterus, most commonly in the fallopian tube) occurs in one in 20 IVF and GIFT pregnancies. This is surprising in the case of IVF, as the procedure bypasses the fallopian tubes. Although the embryo is confirmed by ultrasound to be placed in the uterus, it later moves from the uterus into the fallopian tube. The high rate of ectopic pregnancies may be related mostly to the effects of reduced fertility. Over 100 spontaneous pregnancies in infertile women on our waiting list also resulted in an ectopic pregnany rate of about 7 per cent.

Most ectopic pregnancies are detected by the eighth week of pregnancy; the ectopic pregnancy is surgically removed and in most cases the fallopian tube is conserved. When the fallopian tube is severely damaged, part of it may need to be removed as well. Increased ultrasound monitoring of patients at an earlier stage may prevent damage to the tubes from ectopic pregnancy (Guirgis and Craft 1991).

Premature labor

There is an increased risk of premature labor in patients undergoing assisted reproductive treatments; the causes are not yet understood. In part, they are related to the higher incidence of multiple pregnancy in these patients. However, even in women with a single IVF or GIFT fetus there is a 9 per cent chance of premature labor.

Multiple pregnancy

The result of transferring more than one embryo to increase the chances of pregnancy in an IVF cycle is that 20 per cent of such pregnancies are multiple: 17 per cent are twins and 3 per cent triplets. Very occasionally, quadruplets and quintuplets have been born. The outcome for IVF twins is very good. Although labor commences 3 weeks earlier on average, the degree of prematurity is usually not severe enough to be life-threatening.

Most couples are pleased with the birth of twins. If they are over 35, they may have little chance of another conception. On the other hand, while having twins or triplets might be acceptable to some couples as a way of having an immediate family, multiple births need to be reduced to decrease the possibility of a couple having mentally or physically handicapped children. Most programs therefore are now reducing the number of embryos or oocytes that are transferred in each treatment cycle.

Mode of delivery

There is no reason why some IVF patients cannot have normal deliveries. There are, however, other patients in whom several factors mitigate against this: the increased age of the patient, anxiety of the patient, the obstetricians, or both, the increased risks of premature delivery, and multiple pregnancy. Twins and triplets may require cesarean section delivery to protect the health of the babies and for some women the disease that caused infertility may adversely influence the outcome of the pregnancy. For instance, previous tubal surgery may increase the risk of rupture of the uterus during labor. For these reasons, the cesarean section rate in most programs is around 40 per cent. Cesarean section under epidural anesthetic, which allows the woman to participate in the delivery is now the norm.

Perinatal mortality

Perinatal mortality is increased in both IVF and GIFT, related mainly to the increased risk of multiple pregnancies and prematurity and to the increased age of the parents.

Improving the technology

Changing ovarian stimulation techniques

While there is evidence that producing more oocytes per stimulated cycle is usually associated with higher pregnancy rates, hyperstimulation of the ovaries, when it occurs, increases patient discomfort and morbidity. It has been established in most centers that the use of gonadotropin-releasing hormone (GnRH) agonists is associated with a higher pregnancy rate than the use of clomiphene (Clomid) (Crosignani *et al.* 1988, Frydman *et al.* 1988, Lindner *et al.* 1988), if only because there is a reduced cancellation rate from a failure to respond to ovarian stimulation (Lindner *et al.* 1988).

Collecting immature oocytes

Mature oocytes are necessary for a successful outcome of both the GIFT and IVF procedures, because the fertilization rate of immature oocytes is much lower than that of mature oocytes. It has been reported, however, that incubating a sample of collected oocytes can increase the proportion of mature oocytes, and that subsequent insemination is more likely to lead to fertilization (Osborn, personal communication). This concept was extended by Cha (1991) who collected immature oocytes from whole ovaries, matured them *in vitro*, and reported a successful pregnancy.

Collection of immature oocytes would be an alternative to using ovarian stimulants. Freezing immature oocytes may also be safer than freezing mature oocytes, as chromosomes may be more stable in the immature oocyte. Freezing mature oocytes may increase the risk of aneuploidy.

Improving embryo culture

One of the reasons why the GIFT procedure has a higher pregnancy rate than IVF may be that fertilization occurs in the fallopian tube. The fallopian tube may contribute to embryo development by removing inhibitory factors or by producing embryo growth-promoting factors. There is evidence that oviduct proteins bind to embryos and that oviduct protein extracted from secretions of the oviduct stimulate amino acid uptake by the embryo.

One approach to improve the success of IVF is to study the biochemistry of the embryo and to develop media matching the metabolic needs of the embryo. The embryo may require different nutrients at different stages of development (Gardner and Leese 1990). Further, correlation of an embryo's metabolic needs with its morphological state, shows that lactate production may be significantly higher in healthy embryos (David Gardner, personal communication). One proposal is to use these measurements to select embryos for transfer. A chemical test may be a good predictor of pregnancy outcome and could be used to optimize IVF systems. Increased knowledge about the metabolic requirements of the embryo will enable us to optimize its development and quality in culture and may have important implications for the future success of IVF.

Improving embryo transfer and implantation

Another problem associated with the stimulated cycle is reduced embryo implantation potential. Embryo implantation is affected by multiple factors, including the genetic or chromosomal complement of the embryo, growth factors being produced by the endometrium, and also the early process of endometrial invasion. Pregnancies from stimulated cycles have a lower success rate than pregnancies from natural, unstimulated cycles. The stimulated cycle may affect the production of growth factors from the endometrium, cause a lack of synchrony between the embryo and the endometrium because the embryos are placed in the uterus too early, or disturb the implantation characteristics of the endometrium. The relative contribution of each of these factors has been studied. Selective embryo transfer, based on ultrasound evaluation to determine whether the characteristics of the endometrium are optimal for embryo transfer or whether the embryos should be frozen, has not improved the pregnancy rate.

Reducing multiple pregnancy

As discussed above, reduction in the multiple pregnancy rate associated with GIFT and IVF is a matter of some urgency because of the serious complications associated with high multiple pregnancies. The pregnancy rate for GIFT is related to the number of oocytes transferred but is more dependent on the total number of oocytes collected than the number of oocytes replaced. In GIFT, the pregnancy rate when two selected oocytes are transferred is the same as for five selected oocytes and there is of course no risk of triplets (Calderon, in press). Two-egg GIFT is used in all patients who have five or more oocytes collected. Women who have fewer than five oocytes collected in the original oocyte pick-up have lower pregnancy rates and a very low risk of multiple pregnancy (Calderon, in press).

It is possible to reduce the risk of triplets in IVF by taking into account the quality of the embryos transferred. This has been done by using the number and degree of fragmentation of the cells after 48 h in culture as a predictor score. Couples who have a high predictor score for three normal embryos can be cautioned to have only two of these embryos transferred. One other way of preventing the birth of triplets is to reduce the number of surviving fetuses by selective feticide. It has been found that the babies that survive are better off, being more mature and having fewer neonatal problems. The acceptability of the use of fetal reduction depends on the attitude of the community and the couple to the quantity and quality of life.

Ethical and legal issues relating to the technology

Embryo freezing

One obvious difficulty with storing embryos is the problem of their future use or misuse. In our program, couples are required to sign a form stating what they would do with the frozen embryos should they change their mind about wishing to use them or if they divorce, and what should be done if they die. While this has little legal force, it is a statement of intent which could be used in any future dispute. About 80 per cent of couples prefer to give their unwanted embryos to another infertile couple and a minority wish the embryos to be used for research or to be disposed of.

In the disputes that may arise when couples who have frozen embryos separate or divorce, our sympathies are with the woman, as she has undergone most of the treatment up until this stage and the conception has already started by the time an embryo has been frozen. To force her to dispose of the embryo may be analogous to forcing someone to have an unwanted abortion. The husbands in such situations are concerned about the financial implications of having to support an unwanted child. If one partner wishes to use the embryos, a let-out clause regarding financial responsibility could be considered for the spouse who does not want to use the embryos. The issue of disputed embryos can be analogous to a custody dispute, but raises other questions as well, such as whether or not the embryos are property. Freezing eggs rather than embryos may reduce the occurrence of these types of disputes in the future.

Wastage of embryos

Wastage is a relative term in reproduction. Nature provides a most effective system of abortion. At least 20 per cent—and more likely 40–60 per cent—of embryos abort naturally. The difficulty in determining this figure is that most embryos are lost at fertilization or early embryo development, before a woman is aware that she may be pregnant. There is currently no way of detecting these pregnancies.

The peak incidence of natural abortion coincides with the time of unnatural conception by IVF and ET. The IVF systems in use now may be more wasteful than the natural system. However, the wasted embryos are abnormal and therefore do not implant in the uterus. As the abnormal embryos never had the potential to develop into human life in the form of a fetus, baby, or adult, it is difficult to define their ethical status. The loss of early abnormal embryos in the natural system has never been considered seriously by religious or legal authorities. Supporters of assisted fertilization thus sometimes find it difficult to understand why these authorities are so concerned with IVF human embryo research. It is hoped that IVF and ET will improve to be as good as or better than the natural system in the future.

Embryo research

Embryo research, using a variety of species, has been conducted to develop and improve IVF. Human embryos donated for research by IVF patients have been used in the development of IVF, sperm microinjection, and embryo biopsy. Most research carried out to improve the treatment of infertility involves the use of embryos up to about 4 days after fertilization. In the future, it may be possible to use human embryos to look at the causes of malformations and also to study the early development of different organs in the body. If abnormal development or serious disease processes were better understood, appropriate treatments could be devised. These proposals would require embryo research beyond 14 days after fertilization, but the technology required to grow the embryo to this stage *in vitro* is not available for any species.

There are ethical arguments for and against human embryo research that involve the moral status of the embryo. The views that permit embryo research mostly rely on consideration that moral status is linked to biological development and the importance people place on the developing human being. There is no doubt that the community generally has ignored the first 2 weeks of existence before the the missed period. Throughout this time, the embryos may be insulted by harmful drugs or a mother's acute illness without any recognition or concern, as the woman is usually not aware that she is pregnant. The same lack of concern for the early embryo has been involved in the community's acceptance of the use of the intrauterine device, which was thought to cause early embryo death (see Chapter 8). Acceptance of therapeutic abortion in certain circumstances also makes it inconsistent to object to the choice made by infertile couples to donate their spare embryos for research to improve their chance of having a child. It would seem unjust to discriminate against infertile couples who are wishing to have a child when other couples can kill a fetus for different, but certainly no more acceptable, reasons.

Surrogacy

Surrogacy has been opposed on the grounds that it may be harmful to society, to the surrogate woman, or to the resulting child. Much of this negative feeling has resulted from the media sensationalizing the few instances of surrogacy which have resulted in court cases, while ignoring the majority of surrogacy arrangements which go uncontested (Office of Technology Assessment 1988).

It cannot be denied that surrogacy may be harmful to a woman who regrets her decision to act as a surrogate. However, only 1 per cent of surrogates regret their decision and this low figure may reflect the importance of proper counseling for all parties involved in such an arrangement. Natural conception is followed by regret in a greater number of cases, resulting in therapeutic abortion or in giving the child up for adoption after birth. When giving up the child was the usual outcome of pregnancy for an unmarried mother, 75 per cent of mothers eventually regretted making this decision.

Surrogates are better informed than most women before they commence pregnancy and have counseling to help them consider the issues involved. A let-out clause is made in some surrogacy clinics in the USA so that the surrogate can keep the child if she wishes. This is reasonable on the grounds that pregnancy and birth may alter the woman's attitude to the baby and also that informed infertile couples would understand such a risk if it was explained prior to the surrogacy procedure. The risks of surrogacy are not great and legislation to prohibit it would restrict the reproductive choices available to women who are willing and able to make informed decisions to be involved in such an arrangement. The control of a woman's behavior in this situation implies bias against the female and carries the danger that government may interfere with other freedoms for women or other aspects of reproduction. It would seem more reasonable to enact legislation directed against couples who conceive naturally when it is known that the woman's behavior may harm the child, for example by not having had rubella vaccination, or by excessive smoking, alcohol, or other addictive substance use.

Most of the arguments against surrogacy have been couched in symbolic or emotive language without the accompanying logic to support the symbolism. For instance, it is sometimes claimed that surrogacy represents baby selling. This is a difficult argument to sustain when it is appreciated that the surrogate has made a free choice to be involved in carrying a child for another woman and that the child would not exist were it not for this free choice.

It seems reasonable to provide payment to surrogates. The surrogate uses her brain and body to help someone else have a baby. Why should she not be paid for this freely made decision? Banning commercial surrogacy interferes with a couple's chance of having a child.

Government control

State and federal governments in Australia, as in other countries have been involved in the control of new reproductive technology. The technology affects the federal government in terms of funding and state governments have been involved on the grounds that there are community concerns about reproductive technology and its possible effects on the children born.

Arguments against government control involve consideration of any perceived rights of infertile couples to conceive. Providing the couples are properly informed and are using their own gametes, how they achieve conception is of little moral concern to the government. The normal restriction in health care provided by hospitals and the medical profession would protect couples from poor medical practice.

Infertility treatments have been used over several centuries without special concern about the treatment or special consideration of the children resulting from treatments. Follow-up of children born from infertility treatments has been reported in medical journals and would serve the same purpose in IVF. The legislation in Victoria has laid down conditions for the practice of IVF including the licensing of hospitals for carrying out the procedures, a committee to control the appointment of counselors to IVF clinics, compulsory counseling of all couples, and the recording of the details of treatments to which the government has access. None of these regulations have assisted the practice of IVF in Victoria. The licensing of hospitals has excluded the development of day surgery centers which are better for some patients, compulsory counseling is resented by some patients and the committee determining the practice of counseling has limited the possibility of introducing more innovative methods of counseling.

Perhaps a more basic concern about government control of assisted reproduction is that once the principle is established that government can determine the availability and nature of assisted reproduction, this control may be extended to regulate natural reproduction. If one examined the need for government intervention in reproduction, one could mount much stronger arguments for controlling the natural process than the artificial one. Infertile couples wishing to have a child are well motivated, well informed, and very likely to become adequate and loving parents. The natural system of conception has no way of protecting a child from having inadequate, ill-informed parents who may be drug addicts, chronic alcoholics, or abusive individuals. On these grounds, infertile couples are being discriminated against.

References

AIH National Perinatal Statistics Unit (1991). *Assisted conception: Australia and New Zealand 1989*. Fertility Society of Australia, Sydney.

Behrman, S. J. and Kistner, R. W. (1975). *Progress in infertility*, 2nd edn. Little Brown, Boston.

Calderon, I. Gamete intra-fallopian transfer: the influence of oocyte number and quality on pregnancy rates (in press).

Cha, K. Y., Koo, J. J., Ko, J. J., Choi, D. H., Han, S. Y., and Yoon, T. R. (1991). Pregnancy after *in vitro* fertilization of human follicular oocytes collected from nonstimulated cycles, their culture *in vitro* and their transfer in a donor oocyte program. In *Serono symposium on oocyte donation*. Serono, Melbourne.

Congregation for the Doctrine of the Faith (1987). *Instruction on respect for human life in its origins and on the dignity of procreation: replies to certain questions of the day*. Polyglot Press, Vatican City.

Crosignani, P. G., Ragni, G., Lombroso, G. C., Scarduelli, C., De Lauretis, L., Caccamo, A., *et al.* (1988). Ovarian stimulation of IVF patients: effects of the reversible hypogonadotrophic state induced by GnRH against. *Human Reproduction*, **3**, 39–41.

Dawson, K. (1987). Fertilization and moral status: a scientific perspective. *Journal of Medical Ethics*, **13**, 173–7.

Dawson, K. (1988). Segmentation and moral status *in vitro* and in vitro: a scientific perspective. *Bioethics*, **2**, 1–14.

de Kretser, D., Dennis, P., Hudson, B., Leeton, J., Lopata, A., Outch, K., *et al.* (1973). Transfer of a human zygote. *Lancet* **ii**, 728–9.

Ford, N. M. (1988). *When did I begin? conception of the human individual in history, philosophy and science*. Cambridge University Press.

Frydman, R., Belaisch-Allart, J., Parneix, I., Forman, R., Hazout, A. and Testart, J. (1988). Comparison between flare up and down regulation effects of luteinizing hormone-releasing hormone agonists in an *in vitro* fertilization program. *Fertility and Sterility*, **50**, 471–5.

Gardner, D. K. and Leese, H. J. (1990). Concentrations of nutrients in mouse oviduct fluid and their effects on embryo development and metabolism *in vitro*. *Journal of Reproduction and Fertility*, **88**, 361–8.

Guirgis, R. R. and Craft, I. L. (1991). Ectopic pregnancy resulting from gamete intra-fallopian transfer and *in vitro* fertilization: role of ultrasonography in diagnosis and treatment. *Journal of Reproductive Medicine*, **36**, 793–6.

Handyside, A. H., Pattingson, J. K., Penketh, R. J. A., Delhanty, J. D. A., Winston, R. M. L., and Tuddenham, E. G. D. (1989). Biopsy of human preimplantation embryos and sexing by DNA amplification. *Lancet*, **i**, 347–9.

Heape, W. (1891). Preliminary note on the transplantation and growth of mammalian ova within a uterine foster-mother. *Proceedings of the Royal Society*, **48**, 457–8.

Johnson, G., Robert, D., and Brown, R. (1987). Infertile or childless by choice? A multipractice survey of women aged 35 and 50. *British Medical Journal*, **294**, 804–7.

Kuhse, H. and Singer, P. (1982). The moral status of the embryo. In *Test tube babies*, pp. 57–63. Oxford University Press.

Leeton, J., Rogers, P., King, C., and Healy, D. (1991). A comparison of pregnancy rates for 131 donor oocyte transfers using either a sequential or fixed regime of steroid replacement therapy. *Human Reproduction*, **6**, 299.

Lim, J. H., Kim, S. H., Kim, K. C., Moon, S. Y., Lee, J. Y., and Chang, Y. S. (1990). *In vitro* fertilization (IVF) embryo transfer (ET) program in natural ovulation cycles. *Abstracts of the American Fertility Society*, 0–023.

Lindner, C., Braendle, W., Lichtenberg, V., and Bettendorf, G. (1988). Analysis of 500 GnRH agonist/HMG cycles for *in-vitro* fertilization, IVF and GIFT. *Human Reproduction*, **3**, 2.

McLaren, A. and Biggers, J. D. (1958). Successful development and birth of mice cultivated *in vitro* as early embryos. Nature, **182**, 877–8.

Muasher, S. J., Kruithoff, C., Webster, S., Castillo, K., Wilens, L., Jones, H. W., Jr *et al*. (1990). Natural cycle *in vitro* fertilization (IVF): a simplified treatment method. *Abstracts of the American Fertility Society*.

National Bioethics Consultative Committee (1991). *Access to reproductive technology*. Final Report for the Australian Health Minister's Conference, Australia.

Newman, N. E. and Zoures, C. G. (1991). Emotional experiences of *in vitro* fertilization. *Journal of IVF and embryo transfer*, **8**, 321–8.

Office of Technology Assessment (1988). *Infertility: medical and social choices*. Congress of the United States, Washington DC.

Parliament of South Australia (1988). *Reproductive Technology Act 1988*. South Australian Government Printer.

Parliament of Western Australia (1991). *Human Reproductive Technology Act 1991*. Western Australian Government Printer.

Parliament of Victoria (1984). *Infertility (Medical Procedures) Act 1984*, No. 10163. Victorian Government Printer.

Renou, P., Trounson, A., Wood, C., and Leeton, J. (1981). The collection of human oocytes for *in vitro* fertilization. I. An instrument for maximizing oocyte recovery rate. *Fertity and Sterility*, **35**, 409–12.

Seventh World Congress on in vitro fertilization and assisted procreations (1991). *World Collaborative Report 1989*. Seventh World Congress on in vitro fertilization and assisted procreations, Paris.

Short, R. V. (1979). *Human in vitro fertilization and embryo transfer, Study #10*. Ethics Advisory Board, Dept of Health Education-Welfare HEW, Appendix: HEW Support of research involving human *In Vitro* fertilization and embryo transfer, May 4, 1979. US Government Publication.

Singer, P. and Dawson, K. (1988). IVF technology and the argument from potential. *Philosophy and Public Affairs*, **17**, 87–104.

Steptoe, P. C. and Edwards, R. G. (1976). Reimplantation of a human embryo was subsequent total pregnancy. *Lancet*, **1**, 880–2.

Steptoe, P. C. and Edwards, R. G. (1978). Birth after the reimplantation of a human embryo. *Lancet*, **ii**, 366.

Trounson, A. and Mohr, L. (1983). Human pregnancy following cryopreservation, thawing and transfer of an eight-cell embryo. *Nature*, **305**, 707–9.

Trounson, A. O., Leeton, J. F., Wood, C., Webb, J., and Wood, J. (1981). Pregnancies in humans by fertilization *in vitro* and embryo transfer in the controlled ovulatory cycle. *Science*, **212**, 681–2.

US Department of Health and Human Services, Public Health Service, National Centre for Health Statistics (1988). *National Survey of Family Growth Cycle IV*. US Government Printing Office, Washington DC.

Vessey, M., Doll, R., Peto, R., Johnson, B., and Wiggins, P. (1976). A long-term follow up study of women using different methods of contraception—an interim report. *Journal of Biosocial Science*, **8**, 373–427.

Westmore, A. (1984). History. In *clinical IVF*, (ed. C. Wood and A. Trounson), pp. 1–10 Springer-Verlag, Berlin.

Whitten, R. W. (1956). Culture of tubal mouse ova. *Nature*, **177**, 96.

Wood, E. C. (1992). The current status and future of assisted reproductive technology in the female. In *Serono symposium on implantation in the mammal*, (ed. L. Gianaroli, A. Campara, and A. O. Trounson), pp. 277–88. Serono, Geneva.
World Collaborative Report (1991). *Seventh world congress on in vitro fertilization and assisted procreations*, Paris 1989.

III Maternal Health Care

12 Maternity-related health care in the USA

Lorraine V. Klerman and Irwin R. Merkatz

The four components of maternity-related care are preconception care, prenatal care, labor and delivery management, and postpartum follow-up. The postpartum visit should lead to continuing gynecological care, whether or not further pregnancies are planned. Although in the USA there is general consensus on the value of each component of this sequence, in reality the delivery of these services is often greatly influenced by financial and political considerations. Consequently, the quality and quantity of care that women receive varies according to their economic status, geographic location, and other factors. These inequities contribute to low birth weight and infant mortality, pregnancy outcomes whose rates are higher in the USA than in many countries with similar degrees of industrialization (Liu *et al.* 1992).

The systems providing maternity-related care

Although most women would prefer to have all four components provided by the same clinician, for many—particularly for poor women—different individuals or agencies may be responsible for each phase. Information-sharing among providers is typically limited and resultant communication gaps often lead to poorer quality care.

Preconception care

The idea of preconception care is relatively new in the USA. In 1989, the Public Health Service (PHS) Expert Panel on the Content of Prenatal Care urged that introduction and expansion of preconception care services become a national priority and that these services be reimbursable as an investment in primary prevention. The panel's report defined preconception care as encompassing risk assessment, health promotion, and specific intervention and follow-up when needed. It also specified many of the elements that should be included and mentioned several potential providers and sites for such care. The American Academy of Pediatrics (AAP) and the American College of Obstetricians and Gynecologists (ACOG) have endorsed the concept of preconception care. ACOG (1990) includes a section on preconception health in *Planning for pregnancy, birth, and beyond*, a publication addressed directly to women. The United States Department of Health and Human Services has endorsed preconception care in its publication *Healthy people 2000* (Public Health Service 1991).

The stated national objective for preconception care is that by the end of the century, at least 60 per cent of primary care providers will offer age-appropriate preconception care and counselling. An example of benefits to be gained is reduction in the incidence of neural tube defects resulting from preconception and prenatal folate nutritional supplementation (MRC Vitamin Study Research Group 1991; Centers for Disease Control 1992). For a more detailed discussion of this topic, (See Harrison (1990) and Jack and Culpepper. (1990) in Merkatz *et al.* (1990).

It is not known how many women receive preconception care, but it is presumed to be relatively few, either in the public or the private sector. A large percentage of women of reproductive age do receive family planning services, which are a component of pre- and interconception (between pregnancies) care. The 1988 National Survey of Family Growth found that 37 per cent of women 15–44 years of age had one or more family planning visits in the 12 months before the survey (Mosher 1990). Such existing interactions with the health care system should provide excellent opportunities to incorporate screening, education, and behavioral modification services, which may not only help achieve healthier pregnancies, but also improve women's health in general.

Prenatal Care

The most widely used standards for prenatal care in the USA are those established jointly by AAP and ACOG (1992) in *Guidelines for perinatal care*. The PHS standards differ from these in some respects. There is general agreement, however, that care for the pregnant woman should begin early in the first trimester and that the optimal number of visits depends on each woman's degree of risk, with seven visits considered the minimum. The prenatal care objective in *Healthy people 2000* is to increase to at least 90 per cent the proportion of pregnant women who receive prenatal care in the first trimester.

Unfortunately, the USA is far from this stated objective and in fact appears to have lost ground. According to the National Center for Health Statistics (NCHS), in 1991 (the last year for which data are now available) only 76 per cent of American women started care in the first trimester. The rate of first trimester prenatal care initiation peaked in 1984 at 77 per cent and a frightening 6 per cent of all pregnant women received no care whatsoever or care that began only in the third trimester. This percentage has remained constant since 1983 (NCHS 1993).

The NCHS also reported that the time of initiation of prenatal care varied significantly by socio-demographic characteristics. Among White mothers, 79 per cent began care in the first trimester, compared with 62 per cent of Black mothers. Only 56 per cent of women under the age of 20 began care in the first trimester, while 85 per cent of women aged 30–34 started care that early (NCHS 1993). The Institute of Medicine reported especially low rates of early prenatal care initiation among Hispanics from Mexico, Puerto Rico, and Central and South America, as well as among American Indians. The rates of late or no prenatal care are higher among unmarried women, increase with birth order, and decrease with educational attainment (Brown 1988). The 1982 National Survey of Family Growth revealed that half of the women in families with incomes below 150 per cent of the USA government-defined level of poverty initiated care before the third month of pregnancy, compared with three-quarters of those above the poverty level. Women receiving Medicaid were less likely to begin care this early than those not receiving Medicaid (Pamuk and Mosher 1988). (Medicaid is the federal/state health insurance plan that supports care for low-income people.)

Labor and delivery

The *Guidelines for perinatal care* (AAP and ACOG 1992) and *Standards for obstetric–gynecologic services* (ACOG 1989) also include standards for labor and delivery supervision. In 1991, almost 99 per cent of American births were in hospitals. Most of the remaining mothers delivered at home (0.7 per cent) or in a free-standing birthing center (0.3per cent). Many of these out-of-hospital deliveries were managed by midwives (NCHS 1993). Although the proportion of births attended by nurse–midwives increased from 0.9 per cent in 1975 to 3.4 per cent in 1988, virtually all of this increase (93.2 per cent) was in-hospital births (Declercq 1992). In 1991, certified nurse-midwives attended 167 704 births, of which 158 068 were in hospitals (NCHS 1993). Some non-hospital deliveries are, of course, due to inability to reach the hospital in time; few are due to access problems.

Postpartum examination

Although clinicians uniformly urge a postpartum visit, many women do not obtain this service. The neglect of this care component appears to be related less to financial barriers and more to provider and patient perceptions that such care is not essential and to problems with availability of time, transportation, care for other children, and similar factors.

Access to care

In contrast to most of the industrialized countries of Western Europe, and Canada, Japan, and Israel, the USA has neither a system of universal health care nor a compulsory system of employment-based health insurance. Moreover, the multiple levels of government and the many third parties involved in supporting maternity-related care have led to complex systems of care delivery. Because these systems are often uncoordinated, many women do not receive the care that they need.

Development of the current system

Families with sufficient resources to pay out-of-pocket or with adequate private insurance, usually obtained through the woman's or her spouse's employer, traditionally receive the maternity-related care they need or seek. At the beginning of this century, it was thought that the needs of the poor could be met by charity care, provided at reduced or no cost, and available through public hospitals or through private physicians' offices. Early reports by the United States Children's Bureau, however, indicated that infant mortality was excessively high in this country, particularly among the poor. Later publications emphasized the importance of prenatal care (Bradbury 1962).

Service delivery approaches

The initial response to the problem of inadequate availability of prenatal care was in terms of service delivery. Many localities developed prenatal care programs, usually involving home visits by public health nurses and sometimes care in out-patient clinics (Thompson *et al.* 1990). In 1921, federal grants for maternal and child health were first provided to the states by the Maternity and Infancy Act, usually referred to as the Sheppard–Towner Act. Although this law was allowed to expire in 1929, the idea of federal grants to the states to help provide maternal and child health services, including prenatal care, was incorporated into the Social Security Act in 1935 as the law's Title V.

In the following years, an increasing number of states and localities assumed some responsibility for providing maternity services to indigent women. Nevertheless, in 1962 the Panel on Mental Retardation appointed by President Kennedy reported that inadequate prenatal care was still a major factor in poor pregnancy outcomes. The president recommended, and Congress approved, a program of maternity and infant care projects to demonstrate ways to bring such care to the poor (Bremner 1974).

Soon after, the Office of Economic Opportunity, created by President Johnson as part of the War on Poverty, funded several community health centers to offer medical care to the urban and rural poor. The Public Health Service later funded additional centers and in 1973 these two programs were integrated within the Public Health Service with a mandate to serve pregnant women directly or by referral. Congress continues to support the growth of Title V and community and migrant health centers. Between 1989 and 1992, appropriations for Title V (the Maternal and Child Health Block Grant) increased from $554 million to $650 million and for community and migrant health centers from $482 million to $594 million (Office of Management and Budget 1992).

Financing Approaches

In the late 1950s and early 1960s, the states and the federal government began to experiment with financing approaches to the problem of the medically underserved. Various ways were found to pay for the care of pregnant women who received limited financial support from the Aid to Families with Dependent Children program authorized by the Social Security Act. In 1965, this patchwork of programs was replaced by Medicaid, a medical insurance program jointly funded by the federal government, the states, and in some states by local communities.

Medicaid made a wide range of medical services available to individuals who were recipients of funds under several existing federal programs, including Aid to Families with Dependent Children. Covered services included prenatal care, labor and delivery, postpartum care, and family planning. The intent was to create a seamless system of medical care for pregnancy, with some women paying out-of-pocket, some using private health insurance, and others using Medicaid. Unfortunately, many physicians either refused to accept Medicaid patients or severely limited the number they would serve. The reimbursement rates were considered too low and the paperwork too burdensome; in addition, some physicians were reluctant to treat certain women because of fear of malpractice litigation. Thus, Medicaid did not replace health department clinics, community and migrant health centers, or hospital ambulatory care centers, but rather became an additional source of funding for such facilities.

Family planning services

Family planning services have a similar history (Aries 1987). Contraceptives were illegal in the USA until after 1936. Even then, many health department clinics were reluctant to offer this service. Private agencies, later affiliated as Planned Parenthood Federation of America, operated free-standing clinics which served those who could not or preferred not to seek family planning counseling and devices from private physicians. In 1965, the Office of Economic Opportunity began to fund family planning programs and these soon became an agency funding priority. In 1967, an amendment to the Social Security Act required that a minimum of 6 per cent of Title V grants to the states go toward family planning services. In 1970, the Family Planning Services and Population Research Act (Title X of the Public Health Service Act) was passed and began providing grants to states or other intermediaries for direct support of family planning clinics. As noted earlier, Medicaid pays for family planning services for eligible recipients.

Types of access problems

Despite the web of service and financing programs, not all women receive the maternity-related services they require. Most analysts believe that the principal barrier to obtaining essential maternity-related care remains economic. This belief is supported by studies which find that women who do not receive adequate care most often cite financial factors as the critical impediment (Brown 1988). Currently, the major financial barrier is the absence of health insurance for approximately 15 per cent of the American population and the heavy representation of women and children in this underinsured segment. More than 30 million Americans have neither private nor public coverage, and many millions more are inadequately covered (Bodenheimer 1992; Employee Benefit Research Institute 1992). The generally low reimbursement level of Medicaid persists and contributes to the unwillingness of many private-sector clinicians to accept Medicaid patients.

Not all access problems, however, are financial. Other problems include the poor distribution of maternity care providers, which results in shortages in some areas, inadequate transportation for ambulatory and emergency services, and institutional practices which discourage utilization. Undoubtedly, women and their families share some responsibility for low participation rates. Inadequate education about the need for care, fear or distrust of clinicians, drug-related problems, depression, and other psychological and emotional factors all too often deter women from seeking appropriate care (Klerman 1992). In many poverty-stricken areas, prenatal care is not a priority because immediate needs for adequate food, shelter, jobs, and safety continue to go unmet.

Financing problems

While the complexity of the American health care financing system affects all health care, nowhere is this complexity more likely to result in service inequities than with respect to maternity-related programs.

Private health insurance

Most Americans obtain health insurance through their employer or that of a family member. People who are unemployed or work for companies that do not provide health insurance for employees or family members, and those who are self-employed may purchase health insurance directly, but such policies are considerably more expensive than employer-based group policies. Most private insurance policies cover prenatal care, labor and delivery, and a postpartum examination, although there is often a waiting period between insurance enrollment and initiation of coverage. Such policies, however, do not typically cover preconception care or routine family planning visits. Moreover, private policies increasingly have co-insurance provisions, such as co-payments, deductibles, or maximum reimbursement limits (Alan Guttmacher Institute 1987; Congressional Budget Office 1992). Certain reversible contraceptive measures and oral contraceptives may not be covered (Alan Guttmacher Institute 1994).

Furthermore, existing medical underwriting practices penalize individuals and families with pre-existing conditions such as diabetes, cancer, or heart disease. Women in such families face rapidly escalating insurance premium costs and the threat of being uninsurable with changes in employment. 'Job lock' results from such health insurance practices, which ultimately increase the numbers of people who join the uninsured (Advisory Council on Social Security 1991).

Medicaid

By federal law, all pregnant women with incomes less than 133 per cent of the USA Government-defined level of poverty qualify for Medicaid. Additionally, federal law gives states the option of providing Medicaid coverage to pregnant women in families with incomes up to 185 per cent of the poverty level. As of July 1994, only 25 states had taken full advantage of this option, 6 others were covering women whose family incomes were more than 133 per cent but less than 185 per cent of poverty. Two states were using their own funds exclusively to cover women between 185 and 200 per cent of poverty (National Governors' Association 1994). For eligible women, the Medicaid program must pay for prenatal care services, labor and delivery, and a postpartum check-up, as well as other maternity-related services including family planning.

Grant programs

Most public or quasi-public providers, such as health departments and community and migrant health centers, receive federal subsidies in addition to reimbursements from Medicaid and private insurance and direct out-of-pocket payments from patients. These subsidies permit them to care for clients without any insurance, to cover the difference between insurance and actual costs, and to provide additional health services needed by special populations such as the very young, migrant laborers, and others. State and local health department maternity-related services are supported by federal Title V grants to the states as well as by state and local funds. Through grants authorized by the Public Health Service Act, the federal government directly supports more than 600 community and migrant health centers throughout the country. These offer maternity-related services either on site or by referral. The federal government also supports family planning clinics through grants to the states or other intermediaries under Title X of the Public Health Service Act.

Sources of Payment for Services

The largest proportion of maternity-related care in the USA is received from private sources and covered by private insurance. Almost two-thirds (64 per cent) of women who gave birth in 1985 had maternity care paid for this way. Medicaid paid for an additional 17 per cent, while 15 per cent of women had no coverage at the time of delivery (Alan Guttmacher Institute 1987). In 1988, 64 per cent obtained their family planning services from private medical practices; clinics served most of the rest (Mosher 1990).

Providers of care

Most American women receive prenatal care from physicians in private, office-based practices. These women are attended at delivery by these same practitioners and usually depend upon them for preconception and interconceptional care as well. For the most part, these physicians are specialists in obstetrics and gynecology, but a significant proportion of maternity care is still obtained from generalists. According to the 1989 National Ambulatory Medical Care Survey, 79 per cent of pregnancy-related visits to physicians in office-based practices were to obstetrician–gynecologists, while 21 per cent were to family or general practitioners (ACOG 1991). Although many office-based practitioners are still in solo practice, increasingly they have become part of multipractitioner or multispecialty groups or health maintenance organizations.

Nurses also offer maternity-related care. Nurse–midwives provide prenatal and interconceptional services and labor-delivery care. They sometimes work independently but more often are found in group practices in conjunction with physicians, or in clinics. Nurse practitioners serve in many family planning clinics. A survey by the American College of Nurse–Midwives (1992) carried out in 1990 found that almost one-quarter of certified nurse–midwives were employed by hospitals.

About one in five pregnant women in the USA receives her prenatal care from public or quasi-public clinics operated by hospitals (9 per cent), family planning clinics (5 per cent), state or local health departments (4 per cent), community or migrant health centers (3 per cent), military facilities (3 per cent), or other comparable entities (Alan Guttmacher Institute 1987). Occasionally, these women are delivered by the same clinician who provides the prenatal care, but often labor and delivery are managed by hospital-affiliated obstetricians who do not see the women during the prenatal period. While such clinics almost always offer a postpartum examination as part of their maternity package, they may not always provide preconception or interconception care for the women they supervised during pregnancy. For these women, family planning services are likely to be obtained in a separate family planning or women's health facility.

Number of providers

In 1986, about 28 000 active obstetric–gynecologic specialists were listed in the American Medical Association's (AMA) physician masterfile. Not all of those listed actively practiced *obstetrics*, however. In the same year, the AMA file also listed approximately 68 000 family physicians and general practitioners. In 1986, 35 per cent of the members of the American Academy of Family Physicians, representing slightly more than half of those in the AMA file, included obstetrics as part of their practices. Between 1975 and 1988 the number of obstetrician–gynecologists in the USA had increased by 58 per cent (Klerman and Scholle 1992). In October 1992, almost 32 500 fellows were listed in the ACOG directory. More than 8300 of these were junior fellows (residents in training and new obstetrician–gynecologists who have not yet been board-certified), of whom almost half were women. Women now comprise more than half of obstetrical residents (Pearse 1992). These data indicate that the composition of the pool of obstetrical specialists is undergoing dramatic change.

Between 1982 and 1989, American medical school graduates indicated a decreasing preference for primary care. Those planning a career in obstetrics and gynecology declined from 6.6 to 4.6 per cent and those interested in family practice declined from 15.5 to 11.7 per cent (Colwill 1992). Simultaneously, the high cost of medical malpractice insurance and concern over being sued have prompted significant numbers of practicing obstetrician–gynecologists to curtail their obstetric practices. (The effect of medical malpractice issues on obstetrics is discussed in greater detail in Chapter 27.)

More than 5000 nurse–midwives had been certified by 1992 and more than 4000 are practicing. The number of certified nurse–midwives is limited by the small number of accredited programs (35, including certificate, masters, and precertification programs) and the number of nurse–midwives certified each year (about 350, double the number in 1986). The American College of Nurse–Midwives has a goal of 10 000 by the year 2001 (ACNUM Certification Council 1992; American College of Nurse–Midwives 1992). Some health policy analysts believe that such an expansion would help ameliorate this nation's maternity care access problem. Even if more nurse–midwives were certified, however, practice opportunities might be restricted because some obstetricians are reluctant to allow certified nurse–midwives to practice independently.

These provider data suggest that the absolute number of clinicians available to provide prenatal care and delivery services should be sufficient for the approximately 4 million women who give birth in the USA each year. Yet the uneven geographic distribution of practitioners and the reluctance of many to care for poor women still creates significant access problems in the maternity health system.

Geographic distribution of providers

Across the country, it is generally true that the smaller the population of a county or the more rural, the smaller the ratio of clinicians to population. In 1990, approximately 23 per cent of the population (56 million people) lived in non-metropolitan counties (Bureau of Health Professions, undated). In these areas, specialty care such as high-risk obstetrics is frequently lacking and women must often travel long distances to obtain such care. Moreover, specialists may not be reachable by public transportation, so that owning or being able to borrow a vehicle becomes essential. While women who live in cities may also have to contend with inadequate public transportation, travel-related problems are more frequently associated with rural women.

In 1988, 35 states had sparsely serviced areas with fewer than 20 obstetrician–gynecologists per 100 000 women aged 15–44. Nearly 4 million women resided in these areas, which were primarily rural. Nearly another 400 000 women in this age group lived in areas in 22 states where no obstetrician–gynecologists were available (Klerman and Scholle 1992). Even when other physicians providing obstetric care were included, the ratio of all obstetric care providers to women of childbearing age was lower in nonmetropolitan counties (Summer 1991).

Not only clinicians but also physical facilities are scarcer in rural areas. Between 1980 and 1988, 200 rural hospitals were closed, a rate much higher than among non-rural hospitals. Some analysts believe that the closing of rural hospitals and of obstetric units within surviving rural hospitals has an adverse effect on access. Others maintain that rural hospital closures do not invariably affect access because other hospitals are usually within easy traveling distance (Nadel 1991) and that women's use of the closed units typically declines before the closures (Bronstein and Morrisey 1991).

The shortage of obstetric providers and of facilities may have an adverse effect on pregnancy outcomes. One study found that women who lived in communities with relatively few obstetric providers in relation to the number of births were less likely to deliver in a local community hospital than those in communities with a higher ratio. Women from these 'high-outflow' communities had a higher proportion of complicated and premature births and remained in hospital longer. The closing of obstetric facilities in the high-outflow communities was attributed to decisions by local physicians to discontinue obstetric practice (Nesbitt *et al.* 1990).

In 1983, the Alan Guttmacher Institute (Torres and Forrest 1985) found no family planning clinics in 29 per cent of non-metropolitan counties, placing as many as 300 000 low-income women and 171 000 teenagers at risk for unintended pregnancies. In contrast, only 8 per cent of metropolitan counties had no family planning clinics, placing 117 000 low-income women and 79 000 teenagers at risk.

Women in rural areas not only have problems with access to medical care but also are more likely to be poor and without adequate private health insurance. Moreover, rural states typically have more restrictive Aid to Families with Dependent Children programs and are also less likely to have adopted expanded Medicaid eligibility and service options (Children's Defense Fund 1991). Residence in non-metropolitan areas of the USA thus appears to be a significant barrier to obtaining adequate maternity-related care. This assumption is confirmed by research that finds rural pregnant women are less likely to have initiated care in the first trimester (Hughes and, Rosenbaum 1989; McManus and Newacheck 1989).

Across the USA, inner-city areas also have shortages of office-based obstetric providers. These locales, however, are often the sites of community health centers, health department clinics, or teaching hospital-based prenatal clinics. Some of the private providers who remain in inner-city areas have been accused of running 'Medicaid mills', that is seeing large numbers of women for relatively brief appointments in order to keep their practices profitable despite the low rates of Medicaid reimbursement (Fossett *et al.* 1990). Continuity between such Medicaid mills and the in-patient hospital maternity units is typically poor, leading to fragmentation of care.

Reluctance to serve poor patients

In a 1984 survey, 63 per cent of obstetrician–gynecologists providing obstetric services reported caring for Medicaid patients. Eighty-seven per cent of salaried obstetrician employees of hospitals or health maintenance organizations provided such care, as did 81 per cent of those in multispecialty groups, but only 58 per cent of those in solo practice (ACOG 1988). This is a smaller percentage of Medicaid-participating physicians than that reported by family practitioners or other primary care specialists. Even among providers who accept Medicaid patients, some limit the percentage of their practice devoted to such cases. This limitation in the acceptance of Medicaid patients by private sector physicians forces Medicaid-eligible women into clinics operated by public and quasi-public agencies.

Access in other industrialized nations

Access to maternity-related health services is usually considered to be easier in Western European nations than in the USA. The ten countries studied by Miller (1987) all had lower infant mortality, some form of national health care financing, paid prenatal and postnatal maternity leave, and protective limits on the working circumstances of pregnant women. Home visits, during pregnancy and more often after delivery, were conducted in most of the study countries. A range of benefits was available after delivery, including maternity grants or bonuses, paid employment leave, family allowances, and housing preferences. Miller suggested that these benefits provide incentives for early registration but offered little substantiation. Although the actual number of visits during pregnancy cannot be compared with the USA, since the recommended number for an uncomplicated pregnancy varied from four to 14 between countries, the average number of visits equalled or exceeded that nation's recommendations in several countries. The report did not discuss the number of women who receive no care or late care.

Adequacy of care

In general, the adequacy of the *best* maternity-related care in the USA is probably not surpassed in any other country. Best care, however, is primarily received by women in affluent urban or suburban areas who can afford office-based care and delivery in excellent community or medical school-affiliated hospitals. For this group, the major quality of care issue has become the frequency of cesarean sections, which now exceed 20 per cent of deliveries. Several state and hospital initiatives have begun to address this problem (Dillon *et al.* 1992), which is convered in greater detail elsewhere in this volume.

Unfortunately, women who reside in rural areas, poor women, and certain special populations such as migrant workers, undocumented aliens, and the homeless often do not receive a comparable level of care. Care for these women is often inadequate not only in quantity, but also in content and quality.

Quantity of care

Prenatal care is usually measured in terms of the month or trimester in which care is initiated and the total number of prenatal visits. These two items are often combined into a single index, usually the one developed by Kessner (1973), on the basis of which care is labeled adequate, inadequate, or intermediate. There are obvious problems with a measure that cannot be adjusted for a woman's degree of risk. Women at higher risk should be scheduled for more prenatal visits and healthier, low-risk women may need fewer. Furthermore, the recording on birth certificates of care initiation and of number of visits is often inaccurate, so that conclusions drawn about quantity of care are often incorrect.

Some problems with the Kessner Index are remedied by the Adequacy of Prenatal Care Use Index constructed by Kotelchuck. Using this index, the Alan Guttmacher Institute estimated that in 1986, approximately 16 per cent of women received quantitatively inadequate care. This was defined as care begun in the fifth month of pregnancy or later or care that began within the first 4 months but consisted of fewer than half the recommended number of visits adjusted for the length of gestation (Singh *et al.* 1989).

Content of care

Studies comparing the actual content of prenatal care with AAP/ACOG standards are very rare and no study has compared practice with the PHS Expert Panel recommendations. Several specific practices have been analzsed, however and the results are not encouraging. As late as 1980, some pregnant women were being exposed to X-rays, and newer procedures such as amniocentesis, ultrasonography, and electronic fetal monitoring were not uniformly available geographically or by socio-demographic groups (Kleinman *et al.* 1984). Excessive limitations of weight gain were being advised into the late 1980s (Taffel and Keppel 1986).

One pressing problem which has persisted since the mid-1980s is a shortage of programs and facilities to treat substance-abusing pregnant women. Alcohol and drug treatment facilities often refuse to accept pregnant women, even on an out-patient basis. There are too few in-patient drug treatment facilities and those that do exist can seldom accommodate the previous children of pregnant women (Kumpfer 1991). More pregnant women are affected by the fact that only a limited number of private or public providers offer comprehensive smoking cessation programs. Since smoking and alcohol, cocaine, and other substance abuse during pregnancy are associated with low infant birth weight, preterm birth, placental abruption, and other complications of pregnancy, these prenatal service inadequacies urgently need to be addressed.

Women at high risk for pregnancy complications because of poverty-related social factors frequently require non-medical services in order to achieve healthy outcomes. Translators or bilingual personnel, transportation, on-site child care, and home visitation by nurses, social workers, or paraprofessionals must be incorporated into care for such women. In addition, access to nutritional supplementation and education services, such as the Special Supplemental Food Program for Women, Infants, and Children, is essential. When such services are absent or in short supply, overall care must be considered incomplete.

Several studies have demonstrated that women enrolled in the more comprehensive prenatal care programs have better pregnancy outcomes than those receiving only medical services even when provided by private physicians (Buescher *et al.* 1987, 1991; Lennie *et al.* 1987; Schlesinger and Kronebusch, 1990; Buescher and Ward, 1992; Handler and Rosenberg *et al.* 1992; McLaughlin *et al.* 1992).

Quality of care

Traditionally, the quality of medical care is assessed by structure, process, and outcome (Donabedian 1980), but this has not been true for most studies of maternity-related care. The adequacy of prenatal care has usually been defined by the quantity of care measured in terms of the time of initiation of care and/or number of visits. Yet both these factors are usually determined by the pregnant woman rather than by the provider or facility.

Little attention has been paid to such structural measures as the qualifications of the provider or the equipment available at the site of care. The paucity of studies on the process of care, which would include adherence to recommended standards, has already been noted. Moreover, the outcomes in terms of low birthweight and weeks of gestation attained are more often analyzed in terms of the women's age, race, education, and other characteristics, than in terms of the characteristics of the provider, the 'fit' between the provider and the pregnant woman's risk status, or the capabilities of the provider institution. Nevertheless, a few studies have found that the site of care, for example, may indeed affect outcomes even when controlled for the characteristics of the woman (Morehead *et al.* 1971; Poland *et al.* 1990; Schlesinger and Kronebusch 1990).

The amount of provider time spent with a patient may be an indirect indicator of quality. For example, the 1989 National Ambulatory Care Study found that the average duration of face-to-face contact with an office-based obstetrician–gynecologist was about 15 min (ACOG 1991).

Comparing private and public care

Adequacy may also be addressed by comparing the care received by women in private offices with that received by women attending public or quasi-public clincis. Using private care as the standard, certain deficiencies become evident. For example, in private offices pregnant women are usually assigned a specific time for their prenatal appointment, although some waiting time in the office is usually unavoidable. In comparison, women in clinics are often scheduled in blocks. For example, they are all told to arrive at 8.30 a.m. although the clinic hours may be from 9 a.m. through 1 p.m. Thus, long waiting times are inevitable for many.

More important, such comparisons highlight major differences in continuity of care. Most women in private offices are examined at all prenatal visits by one provider or by a relatively small team, and are delivered by the same provider or by one of the team members. Women in clinics are typically seen by whichever clinician is next available and little effort is made to achieve continuity except through the written record. In addition, clinic patients are often delivered by a clinician whom they never have seen during the prenatal period. There is no evidence that this lack of continuity has a negative effect on outcomes, but many women are distressed by such practices. Moreover, it is likely that important but subtle pieces of information are not always communicated and some components of care are duplicated unnecessarily. When vital pieces of data are unavailable, the quality of care may be compromised. To avoid these problems, many forward-looking ambulatory care settings and obstetrical residency programs have reoriented their programs to ensure continuity of care (American Medical Association 1992).

The effectiveness of prenatal care

This section will focus on the effectiveness of prenatal care as a whole rather than on specific components, which are covered in more detail in Public Health Service (1989), and Chalmers *et al.* (1989).

Every major American public health report since 1982 has emphatically stated that prenatal care is the most effective strategy for reducing low birthweight and other adverse outcomes of pregnancy. Many of the studies on which this assertion is based depend on data from birth certificates. These studies showed that women who received quantitatively adequate prenatal care were more likely to have positive pregnancy outcomes than those who received quantitatively inadequate or no prenatal care. Such studies are probably biased by self-selection, in that women who are most likely to have favorable outcomes regardless of care are more likely to seek care in the first trimester and adhere to the schedule of prenatal visits recommended by their provider. Many studies have attempted to control for variables that cause these biases, such as age and education; the success of these efforts can not be proven, however.

Other studies have compared outcomes among women who receive standard care with outcomes among women participating in an augmented program of prenatal care. Most of these studies show positive impacts for augmented care (Buescher *et al.* 1987, 1991; Lennie *et al.* 1987; Schlesinger and Kronebusch, 1990; Buescher and Ward, 1992 *et al.*), but they usually employ comparison groups rather than randomization, which again makes their results questionable. An exception is a study in which pregnant women were randomly assigned to standard prenatal care provided by obstetric residents or to comprehensive prenatal care provided by a multi disciplinary team of nurse–midwives, social workers, a nutritionist, a home visitor, and a psychologist. Comprehensive care had a favorable effect on birth weight for primiparous but not multiparous women (McLaughlin *et al.* 1992). For an extended discussion comparing studies based on large databases, usually birth certificates, with evaluations of specific programs of prenatal care, see Institute of Medicine (1985).

Not all published studies on prenatal care have been positive. Tyson *et al.* (1990) found that indigent women benefited substantially, in terms of reduced mortality and morbidity, from prenatal care received after 30 weeks gestation but not from earlier care. Nevertheless, most American experts agree that overwhelming evidence suggests that prenatal care *is* effective in reducing adverse pregnancy outcomes for mother and infant. Additional research is needed to determine which elements of prenatal care make a difference, the mechanisms by which these elements improve outcomes, and the amount and timing of prenatal care necessary for it to be effective.

Recommendations

Rates of low birthweight and preterm labor in the USA imply that maternity care is less than optimal, yet the qualifications of most clinicians and the technology at many facilities are considered superb. The over-riding problem is that many women are underserved because of economic conditions, geographic location, or special circumstances such as being a migrant worker or undocumented alien. Personal factors such as lack of motivation for care, inadequate knowledge about the importance of care, and substance abuse also contribute to these adverse pregnancy outcomes.

The first and perhaps easiest way to address these problems is to remove financial obstacles to care. This might include raising Medicaid eligibility for maternity-related health care to 200 per cent of poverty and requiring private health insurance policies to cover maternity services without waiting periods or co-insurance provisions. These changes by themselves may not be enough, however. The process of Medicaid certification remains arduous in many areas and women across the country report being hassled by welfare workers. Simplification of forms and placement of eligibility workers in hospitals would increase enrollment (Breyel 1990).

In addition, providers of maternity services must be better distributed. Raising provider reimbursement and reducing required paperwork might help increase the number of physicians in private practice who will accept Medicaid patients. Medical malpractice liability reform is critical to the future of the maternity health care delivery system in the USA. Rural areas require more targeted initiatives, including increased assignment of National Health Service Corps physicians and nurses, more innovative use of certified nurse–midwives in outlying areas under the supervision of physicians from central areas, the development of mobile units, and increased availability of helicopter and fixed-wing aircraft.

The content of care, particularly for poor women and those from different cultures, needs specific attention. These women may not be served best in private provider offices, but rather may benefit substantially from multidisciplinary teams which can be assembled in hospital-based, health department, and community or migrant health center clinics. Collaborative arrangements between private physicians and such facilities may be effective and efficient means of improving care.

Certified nurse–midwives have been especially valuable in caring for young and poor inner-city women. Public facilities, as well as voluntary hospital ambulatory clinics, which are willing to provide the necessary wide range of services for needy women require additional financial and political support. This would enable them not only to serve adequately the women who come to them, but also to employ outreach workers who can bring into care those women who are uninformed or indifferent about their pregnancy needs. Many women are reluctant to seek care because they are fearful or feel otherwise unsupported.

Both private offices and clinics need to increase their awareness of factors that create barriers, such as long waiting times for appointments or while in the facility, insensitive personnel, and an absence of translators, child care, or educational materials. These barriers can only be reduced if physicians, nurses, and other health personnel believe sincerely that their function is to serve *all* women with maternity-related needs.

Finally, a massive public education campaign could help to convince American women, their male partners, and their families of the benefits and importance of maternity-related care, beginning before conception. For many, pregnancy still seems to be something that 'just happens' rather than an event that is planned. Prenatal care is not always perceived as being essential. This perception must be changed. Pregnancy should be viewed as a healthy condition rather than as a disease, but the general public—and especially women in the childbearing years—should know that they can do much to improve the likelihood of a healthy pregnancy and infant.

A partnership between families and the network of maternity-care providers needs to be fostered in order to protect and improve the health of future generations.

References

Advisory Council on Social Security (1991). *Commitment to change: Foundations for reform*. US Government Printing Office, Washington DC.

Alan Guttmacher Institute. (1987). *The financing of maternity care in the United States*. Alan Guttmacher Institute, New York.

Alan Guttmacher Institute. (1994). *Uneven & unequal. Insurance coverage and reproductive health services*. Alan Guttmacher Istitute, New York.

AAP and ACOG (American Academy of Pediatrics and American College of Obstetricians and Gynecologists) (1992). *Guidelines for perinatal care*, (3rd edn). American Academy of Pediatrics, Elk Grove Village.

American College of Nurse–Midwives (1992). *Fact Sheets*. Washington DC.

ACOG (American College of Obstetricians and Gynecologists) (1989). *Standards for obstetric–gynecologic services*, (7th edn). ACOG, Washington DC.

ACOG (American College of Obstetricians and Gynecologists) (1990). *Planning for pregnancy, birth, and beyond*. ACOG, Washington DC.

ACOG (American College of Obstetricians and Gynecologists) (1991). Office visits to U.S. obstetrician–gynecologists: 1975 and 1989. *Economic Impact*, July.

ACOG (American College of Obstetricians and Gynecologists) and Committee on Health Care for Underserved Women. (1988). *Ob/Gyn services for indigent women: issues raised by an ACOG survey (1987)*. ACOG, Washington DC.

American Medical Association (1992). *Directory of graduate medical education programs 1992–1993*. AMA, Chicago.

Aries, N. (1987). Fragmentation and reproductive freedom: federally subsidized family planning services, 1960–80. *American Journal of Public Health*, **77**, 1465–71.

Bodenheimer, T. (1992). Underinsurance in America. *New England Journal of Medicine*, **327**, 274–8.

Bradbury, D. E. (1962). *Five decades of action for children: a history of the Children's Bureau*. US Department of Health, Education, and Welfare, Washington DC.

Bremner, R. H. (1974). *Children and youth in America: a documentary history*, Vol. III: 1933–1973. Harvard University Press, Cambridge.

Breyel, J. (ed.) (1990). *Improving state programs for pregnant women and children: Conference proceedings*. National Governors' Association, Washington DC.

Bronstein, J. M. and Morrisey, M. A. (1991). Bypassing rural hospitals for obstetrics care. *Journal of Health Politics, Policy and Law*, **16**, 87–118.

Brown, S. (ed.) (1988). *Prenatal care: reaching mothers, reaching infants*. National Academy Press, Washington DC.

Buescher, P. A. and Ward, N. I. (1992). A comparison of low birth weight among Medicaid patients of public health departments and other providers of prenatal care in North Carolina and Kentucky. *Public Health Reports*, **107**, 53–60.

Buescher, P. A., Smith, C., Holliday, J. L., and Levine, R. H. (1987). Source of prenatal care and infant birth weight: the case of a North Carolina county. *American Journal of Obstetrics and Gynecology*, **156**, 204–10.

Buescher, P. A., Roth, M. S., Williams, D., and Goforth, C. M. (1991). An evaluation of the impact of maternity care coordination on Medicaid birth outcomes in North Carolina. *American Journal of Public Health*, **81**, 1625–9.

Bureau of Health Professions (undated). *Rural health providers: supply and distribution*. BHP, Rockville.

Centers for Disease Control (1992). Recommendations for the use of folic acid to reduce the number of cases of spina bifida and other neural tube defects. *Morbidity and Mortality Weekly Report*, **41**, RR-14.

Chalmers, I., Enkin, M., and Keirse, M. J. N. C. (ed.) (1989). *Effective care in pregnancy and childbirth*. Oxford University Press.

Children's Defense Fund. (1991). *Falling by the wayside: children in rural America*. CDF, Washington DC.

Colwill, J. M. (1992). Where have all the primary care applicants gone? *New England Journal of Medicine*, **326**, 387–409.

Congressional Budget Office (1992). *Projections of National Health Expenditures*. US Government Printing Office, Washington DC.

Declercq, E. R. (1992). The transformation of American midwifery: 1975 to 1988. *American Journal of Public Health*, **82**, 680–84.

Dillon W. P., Choate, J. W., Nusbaum, M. L., McCarthy, M. A., McCall, M., and Rosen, M. G. (1992). Obstetric care and cesarian birth rates: a program to monitor quality of care. *Obstetrics and Gynecology*, **80**, 731–7.

Donabedian, A. (1980). *The definition of quality and approaches to its assessment*. Health Administration Press, Ann Arbor.

Employee Benefit Research Institute (1992). Source of health insurance and characteristics of the uninsured, analysis of the March 1991 Current Population Survey. *EBRI Special Report and Issue Brief*, no. 123.

Fossett, J. W., Perloff, J. D., Peterson, J. A., and Kletke, P. R. (1990). Medicaid in the inner city: the case of maternity care in Chicago. *Milbank Quarterly*, **68**, 111–41.

Handler, A. and Rosenberg, D. (1992) Improving pregnancy outcomes: public versus private care for urban, low-income women. *Birth*, **19**, 123–30.

Harrison, E. A. (1990). Preconception and postconception care of women with medical illnesses. In *New perspectives on prenatal care* (ed. I. R. Merkatz and J. E. Thompson), pp. 89–107. Elsevier Science Publishing, New York.

Hughes, D. and Rosenbaum, S. (1989). An overview of maternal and infant health services in rural America. *Journal of Rural Health*, **5**, 299–319.

Institute of Medicine (1985). *Preventing low birthweight*. National Academy Press, Washington DC.

Jack, B. and Culpepper, L. (1990). Preconception care. In *New perspectives on prenatal care*, (ed. I. R. Merkatz and J. E. Thompson), pp. 69–88. Elsevier Science Publishing, New York.

Kessner, D. M. (1973). *Infant death: an analysis by maternal risk and health care*. National Academy of Sciences, Washington DC.

Kleinman, J. C., Cooke, M., Machlin, S., and Kessel, S. S. (1984). Variations in use of obstetric technology. *Health United States and prevention profile, 1983*. National Center for Health Statistics, Hyattsville (DHHS Publication No. [PHS] 84–1232).

Klerman, L. V. (1992) Non-financial barriers to the receipt of medical care. *The Future of Children*, **2 (2)**, 171–85.

Klerman, L. V. and Scholle, S. H. (1992). Issues in the provision of maternity care. In *A pound of prevention: the case for universal maternity care in the U. S.* (ed. J. B. Kotch, C. H. Blakely, S. S. Brown, and F. Y. Wong), pp. 138–58. American Public Health Association, Washington DC.

Kumpfer, K. L. (1991) Treatment programs for drug-abusing women. *The Future of Children*, **1 (1)**, 50–60.

Lennie, J. A., Klun, J. R., and Hausner, T. (1987). Low-birth-weight rate reduced by the obstetrical access project. *Health Care Financing Review*, **8**, 83–6.

Liu, K., Moon, M., Sulvetta, M., and Chawla, J. (1992). *International infant mortality rankings: a look behind the numbers*. The Urban Institute, Washington DC.

McLaughlin, F. J., Altemeier, W. A., Christensen, M. J., Sherrod, K. B., Dietrich, M. S., and Stern, D. T. (1992). Randomized trial of comprehensive prenatal care for low-income women: effect on infant birth weight. *Pediatrics*, **89**, 128–32.

McManus, M. and Newacheck, P. (1989). Rural maternal, child, and adolescent health. *Health Services Research*, **23**, 807–48.

Merkatz, I. R., Thompson, J. E., Mullen, P. D., and Goldenberg, R. L. (ed.) (1990). *New Perspectives on Prenatal care*. Elsevier Science Publishing, New York.

Miller, C. A. (1987). *Maternal health and infant survival*. National Center for Clinical Infant Programs, Washington DC.

Morehead, M. A., Donaldson, R. S., and Seravalli, M. R. (1971). Comparisons between OEO neighborhood health centers and other health care providers of ratings of the quality of health care. *American Journal of Public Health*, **61**, 1294–1306.

Mosher, W. D. (1990). Use of family planning services in the United States, 1982 and 1988. *Advance Data*, **184**, 1–8.

MRC Vitamin Study Research Group. (1991). Prevention of neural tube defects: results of the Medical Research Council Vitamin Study. *Lancet*, **338**, 131–7.

Nadel, M. V. (1991). *Rural hospitals: closures and issues of access*, testimony of US General Accounting Office before US House of Representatives Task Force on Rural Elderly, Select Committee on Aging, 4 September 1991.

NCHS (National Center for Health Statistics) (1991). Advance report of final natality statistics, 1989. *Monthly Vital Statistics Report*, 40, 8, Supplement (DHHS Publication No. [PHS] 92–1120).

National Governors' Association (1992). *State coverage of pregnant women and children—January 1992*. NGA Center for Policy Research, Washington DC.

Nesbitt, T. S., Connell, F. A., Hart, L. G., and Rosenblatt, R. A. (1990). Access to obstetrical care in rural areas: effect on birth outcomes. *American Journal of Public Health*, **80**, 814–8.

Office of Management and Budget Executive Office of The President of the United States (1992). *Budget of the United States Government. Fiscal Year 1993*. Superintendent of Documents, Washington DC.

Pamuk, E. R. and Mosher, W. D. (1988). Health aspects of pregnancy and childbirth: United States, 1982. *Vital and Health Statistics*, **23** (16), 1–74.

Pearse, W. (1992). *ACOG fellowship statistical report*. American College of Obstetricians and Gynecologists, Washington DC.

Poland, M. L., Ager, J. W., Olson, K. L., and Sokol, R. J. (1990). Quality of prenatal care; selected social, behavioral and biomedical factors; and birth weight. *Obstetrics and Gynecology*, **75**, 607–11.

Public Health Service (1991). *Healthy people 2000*. US Government Printing Office, Washington DC.

Public Health Service. (1989). *Caring for our future: the content of prenatal care*. PHS, Washington DC.

Schlesinger, M. and Kronebusch, K. (1990). The failure of prenatal care policy for the poor. *Health Affairs*, **9**, 91–111.

Singh, S., Forrest, J. D., and Torres, A. (1989). *Prenatal care in the United States: a state and county inventory*. Alan Guttmacher Institute, New York.

Summer, L. (1991). *Limited access: health care for the rural poor*. Center for Budget and Policy Priorities, Washington DC.

Thompson, J. E., Walsh, L. V., and Merkatz, I. R. (1990). The history of prenatal care: cultural, social, and medical contexts. In *New perspectives on prenatal care*, (ed. I. R. Merkatz and J. E. Thompson), pp. 9–30. Elsevier Science Publishing, New York.

Taffel, S. M. and Keppel, K. G. (1986). Advice about weight gain during pregnancy and actual weight gain. *American Journal of Public Health*, **76**, 1396–9.

Torres, A. and Forrest, J. D. (1985). Family planning clinic services in the United States, 1983. *Family Planning Perspectives*, **17**, 30–5.

Tyson, J., Guzick, D., Rosenfeld, C. R., Lasky, R., Gant, N., Jiminez, J., *et al*. (1990). Prenatal care evaluation and cohort analyses. *Pediatrics*, **85**, 195–204.

13 Maternal health care in the developing world

R. H. Philpott

Maternal health care in the developing world is one of the most neglected subjects in the field of human reproduction. This fact is an indictment against all who purport to be concerned about the health of mothers. There are many who believe that the problem will always be with us, that the astronomically high mortality and morbidity are due to something inherent in the developing world, like the heat, which is beyond our control. Worse, some believe that women in the developing world are so accustomed to suffering and loss that they accept the poor quality of care and its consequences without experiencing the grief that would be expected in developed countries.

Many policy makers and over-extended health workers in the developing world treat maternal health as an isolated issue, such as oral health or leprosy control, failing to recognize its complexity and the need for a comprehensive approach. When I joined two other doctors in a busy mission hospital in West Africa in the early 1950s, I was given charge of the maternity unit because I had done a 6 month obstetric job since qualifying 18 months previously as a doctor. That was 6 months more experience than either of my colleagues, but woefully inadequate for the enormity of the task. Fortunately, a team of midwives was kind enough to protect their patients from me and at the same time introduce me to both obstetrics and the much wider concepts of motherhood and quality of life.

What do we expect of maternal health?

The standard of maternal health in a community could well be used as the index for measuring the quality of life in the whole community. Unfortunately, in the developing world it has often been out of the hands of that community, let alone its mothers, to determine what those standards should be. There must be a gold standard against which all concerned—whether health workers, policy makers, economists, or the mothers themselves—can measure their expectations and plans for maternal health. The gold standard will not always or often be met, but it will never be met if we do not set it before us. Here are a set of standards that a group of mothers in Zululand described as optimal for their community:

1. A couple enter marriage in commitment to a lifelong partnership based on their mutual love for each other.
2. They are equal partners in the marriage.
3. They complement each other in what they give to the partnership.
4. They create space for their personal and mutual development.
5. Their sexuality is a response to their mutual love, respect, and commitment to each other.
6. Contraception should be available to enable them to determine the number and timing of their pregnancies.
7. Ideally they should limit their family to two children and not more than three and these should be born when the mother is between 20 and 35 years of age.
8. There should be adequate prenatal care and a safe delivery attended by a well-trained midwife.
9. Health care and support should be available for the mother and the child during the child-rearing years.
10. Health care should be provided for the mature years.

These criteria imply preparation for marriage and motherhood. They also imply attention to the factors which deny women the option of true maternal health.

The plight of many women in southern and central Africa illustrates how it is nearly impossible for some women to survive the reproductive years, let alone experience motherhood in the manner outlined above (Bassett and Mhloyi 1991). Colonialism and racial domination, with the iniquities of the migrant labour system and land acquisition for commercial farming, destroyed traditional society structures and standards of maternal health, leaving a vacuum of broken families and a divided society. Many women only see their husbands 2 weeks in a year; for the rest of the year, the men find sexual satisfaction in the market-place. At one time, the worst consequences were a high birth rate in September (9 months after the mines closed for Christmas) or possibly infertility from sexually transmitted diseases. Now, the men bring AIDS home at Christmas or transmit the virus along the commercial truck routes and the epidemic is destroying all vestiges of family life on the African continent.

The magnitude of the social pathology that has disrupted family life throughout the world may well be the catalyst that challenges us to look at maternal health more holistically. In the ensuing text, I will consider safe motherhood as one component of this comprehensive picture and in examining it will illustrate what holistic maternal health demands. If we fail to consider this wider context, we will have missed our vocation and deserve only to be classified as technicians.

Safety in maternal health

Safety is only a token of what motherhood is about. Maternal mortality, although a crude parameter, is nevertheless a very evident index of safe motherhood. In developed countries, a maternal death is now very rare, but in many countries of the developing world not only is maternal death common but the rate has failed to decrease over many years. In 1987, the World Health Organization published tables of maternal mortality around the world (Boerma 1987). The report shows that in those parts of the developing world where mortality is highest, deaths are often not registered or their cause is not specified.

On the basis of the WHO survey, it is possible to estimate that each year at least half a million women die from causes related to pregnancy and childbirth. All but about 6000 of these deaths are in developing countries: 150 000 in Africa, 308 000 in Asia, and 34 000 in Latin America. In Africa, high mortality is compounded by high birth rates, so that women are exposed to these high mortality risks up to ten times in their life. Thus, for a woman in Africa, the life time risk of dying from pregnancy-related causes is often greater than one in 20, whereas for women in the developed world, there is a much lower risk of one in 2000.

Maternal death in the developing world

The obstetric causes of maternal death are similar in all countries of the developing world, although their proportions may vary. Hemorrhage is the leading cause, followed by illicit abortion, hypertension (including eclampsia), sepsis, obstructed labor, and ruptured uterus. Nearly all of these problems are preventable and certainly maternal death from any one of them can be avoided. There must then be other reasons why these conditions commonly cause death in the developing world; this will be explored in the next section of this chapter.

Maternal death rates in the developing world are comparable with rates for northern Europe and North America at the end of the last century, whereas rates in the developed world are now 100 times lower. The information that follows suggests that the developed world is not serious about its commitment to the problems of the developing world and in particular to the problems faced by women and the quality of family life.

Maternal health care in the developing world

Many health problems are primarily the result of socio-economic factors; when those are resolved, the prevalence of disease is diminished. Gastroenteritis and pneumonia in children are examples. It is important to recognize the socio-economic factors that influence maternal mortality and morbidity, acknowledging at the same time that mothers cannot deliver safely without a quality maternity service. The services provided in the developing world must be analyzed in light of socio-economic factors. The following integrated factors determine the difference between maternal health in the developing and the developed world; each of these factors is influenced by social, political, and economic determinants.

Maternity services in the developing world

Insufficient provision of services

Provision of services is very uneven; many cities and large towns have maternity hospital services, although these are usually seriously overcrowded. In the rural, poorer parts of the same country, where the majority of women live, the primary health care clinic facilities are inadequate for maternity care.

Access

Even when services exist, they are often not fully used because they are difficult to reach and many women deliver at home, unattended. Transport to the nearest maternity clinic can be prohibitively expensive and unsuitable for a woman in labor. This problem is worse in parts of the world where there has been constant warfare for many years. The problem of access is so severe that in many communities, roads and bridges are mentioned before hospitals as priorities in primary health care.

Women who deliver at home are often labeled by health workers as 'unbooked' or 'defaulters', even though the negligence is the fault of a poorly planned health service, designed and managed without consulting the potential users. The location of maternity clinics is seldom determined by the women who need the services. Instead, influential men in the village or town make a unilateral decision to boost their own prestige. The credibility of midwives in these peripheral clinics is often challenged by the local community when there is no telephone to enable them to consult or call for an ambulance.

Many countries have dealt with the communication difficulties by providing maternity villages next to hospitals or clinics, where women at high risk are housed at low cost as they approach delivery. Another solution has been for a clinic advisory board to establish a transport fund to provide cheaper means of transfer to hospital for referrals.

The impact of the world economic crisis has been felt most severely in the developing world and particularly in the already impoverished rural areas. Where governments have responded by privatizing health care, the already inadequate maternity services for the poor have worsened. Many health providers presume that poorer women do not mind waiting all day for an antenatal visit. Poor women are presumed to enjoy the social outing, whereas in truth such inconveniences are detrimental to the economy and survival of the family.

Quality

The quality of a maternity service has a direct bearing on pregnancy outcome. In addition, the quality of a health service and the attitude and training of its personnel have a significant influence on its utilization. Unfortunately, in many clinics and health centres in the developing world, the standards of clinical care are seriously inadequate. This is partly due to severe limitations in trained staff, insufficient laboratory facilities for even the few essential tests, and inadequate equipment for operative deliveries. Ironically, it is in the developing world where high-quality service is particularly needed, because obstetric complications such as severe hypertension, cephalo-pelvic disproportion, prematurity, and fetal growth retardation are far more common. In well-nourished, healthy communities in the first world, many women could deliver safely without the sophisticated service that is available to them.

In any community, it is essential to assess, on the basis of prevalent complications, the level of quality below which no service may be permitted to deteriorate. There are certainly levels of quality below which it would be safer to have no service at all, for poor service is not only ineffective but it also predisposes to a dangerous complacency, whereas the absence of a service can be a challenge for suitable provision.

In the developing world, where the struggle to provide basic services for all women is constant, there is seldom a chance to consider the important aspect of quality of the care-giving process. A study in Zimbabwe showed that the majority of women, whether in urban or rural areas, desired to deliver in the safety of a hospital or clinic, but when asked who they would choose to attend them at their delivery, they chose a traditional birth attendant ahead of a midwife or doctor. This was a clear expression of their appreciation of the understanding of the traditional attendants for the cultural values of their clientele, the care and attention given throughout the labor, and the attention paid to the needs of the whole family at the time of the delivery. It would be good if we could combine the caring of the traditional birth attendant with the clinical skills of the midwife and doctor.

Acceptability

In addition to the quality of interpersonal care, acceptability is influenced by the accommodation provided for women in labor. This is true everywhere, but particularly for women who have never seen a white-walled, sterile, Western-type labor ward. The Western practice of requiring that women lie flat on a bed is not only physiologically incorrect but also violates the woman's traditional expectations.

Antenatal clinic hours are usually determined to suit the providers of the service rather than the recipients. Many rural women work in the fields during the day and cannot attend clinics during the daytime. If they were consulted about clinic schedules, they could well suggest more appropriate hours.

Inadequate information

Again, traditional birth attendants score higher when it comes to communicating with pregnant women. They share the same cultural values and have the same knowledge base as those they serve and so can gain the women's trust and inspire confidence and reliance. I recall being taken by Dr Colin Bullough to visit a traditional birth attendant in a village on the western border of Malawi. The men of the village had built a series of huts for her maternity service, one for the labor ward, others for the antenatal clinic and mothers with premature babies, a waiting area, and so on. In the antenatal clinic, a crowd of women was viewing a demonstration on how to prepare nutritional meals for their family. On the return journey to Lilongwe, we passed a government clinic with a young White uniformed midwife who had no patients. The difference was that the traditional birth attendant had been chosen by the community for her sensitivity to their needs. Dr Bullough had been able to assist traditional attendants by expanding their knowledge base. The picture becomes complete when we invite them to share with us their knowledge of the local cultural values and their communication skills, so that we can add those dimensions to our clinical skills.

The quality of information that we provide to our clients can be measured by their participation in the health programmes we plan together and in the standards of reproductive health in the community. If we do not review these programmes regularly, inadequate use of a service can persist for years. In our antenatal clinics, we decided to ask women why they did not book until about the thirty-second week of their pregnancy. They responded that they thought the purpose of an antenatal visit was to pay the deposit for the cost of their delivery. When we explained the purpose of antenatal care, they readily accepted the benefits of early booking.

Health personnel

In the developing world, only about half of women deliver with the assistance of a trained midwife. This figure is even lower among the rural poor, among whom mortality is disproportionately high. Many of these women are attended by traditional birth attendants, who are often not recognized by other health professionals and are seldom included in an integrated health service. In fact, they tend to be regarded as charlatans by the medical profession. Consequently, they receive little further training—in spite of the fact that they are the community's first choice as birth attendants.

Not only are the traditional attendants not recognized by other health personnel, but doctors and nursing councils impose restrictions on trained and highly experienced midwives, even though there are not—and will not be, for many decades—enough trained doctors to deal with the obstetric needs of women.

The training given to midwives and doctors for that matter follows a curriculum devised in Western countries decades ago. It is no longer appropriate in the West, but in developing countries its deficiencies become even more apparent. The training tends to be didactic and compartmentalized. Clinical teaching must always be of high quality, but doctors and midwives must also be open to an understanding of the sociological and other factors that affect the health of women. They need a strong, comprehensive primary health care approach.

Education

The level of education in a community and particularly among the women has a major influence on reproductive health. Educational opportunities influence a woman's choice regarding the timing of marriage and childbearing and also the size of her family. Adequate education in sexuality and reproductive health help her to make informed decisions. When this education is supported by discussion of moral and ethical standards, the woman and her partner are more likely to take responsibility for their own healthy life-style.

Where the general level of education of the community is promoted, their societal structures are stronger, their expectations are higher, their awareness of the options for health care are broader, and all of this has a significant impact on health and the quality of life.

The status of women

In many countries, women have less say than men in determining health policy at national and local community levels. This inequality is accentuated in most developing countries and has been a significant factor in delaying the improvement of health services. At the individual level, male dominance in decision making has often prevented women from availing themselves of available maternal services and participating in family planning programmes. Many cannot obtain permission from their husbands for sterilization, even when it is for life-threatening medical indications.

The solution to this problem is not necessarily to conduct campaigns to deal with the status of women but rather for health workers to use health issues as a focus for participation in communities and, in so doing, help people to see that the dignity of women is an essential component of achieving health for all.

Poverty

The factors cited as reasons for maternal health differences between the developing and the developed countries are really but the consequences of a much deeper problem and that is poverty. Health workers need to probe still further and understand why some countries and even some people in those countries are poorer than others. At this fundamental level, I take issue with the title of this chapter, for in understanding the terminology used to describe the poor nations, we recognize the underlying reasons for mass poverty. Sanders (1985) uses the term 'underdeveloped' rather than 'developing' and quotes Berger (1975) who states:

> the only serious contribution to this semantic discussion has been made by the Cubans, who have pointed out that there should be a transitive verb: underdevelop. An economy is underdeveloped because of what is being done around it, within it and to it.

That the problems of equity in health, development, and underdevelopment are intimately linked is illustrated in the following very typical example. I was asked to evaluate the quality of health care provided by a clinic in Swaziland, which had been built and equipped by a multinational sugar company for its workers and families. The clinic, its nurses, and doctor were the very best, but the health of the people was poorer than it had been before the sugar company and the clinic had arrived. The reason was obvious, although not to the health workers. The multinational company had bought up all the land in that region of Swaziland, including the farms of the peasant farmers, which had been their adequate source of food. All the arable land was planted with sugar cane and some, but not all, of the peasant farmers were employed in the plantations at wages too low to feed their families. The obstetric consequences of the resultant undernutrition included intrauterine growth retardation, prematurity, abruptio placentae, none of which could be corrected by the beautiful clinic but all of which were due to the poverty resulting from land and economic exploitation.

Other countries have different reasons for their poverty and it is difficult to understand why most health workers fail to make the logical links and incorporate such awareness into a comprehensive health care program. Few South African health workers have taken note of their history. Prior to 1870, the African peasant farmer was much more industrious and productive than the White settler farmer, to the extent that they sold excess produce to the Whites. After 1893, two changes took place as a result of exploitation by a colonial power: the development of the mining industry and the granting by Britain of 'responsible government' to the White settlers.

From then on, the colonists invoked the state on the side of White agriculture and instituted state pressure upon African peasants. The Africans were squeezed off the lands and forced into the labor market. The wages were pitifully low and poverty descended upon a proud people. In the decades that followed, oppression and discrimination was institutionalized by legislation and from then onwards to be Black was to be poor. Fortunately, within the South African liberation struggle, new progressive health groups have been formed and these health workers have given new meaning to comprehensive primary health care. They have tackled both the root causes of poverty within the politico-socio-economic inequities of the country and the well-recognized preventive, promotive, and curative aspects of health care.

Principles of management of maternal health care in the developing world

One of the greatest hindrances to improvement in maternal health care in the developing world has been the way in which medical and nursing students are socialized during their training. Their learning takes place in teaching hospitals that are mostly clones of their counterparts in the cities of the Western world and far removed, literally and figuratively, from the realities of life for the rural and periurban poor of the developing world. The concepts of primary health care and the principles of sociology, politics, and economics do not appear in nursing and medical curricula, when in fact these disciplines have more to say to us as health care workers than much of the didactic teaching that we present in the classrooms of our teaching hospitals. It is little wonder that our graduates are skilled at the clinical and laboratory diagnosis of intrauterine growth retardation and the neonatal care of the very small baby, but have little understanding of the cause and prevention of the problem.

Here are a set of principles that need to be addressed, alongside the clinical skills of modern obstetrics, in planning maternal health care programmes in the developing world.

Community-based programmes

In the past, the hospital has been regarded as the focus of an obstetric service and all the decisions have been taken by doctors, with the result that obstetrics is rather clinical and driven by statistics. The service can be humanized without lowering the standard of clinical care, by moving the focus to the family and the community, giving them the opportunity to participate in planning. There will be issues that are entirely within the expertise of the health personnel and others that are dependent on the experience of the community, with a number of decisions being made as a result of joint discussion.

The members of health committees at local, community levels can play important roles when health personnel recognize and accept that members of the community have a valuable perspective to contribute and that all members of the committee have much to learn from each other. This is the ultimate forum, where accountability for meeting the health needs of the community must be assigned and accepted.

Comprehensiveness of care

In no circumstances may we ever lower the standards of the obstetric skills we expect of the practitioners we train, whether they be doctors or midwives, but let us ensure that those skills are provided in the context of a comprehensive service that attends to the preventive, promotive, curative, rehabilitative, and palliative components of health care on a basis of equity and community participation, and includes the following.

Nutrition of young girls

The nutrition of the female fetus *in utero* and the food provided during her growing years will have an influence on her eventual pelvic size and also the successful outcome of her own pregnancy. In turn, there are many factors that will determine female nutrition, from national and international policies to cultural practices within families. These are essential issues that need to be addressed by health personnel in consultation with community and families. Examples of the type of problems that may need to be tackled include national policy on food storage and distribution as well as the tendency in some societies to give the females the leftovers of the family meal.

Family life teaching

This is the first and most important step in dealing with teenage pregnancy, which is one of the really serious complicating factors in pregnancy outcome among the poor. When teenage pregnancies occur, they are often hidden and only are revealed when a major obstetric crisis occurs. In addition, teenage mothers suffer sociological consequences that affect the rest of their lives. Most of them have to drop out of school and lose out on career training and a normal family life. Family life teaching is best provided by example in the home and backed up by teaching at an early age in school, church, and health center.

In some societies, the disruption of family life has economic and political causes, as in South Africa, where the father is away from the family for 11 months of the year as a migrant laborer in the mines. No amount of family life teaching will solve problems of this nature, which are due to exploitative labor practices and which must be challenged and dealt with at the root cause.

Family Planning

This service is best established in a primary health care center for all sexually active young people and as an integral part of a comprehensive maternal service where mothers are prepared for future family planning during their pregnancy and a suitable choice of methods is available. Special attention must be given to women with medical conditions such as cardiac and renal disease; pregnancies in these women require very careful planning or even complete prevention.

Avoidance and management of sexually transmitted diseases

In many societies, gonorrhoea is the most common cause of infertility and syphilis one of the most common causes of perinatal mortality. Prevention lies in adequate and appropriate education and in early detection and treatment in accessible primary health care. The prevention of AIDS will depend on the adoption of new moral standards in human sexuality, backed up by the provision and use of condoms, community education programmes, and attention to the social factors that predispose to the spread of the disease.

Accessible antenatal care

To ensure that an antenatal clinic is used by all the pregnant women in the area, the community must be involved in deciding its location and also the times when it will be open. The community should also be able to select the midwives who will work in the clinic and to comment on the acceptability of the service they render. These factors will determine 'compliance', but there must also be medical standards below which the poorest clinic service cannot go. Each country must clearly identify these minimal standards and maternal and child health coordinators need to review the clinics in light of these standards.

Delivery attendants

Each mother must be able to depend on having a trained assistant during her labor and delivery. The assistant must be able to recognize obstetric risk factors and work within clearly defined protocols of management. A major determinant of successful delivery outcome in peripheral clinics is the availability of two-way radio or telephone communication with doctors in the nearest hospital. Unfortunately, this is not always possible, but it must be a high priority in developing a quality service and in establishing due credibility to the work of the isolated midwife. In-service training, particularly through review of clinical problems and a perinatal audit, is essential if quality and community acceptance are to be maintained.

Transport for referral

A number of disciplines in clinical medicine can be practiced entirely at the peripheral clinic level. Obstetrics is not one of these and if adequate provision is not made for timely transfer of high-risk patients to a secondary level facility for possible operative intervention, then the peripheral clinic will understandably fall into disrepute. As it is not always possible to provide an ambulance for such transfers, the local health committee must ensure that patients are not exploited by those who would make excessive profit out of their misfortune. This can be prearranged on a contract basis.

The referral hospital

The comprehensive service should be organized at district level so that the referring clinics and the base hospital are recognized as integral parts of the entire service. There are too many examples of poor relationships between the hospital and the surrounding clinics with consequent deleterious effects on the maternal service. Respect for each other's value has to be built and maintained or the patients suffer.

Affordability

The tension between ensuring that the service is adequately financed and that no patient is excluded from the full comprehensive care she deserves must be addressed. It will be tackled in different ways in different areas. This could mean that it is part of a national health service or that an insurance scheme is devised. A financial arrangement that covers antenatal care, delivery, and postnatal care is usually the best way to ensure continuity.

Proper use of human resources

The advanced midwife

Since the early 1980s, a new category of health worker has become established; its members are the key people in the organization of maternal health services in Natal, South Africa. This commenced as a research project, but now the advanced midwife has proved herself by transforming a third-rate regional obstetric service into one that is improving remarkably each year with the expansion of this new concept. The details of selection and training will be described later in this chapter, but the context in which the advanced midwife functions needs to be described here.

In many parts of the developing world, there are insufficient doctors and the few that are available tend to be in the larger towns and cities. Maternal health care lends itself to an alternative to dependence on doctors, because there are many midwives with more experience than their medical counterparts. By selecting the best of the midwives and giving them advanced training, it has been possible to have them do everything in the maternity service short of intra-abdominal surgery. They have in fact developed a district-wide service. The gap between the few overworked doctors and the midwife with limited training must be bridged and the advanced midwife has proved to be the answer, as long as doctors and administrators accept her role and qualifications for fulfilling that role.

The traditional birth attendant

Whatever approach we take to the traditional birth attendants, we must accept that they attend more women in the developing world in childbirth than do nurse–midwives and doctors and that for a long time to come there will not be sufficient nurse–midwives and doctors to take their place. Furthermore, with the poor reputation that health professionals have in many parts of the world, many women would choose traditional birth attendants because of the emphasis they place on caring and understanding of traditional values.

Some maternity services have established good working relationships with traditional birth attendants and linked together in a joint service. The ideal situation is one in which these attendants and nurse–midwives are incorporated in a single integrated maternal service with an advanced midwife as the coordinator.

Nurse–midwives

None of what has been said above should in any way detract from the important role of the nurse–midwife, who is essential to a successful maternal health service. In the developing world, nurse–midwives will carry greater responsibility than their counterparts in the developed world and their training must equip them for that role.

Medical doctors

There are some outstanding physicians in the developing world, but unfortunately there are others who are not only dangerous but who defensively prevent highly skilled midwives from rendering the service for which they are well equipped. To a large extent, those responsible for the doctor's training are culpable, for while that training may well be sufficient for privileged parts of the world where there is little pathology, it does not equip a doctor for service in the developing world. Medical students who have received traditional Western undergraduate obstetric training should spend time in postgraduate training in one of the few well-supervised teaching hospitals in the developing world before moving to a more peripheral hospital. Their ideal role would then be to assist in the training of advanced midwives who will carry the major responsibility for the maternity service in the area while the doctor is released for other medical activities.

Listening to women

The health profession received a big jolt in the early 1970s when women let it be known that they did not approve of escalating rates for induction of labor, cesarean section, and other interventions, particularly because they had never been consulted about these changing trends. Unfortunately, lack of sensitivity to the concerns of women has persisted in maternal health practice in the developing world, possibly because most professionals presume that a lack of formal education makes it impossible for women from poorer communities to debate their reproductive needs. This is far from the truth and lack of consultation is a serious form of professional negligence. If we are to establish effective and efficient maternal health services, we need to spend time in listening and discussion.

Listening to women is not easy if we ask the questions from the vantage point of our health institution or as sporadic visitors to their community, particularly if they are poor and we are not. The most successful listeners are those who identify themselves with the poor and the oppressed and are prepared to ask about their perceived needs before imposing a program from outside. This can often be best accomplished through the existing social structures in the local society, which sometimes need to be supported and strengthened to enable the women to negotiate on an equal footing.

If we are prepared to take the first step of asking questions and listening to the answers, we must be ready for surprises, for their priorities may be different from our own and possibly not even on our agenda. One squatter community asked for a bridge over a river so that they could get to the nearest health facility and another asked for a clean water supply to ensure that the children did not die from diarrhea.

We gain a new perspective when we listen carefully and work with people rather than for them in improving their health status. Our educational background has compartmentalized our knowledge and understanding of people's health needs, not only into medical specialties but, more seriously, into a presumption that the biomedical approach is the only solution that matters. The women in the village who speak to us first of a clean water supply are opening up issues of sociology, engineering, economics, and political justice, which are as much a part of maternal health care as the external cephalic version of a breech presentation.

None of these concerns indicate an undervaluing of a high-quality obstetric service. Instead, there is a call to place it in the context of a comprehensive understanding of women's health, which can only be done if the participants are members of a multidisciplinary team functioning in partnership with the women of the community.

Politico-economic awareness

This is best assimilated when students are assisted in unraveling all the facets of a health problem rather than by teaching political and economic theory, for it is in grappling with etiology that we get into the habit of comprehensiveness. Politics is no longer a dirty word when we define it as the study of people in community and no-one can deny that this must be on the agenda of every health worker, particularly in the developing world.

Ethics in human reproduction

The ethical responses of society and government to maternal care have been dealt with, but the individual's ethical standards in human sexuality and reproduction must also be well informed if maternal health is to reach its optimum. Human choice plays a major role in maternal health and, in facing conditions like AIDS, it is the only variable that can be controlled by the individual. Health workers themselves must adopt their own ethical standard that, when offered to others, ensures the best in reproductive health. A tested set of standards were presented at the beginning of this chapter.

The implementation of a comprehensive maternal health care program

The practicalities of implementing a comprehensive maternal health care program in the developing world require that it be done within the context of a national health service that emphasizes comprehensive primary health care. This does not exclude private services, but they alone can never redress the present gross inequities and deficiencies in health care. Within a national health service, there will be regional and district health services. The district refers to the most peripheral level of local government and is therefore most capable of ensuring community or public involvement in planning and decision making. Within a district, which usually serves 200–500 000 people, there will be one or two hospitals and a number of clinics and health centers.

True comprehensive primary health care includes both the front-line service in the health center and the secondary referral hospital in an integrated program. The comprehensiveness of the program is practiced mainly at the site of first contact, the health center, but needs to be reinforced by those who practice in the referral hospital. At district level, the headquarters for the health service—and therefore the maternal health service—should be the largest of the health centers in the district, rather than the hospital, because this will show that the hospital is not the most important component of comprehensive health care.

A similar shift in perspective is needed in defining the key health worker in maternal health care services in the developing world. In the past, this role has been filled by the over-worked, over-stretched doctor in the district hospital with his or her faithful band of inadequately trained midwives and usually neglected traditional birth attendants. We in Natal, South Africa, have promoted the advanced midwife to fill the role of key health worker in maternal health care. As a result, we are seeing lowered maternal and perinatal mortality, more satisfied clients, and doctors released to attend to other pressing needs in the health service.

The health center

Standards and the quality of care

The quality of maternal health care in a country is best measured by the standards set in the most peripheral health center. In many countries in the developing world, politicians and health planners have got away with a 'second class service for second class citizens', but with the gradual demise of colonialism and racial discrimination there is a call for more democratic practices and greater equity in society. While accepting that a service must be affordable, national and district planners must pay special attention to the hitherto under-served, if for no other reason than that it is within the poorest communities that pathology is most prevalent.

In planning a health center, standards are best set and attained when there is joint community and health service partnership and involvement in its management. The health service will bring expertise and understanding of clinical aspects and the community will help in setting the priorities and the context of the service. With such a partnership, better decisions will be made regarding the appropriate provision of antenatal care and intrapartum services and the siting and design of the health center. Antenatal care, if it is to be well used, must be within reasonable walking distance of all mothers and community education on health must be provided to ensure that women are in a position to make the best choices regarding their health. In densely populated areas, the antenatal clinic at the health center will be sufficient, but in rural areas, where the distances are greater, antenatal clinics can be conducted in mobile clinics or visiting points.

There will always be a debate as to whether women should deliver in a health center or at home. The strongest reason that women have for wanting to deliver at home is the familiarity of the surroundings and the desire for delivery to be an event that is shared by the family. The very design of our clinics and health centers adds to this sentiment and, if we are to promote our concern for the mother's safety, we need to consult with women in the community in making our birthing units more like home and make provision for the mother's chosen attendant to be present during her labor. It is usually possible for the mother to go home soon after the delivery if it can be arranged for a trained attendant to visit her daily as she establishes lactation and to help with the housework while she has adequate rest and renews her strength.

The purpose of involvement of communities in planning the maternal health service is 2-fold. First, if women do not take well informed responsibility for their own health care, the best of obstetric care will remain a last resort to be turned to after less well-substantiated alternatives have failed. Thus, a well-planned and tested system of health education for the community must originate from the health center, with learning opportunities based on actual problems raised by the women of the community, but taken to the women in their homes and community organizations. Then, secondly, well-informed community health committees are able to make significant contributions to the planning of the service, which thereby becomes a service that they own and use.

Community involvement in health service planning is a new and sometimes strange concept to many health personnel, who believe they know what is best for the women of the community. As a result, women make their own plans and often lose out on the benefits that could be provided by the health service.

To bridge this gulf of trust, health workers need to be trained in the principles and dynamics of working in partnership with the community they serve. For some this is tantamount to a conversion experience. After initial training, they really learn what partnership means once they open themselves to its practice and implementation. Then, because the poorer communities have seldom been given the opportunity to become involved with health institutions in health service planning, an active program of health education and even education in how to engage with authorities in an assertive way is essential if partnership is to be more than just rhetoric.

The ideal community structure to work with is the civic association or its counterpart and in particular the local health committee. Where such structures do not exist, communities need to be assisted in setting them up and training them to fulfill their functions. The establishment of true primary health care will be the catalyst for on-going community development.

Measuring the quality of care

Maternal health in the developing world has been measured statistically by looking at outcomes such as maternal or perinatal mortality. As stated above, a number of factors outside the health care system determine maternal health; these include economics, social status, and political systems. Within the health care system, we have tended to limit our analysis to the quantity or coverage of the system and paid little attention to measuring the quality. Family planning services have probably been studies in greater depth than any other health service in recent years (for varying reasons) and it is not surprising that it is in this field that work has been done on the analysis of quality of care. Bruce (1990) has produced a conceptual framework for the analysis of quality of care in family planning and Jain *et al.* (1992) has applied this to a definition of quality of care in women's health care overall. Jain provides the following suggested list of elements and their corresponding indicators.

1. *Provider–woman information exchange* Information which should be conveyed to women includes an explanation of the diagnosis, information (where medically appropriate) on treatment options, information on the therapeutic regimen, information on contraindications to and side-effects of all medications and drugs. The provider should also listen to and understand women, including their background, preferences for treatment, and medical history.

2. *Provider competence* This requires accurate knowledge about the disease, problem, or condition, technical proficiency in providing safe and appropriate clinical treatment known to produce an impact on mortality, morbidity or the existing condition, and knowledge of procedures for referring cases which cannot be adequately managed.

3. *Interpersonal relations* There should be sensitive treatment of women, including privacy, respectful and responsive provider behavior, encouragement of women's participation in decision making, avoidance of moral judgements, confidentiality, limited waiting time, and spending enough time with the woman.

4. *Mechanisms to encourage continuity of medical care* These include information about when to return and, if possible, other locations where services and medications can be obtained and specific follow-up procedures including, when deemed necessary, future appointments and home visits.

Mensch has purposely left out two other criteria of quality of care that deserve consideration. She has not included constellation of services, as she does not feel that it is possible to state which health care delivery systems are most appropriate in every circumstance; rather, she feels this must be defined for a particular area. Nor does she include access to care, not because it is unimportant, but because she sees quality as describing what happens on arrival at the point of service. In maternal health care, both the quality of the health delivery system and access to it, including acceptability as perceived by the client, need to be included in the above list of elements of quality of care, particularly in defining a list for a specific area or region.

Mensch takes the consideration of quality of care a step further by proposing that, using the above descriptive elements, it is necessary to establish standards which are acceptable and achievable within the context of each country. This still requires identification of important levels or standards below which no service may fall, regardless of the available resources, if it is to retain legitimacy, let alone credibility.

Auditing quality of care

Accountability in the delivery of a maternity service must be built into the standard practice of a health center. This requires accurate record keeping and the provision of a weekly statistical report with a detailed account of maternal or perinatal deaths and of patients referred to the hospital. At a weekly meeting of all staff members, these statistics should be reviewed as a learning exercise that will lead to continuing improvement in the quality of service rendered by the team. Less frequent meetings should be held with the health committee to report on the work being done by the center and to hear recommendations from the community.

The training of the advanced midwife

As already mentioned, it is proposed that this new category of health worker be the key to the reorientation of maternal services in the developing world. It is therefore necessary to present some of the principles used in their training. Advanced midwives have been trained in Natal, South Africa for the past 10 years. Over that period, as a result of research that has sought to find correlations between selection, mode of teaching, learning progress, and impact on the health of women served, evolutionary changes in the educational process have resulted in the present model. The course has the cumbersome but descriptive title of Decentralized Education Program in Advanced Midwifery and Neonatal Science (DEPAM) and has evolved under the guidance of the nurse–midwives, Ross and Mzolo.

Job description

The advanced midwife is sufficiently skilled as a clinician to be a consultant to midwives serving in the hospitals and clinics in her area and, as an educator, to provide in-service training for others who are responsible for maternal health care. She is able to initiate new maternal health services and evaluate and reorganize existing services at hospital, clinic, and community levels. Her training in educational skills enables her to give health information and become involved in the health concerns of her community. In this way, she is able to help people take responsibility for their own health and to contribute to the health of society.

The conceptual framework of the course

In the early days of the program, students came for their training to a teaching institution that was often far from their home. This caused major family disruption, as these were often married women with young children. Also, there was the likelihood that the learning experience would be divorced from the type of demands they met in their community environment. The term decentralized is used to describe the program in preference to distance learning, as there is a strong practical component that requires skilled facilitation by experienced practitioners. With the bulk of the education taking place in the base hospital and surrounding clinics where the midwife will eventually work, there is no break in her employment. The learning experience also relates to her work and benefits her work immediately and there is the opportunity for the entire maternal health service at the local level to improve as it becomes part of her learning development.

'**Education**' refers to the collaborative venture between student and facilitator, with the emphasis on growth toward self-directed learning that will continue throughout her life. The facilitators provide liberating support structures, within which students gain increasing self-confidence and educational independence. The program is sufficiently flexible to recognize that each student has a different learning history and also a different task to fulfill on completion.

'**Advanced midwifery**' refers to her experience and expertise in maternal health, starting at the community and family level, where she is able to support and equip people for initiatives that address the socio-economic and environmental factors that affect women's health, and including the organization and management of a maternal service at district level.

Organization of the course

Selection

An advanced midwife is a qualified nurse–midwife with at least 4 years of practice experience. She is then trained to provide a full range of obstetric care in her district. Students are recommended by their employing authority and local community health committee and are selected on the basis of a variety of tests which assess present knowledge, personal qualities, motivation, and evidence of a caring nature.

Length of the course

The course takes a minimum of 18 months and a maximum of 30 months, accepting that the standard to be obtained should be the constant and the length of time to reach that standard the variable. Students are required to achieve a specific standard of clinical competency before being permitted to sit the examination for advanced midwives that is recognized by the Nursing Council. During the program, the student remains in her full-time post, but the employing institution is expected to provide release time for study and for formal blocks at the base hospital.

Self-directed learning with individualized learning contracts

Students identify their own goals and learning needs by assessing their knowledge and experience base and negotiating with the home insitution and community to determine expectations on graduation. This enables them to determine their personal curriculum, which is formulated on the basis of a series of problem-based exercises that consist of real problems of patients, administration, or the community. These exercises integrate theory and practice and provide advanced knowledge from the natural, biological, social, and educational sciences. As part of their learning contract, students negotiate their own self-assessment procedures at the commencement of the course.

Clinical experience

This takes place during the normal working day, but it is carefully structured in consultation between the student and her clinical supervisor in order to cover the full range of the curriculum by rotating through the various components of the service, the identified tasks, and skills under supervision, until both the supervisor and the student are confident that the skill has been developed to a degree that the student is able to function alone safely and confidently. The competency assessment tool (CAT) that is used is an invaluable educational instrument to monitor the progress of students in a distance learning programme.

Resources for the course

The students do assignments and are provided with detailed feedback. They are given manuals on each of the major components of the course, and there is a library at each of the base hospitals. Each base hospital has a clinical supervisor who is herself an advanced midwife, and there are peripatetic facilitators who spend a week at a time with pairs of students.

The role of the facilitator

The program started off with one peripatetic facilitator who visited all the students on a regular basis, helping to supervise their practical work, moderating their theory studies, and carrying out formative assessments. This facilitator has since helped to train other advanced midwife graduates as facilitators for courses in different parts of the country.

The facilitators administer the DEPAM course in their region. They are responsible for the selection process and for conducting the orientation course for new students, during which they do baseline assessments of knowledge and skills, facilitate self-directed learning and group dynamics, help students develop their learning contracts and subsequent study blocks, and plan their formative assessment activities. They facilitate the block learning programs and visit the students in their home base to carry out skill competency training and assessments before admitting the student to the summative assessment.

The facilitator must provide close support in the initial stages but must identify a strategic time for phased withdrawal to enable the student to become an independent learner. The final role of the facilitator is to evaluate the epidemiological markers in the health ward over a few years, to ensure that the education of the advanced midwife has really improved maternal and neonatal health.

References

Bassett, M. T. and Mhloyi, M. (1991). Women and AIDS in Zimbabwe: the making of an epidemic. *International Journal of Health Services*, **21(1)**, 143–56.

Berger, J. and Mohr, J. (1975). *A seventh man*. Penguin, Harmondsworth. p. 21.

Boerma, J. T. (1987). Levels of maternal mortality in developing countries. *Studies in Family Planning*, **18(4)**, 213–21.

Bruce, J. (1990). Fundamental elements of the quality of care: a simple framework. *Studies in Family Planning*, **21(2)**, 61–91.

Jain, A., Bruce, J., and Mensch, B. (1992). Setting standards of quality in family planning programs. *Studies in Family Planning*, **23(6)**, 392–5.

Sanders, D. (1985). *The struggle for health*. MacMillan, London. p. xii.

14 An evaluation of maternity services

R. W. Beard and Jean Chapple

Pregnancy has become a relatively safe event for the mother and her baby, so why is it that Western societies continue to make a substantial investment in providing health care? This question highlights an ambivalence of approach that spreads from government to all professions involved in maternity care and to the public. Pregnancy is a natural and important event and most women remain well throughout their pregnancy. Yet unpredictable complications still occur which can kill or maim for life a baby and even the mother. It is this uncertainty in the developed world, with its high expectations and concern for the individual, that drives us all to do better. With this has come the emergence of the voice of women demanding the right to have a major say in their management during a major life event such as pregnancy. These two factors—the improved safety of pregnancy and the greater involvement of women in their care—have led to a questioning of decisions made by obstetricians and, to a lesser extent, midwives. An intervention in pregnancy has to be justified, for if it is well chosen the risk to mother or baby is reduced, but if it is not then a potentially normal outcome may become very abnormal.

These are some of the issues that are shaping the development of maternity care in a Western country like the UK. Technology, natural childbirth, audit, and litigation are some of the possible solutions which are being tried with variable success.

History of the maternity services in England and Wales

Midwives have until recently been regarded as the appropriate people to supervise care in pregnancy. In 1567, licenses to practice were granted by the bishops. The license specified a code of conduct but did not require any skill as a requirement to practice. It was not until the late seventeenth century that obstetricians, or 'man-midwives' as they were known, appeared with increasing numbers at the same time as the invention of the obstetric forceps. From the start, there was a schism which exists to this day between the long-established midwives and the newly arrived obstetricians. In the eighteenth century, lying-in hospitals were established for women who developed life-threatening conditions such as uncontrolled hemorrhage, toxemic convulsions, and obstructed labor. In 1835, the Society of Apothecaries granted a license in midwifery to doctors and in 1886 the General Medical Council required midwifery to be part of the curriculum for doctors in training. It was not until 1902, with the passing of the first Midwives Act, that midwives were required to receive some formal training before they could practice. This coincided with the formation of the Central Midwives Board to regulate their training and certification. Interestingly, the independent practitioner status of midwives was granted at that time because midwives had to conduct the majority of deliveries without any kind of medical supervision or support.

Home delivery was the norm at the turn of the century for up to 90 per cent of women in rural areas and 50 per cent in major cities (Infant Mortality Committee 1870). In 1918 the second Midwives Act made it compulsory for midwives to summon medical aid in the event of a pregnancy or labor becoming abnormal. No doubt this further fueled the conflict between midwives and doctors, with the midwives trying to protect their patients from unnecessary intervention (and also trying to protect their fees, which were lost if a doctor took over the case).

Until 1936, midwives either worked for an association or were in private practice, but the third Midwives Act empowered local Supervising Authorities to employ midwives full-time, eventually in local authority hospitals. This and the Local Government Act 1929 set the scene for creating a permanent rift between the midwife as an independent practitioner and the doctor as the individual responsible for clinical practice in hospital.

In 1929 the College (later Royal College) of Obstetricians and Gynaecologists was founded with powers to examine and to confer diplomas, memberships, and fellowships. There is little doubt that this played an important part in the sharp rise in hospital confinements that followed. In 1927 only 15 per cent of women had a hospital delivery, in 1937 it was 40 per cent, and 50 per cent by 1946. The recommendation by the Peel Committee (Peel 1970) that all women should give birth in hospital to prevent avoidable maternal deaths led to the present position where all but a few women are delivered in hospitals.

It was recognized that there was wide variation in the quality and standards of practice, and in response to the concern about this, the Confidential Enquiry into Maternal Deaths was set up in 1952 by the Government. Reports have been issued every 3 years since then. Figures 14.1 and 14.2 show the maternal and perinatal mortality rates over the years with a marked fall starting in the early 1930s.

General practitioners have had a variable involvement in maternity care. Up until the time when most women delivered in hospital they played an important part in providing support for the midwives involved in confinements at home or in general practitioner maternity units. Under the 1946 National Health Service Act, general practitioners wishing to practice obstetrics had to be on the local 'obstetric list' which was established to ensure that they possessed an acceptable

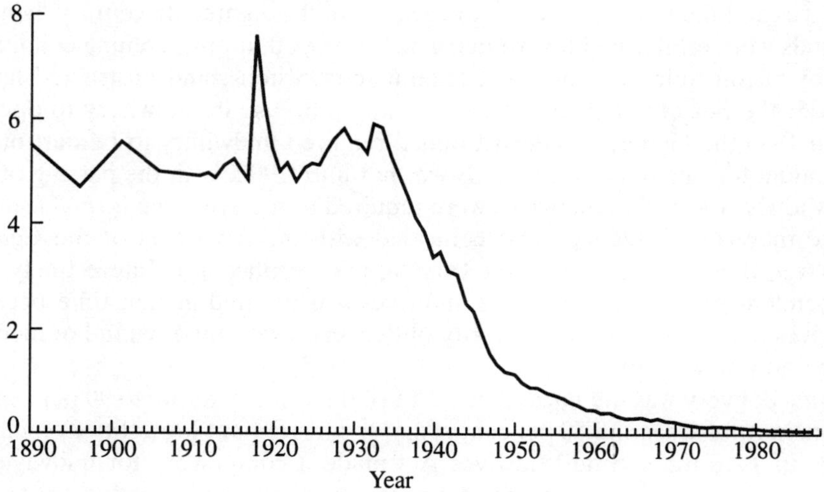

Fig. 14.1 Maternal mortality per 1000 maternities in England and Wales, 1890–1987.

degree of obstetric expertise. This proved to be a relatively ineffectual means of ensuring such expertise and was criticized by the Parliamentary Social Services Select Committee (1980) which noted that in some localities more than 90 per cent of general practitioners were on the obstetric list. Nevertheless, general practitioners continue to play an important part in maternity care, particularly in some rural areas which are distant from hospital services. Most would argue that pregnancy is a family event and that general practitioners should be involved in providing care, at least during the months leading up to and after delivery.

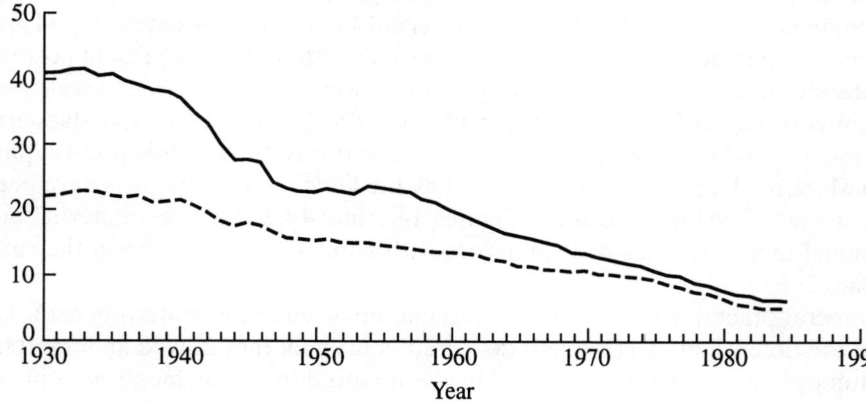

Fig. 14.2 Stillbirths (– – – – – –) and neonatal deaths (———) per 1000 births in England and Wales, 1930–1989.

What have maternity services achieved?

In the twentieth century, obstetricians in the UK have taken care to look at what the services have achieved. Three national perinatal mortality surveys were carried out in 1947, 1958 and 1972. Since the Second World War numerous surveys have been done by health regions and it remains customary for individual maternity units to produce an annual report. Such detailed analysis of the quality of clinical practice in the maternity services has contributed to the sharp fall in perinatal mortality during this time. The 4-fold fall between 1956 and 1990, from 32 to eight per 1000 births (Fig. 14.2) would suggest that clinical care in pregnancy is beyond reproach. However, closer inspection of outcomes in individual cases reveals that the quality of care can be variable, with poor quality of care occasionally resulting in avoidable death or disability. This philosophy has been adopted in the Confidential Enquiry into Maternal Death carried out jointly by the Department of Health and the Royal College of obstetricians and Gynaecologists. Deaths associated with some aspect of care which the assessors regard as falling below the expected level of professional competence are classified as substandard.

Fig. 14.1 shows an impressive fall in maternal mortality which started as early as 1936, coinciding with the introduction of antibiotics, a national blood transfusion service, and improved general anesthesia. It is likely that the continued downward trend owes much to the audit of maternal deaths by the profession.

Modern maternity care

Maternity services in the UK today

Under the National Health Service, with few exceptions, all pregnant women in the UK are entitled to free care for themselves and their babies. About 95 per cent are cared for in this way, the remainder opting for private care. Women are encouraged to see a doctor before the end of 3 months of pregnancy and most are referred to a hospital maternity unit where they are booked for delivery. Antenatal care is provided either by general practitioners and midwives, by the hospital staff, or by both (shared care). In general, obstetricians look after women with any form of pregnancy complications who are regarded as high risk, while midwives and general practitioners care for low-risk women.

Care in hospitals is provided by obstetricians and midwives. The delivery unit is staffed 24 h a day by a team consisting of midwives, obstetricians, a pediatrician, and an on-call anesthetist. Team care is generally regarded as the safest and most cost-effective way to look after a pregnant woman, although it is obviously less personal than care by one individual throughout pregnancy. Maternity units usually provide a midwife who stays with a woman in labor until she has delivered. Husbands, members of the family, and close friends are encouraged to be present if the mother wishes. Most women leave the hospital within 24 h after an uncomplicated delivery.

Some women opt for a 'domino' delivery, in which prenatal care is provided by a midwife or general practitioner, who will perform the delivery in the hospital or, less commonly, at home. In the UK, a doctor or midwife must be present at a delivery by law. When a midwife plans to deliver a woman at home, she will usually ensure that a general practitioner or the local maternity unit will provide back-up support. Professional attitudes to home confinement vary, with obstetricians being far less enthusiastic about it than midwives. A recent report by the Parliamentary Health Committee (1992) recommended that women be given greater choice in where they deliver and it seems likely that there will be a small increase in the demand for home confinements.

Recent developments

It is easy to forget when reading the history of medicine that change, when it occurs, is often rapid and that each change brings its own set of problems. This is true for the maternity services in the last 60 years and particularly for the last 30 years. The fall in perinatal deaths (viable babies dying before and in the first week after birth) followed the introduction of rhesus immunization (Clarke *et al.*, 1963; Chown *et al.* 1969) and then of neonatal intensive care. The effect of this latter advance on the survival of low birthweight babies is shown in Fig. 14.3 over a 32 year period.

The contribution of medical science to fertility and the safety of pregnancy has been particularly evident in recent years. Assisted fertilization techniques (see Chapter 11) now offers hope of a normal child to women who had no chance 20 years ago. The chance of successful pregnancy in women with diseases such as diabetes, high blood pressure, and kidney disease has changed beyond recognition. Before insulin was discovered it was rare for any woman with diabetes to have a pregnancy progressing beyond the first 3 months. Now the chance of such a woman delivering a healthy mature baby are virtually the same as for any normal non-diabetic woman. It is sometimes said that advances in medicine have had little to do with the dramatic improvement in mortality for mothers and babies and that it is all due to the improved health of pregnant women. While no-one would deny that good general health makes an important contribution to a successful pregnancy, it is not by chance that the steep fall in maternal mortality from the 1930s, accompanied by a fall in damage to mothers who survived a 'near-miss', coincides with the introduction of some of the major advances in medicine of this century.

These improvements in the care of pregnant women have not been without their problems. A good example of this is the greater facility to detect fetal abnormalities (Wald *et al.* 1992). This has come about as a result of the introduction of techniques to detect genetic and metabolic diseases in early pregnancy such as the collection of fetal cells by chorionic villus sampling and amniocentesis. Routine ultrasound scanning of all women ensures that the majority of structural abnormalities that can affect the baby are detected by mid-pregnancy, when termination of pregnancy carries a low risk. In the UK, as in most Western countries, the law allows a woman with a seriously malformed baby to have an abortion if she wishes. However, no woman can easily decide to destroy a baby she has been thinking about, often for much longer than the duration of the pregnancy. Many women prefer to avoid this decision and in the North West Thames Region, less than half of women more than 37 years old accept the offer of amniocentesis to detect Down syndrome.

The problems do not end there. Modern technology such as ultrasound can reveal an abnormality which is not severe enough to interfere with life, but is not alway correctable. An example is talipes, a deformity of the feet. Should this be accepted as sufficient grounds for a termination of pregnancy if the mother requests it? Another issue is that some babies are born with a more serious malformation than was originally suspected. This may give rise to considerable resentment and even litigation on the part of the parents who may suspect that an error was made at the time of ultrasound scan for malformation.

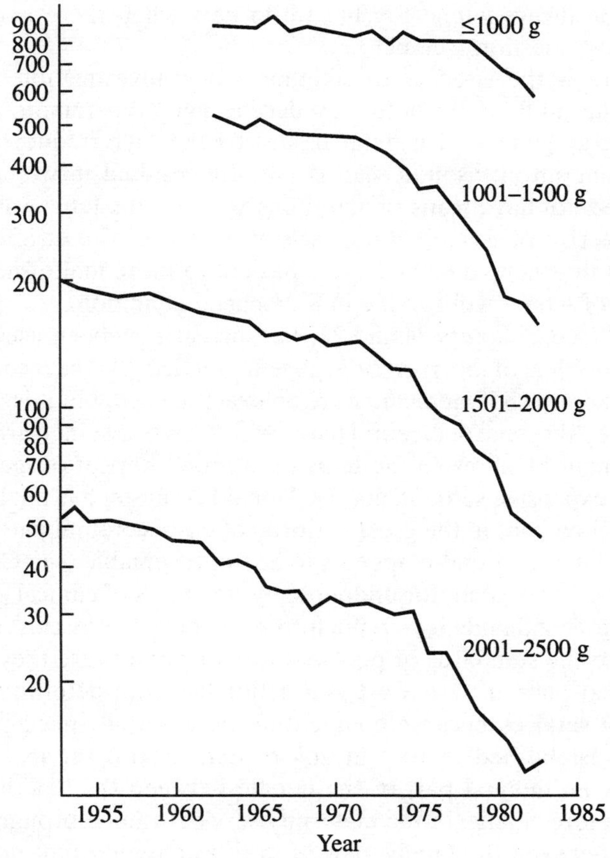

Fig. 14.3 Neonatal mortality rates per 1000 live births relative to birthweight in England and Wales 1953–1983. (Reproduced with permission from Pharaoh (1986).)

Human, medical, ethical, and political issues

In recent years, all these issues have had a profound effect on the value placed on maternity services and the debate about their future development. Nowadays, women and their partners are better educated. With this change has come the understandable wish to be more involved in what for them is a major life event (Brown and Harris 1978). This has meant a shift from the total responsibility for decision making that the obstetrician used to have, to one of greater equality in the relationship between patient and professional. Advances in technology have led to an improved knowledge of the condition of the fetus. A pregnant woman normally wishes to know the results of all investigations, particularly if there is any threat to the normality of her baby. This leads to a dialogue between her and her obstetrician which has to be conducted with considerable care and sensitivity if misunderstanding and unreasonable anxiety are to be avoided. In some cases, such a dialogue inevitably leads to a decision to deliver the baby prematurely because of the risk of intrauterine death if the pregnancy continues. The best outcome is for the mother and her physician to agree on a course of action, but this does not always happen. What to do next when there is disagreement is an unresolved question (see below).

Then there is the issue as to whether a new investigation or treatment is potentially harmful to the fetus. A decade ago, the remote possibility that physical energy generated in fetal tissues by the high-frequency sound waves emitted during an ultrasound scan is harmful resulted in women in the USA being advised not have scans to determine whether the fetus was normal. More recently, the risk of litigation and lack of evidence of cost-effectiveness have perpetuated this view. Inevitably, this has led to more malformed babies being born, some of whom will survive in a damaged condition.

Litigation (see Chapters 24 and 27) has increasingly been used as a means of solving the problem of incorrect or negligent practice. On the face of it, this would be a logical approach if medicine were an exact science, but it is not. This is well examplified by the issue of cerebral palsy, which it was assumed arose mainly from mismanagement by allowing the fetus to become short of oxygen during labor. After many expensive settlements, Sir Donald Acheson has finally collected the evidence to show that in the great majority of cases cerebral palsy occurs before the onset of labor and that it appears to be unpreventable (see Chapter 24). But all litigation is not wasted, for undoubtedly standards of clinical practice do vary widely. Doctors and midwives in the future will have to pay closer attention than in the past to the standards of personal and corporate care they provide.

Politics also plays a part. Cost is a major factor in determining the quality of maternity services because competition between all specialities for limited funds is an established feature in any modern health service. Issues such as this are now an integral part of the debate between the health managers and the public before change in the maternity services can be brought about. There is a conflict between the family view of birth as an important normal life event against the more general view of politicians, tax payers, insurance companies, and professionals that it is an event where safety and value for money are paramount.

In our egalitarian society, public debate is regarded as entirely acceptable, but there are undoubtedly drawbacks in compromise solutions which attempt to satisfy all parties. The remainder of this chapter is devoted to considering some of these issues and possible solutions.

The human issues—the needs and feelings of pregnant women

Ask a pregnant woman what her priority is and she will most likely say, 'that I should have a normal, healthy baby'. Inquire further and she will say that the experience of pregnancy and delivery should be a happy one. The twin objectives of safety and happiness, if achieved, contribute to the sense of security that most doctors, midwives, and mothers recognize as vital to the well-being of any pregnancy. It is not often that a woman who feels both physically well and has a sense of contentment about her pregnancy has a complicated pregnancy. It must be the primary aim of all who are responsible for maternity services to achieve these objectives.

Much of the debate is over such issues as women's choice in pregnancy, long waiting times in antenatal clinics, thoughtless remarks by doctors or midwives in front of patients, and whether it is a better to deliver a baby at home or in hospital. All these issues are relevant to personal security and happiness. The Parliamentary Social Services Select Committee (1980) and the Parliamentary Health Select Committee (1992) recommended that 'cattle-market' conditions in antenatal clinics should be improved by reducing waiting time at the clinics. The Committee also proposed that the hospital environment in which pregnant women are cared for should be improved by making the decor more homely and less like an operating theatre (Parliamentary Health Select Committee 1992). Today, most maternity units feature soft furnishings and attractive colors in delivery rooms and antenatal clinics. This trend has been accelerated by competition between hospitals to attract new customers, generated by the 'internal market' of the new National Health Service. Increasingly, attention is being paid in maternity units to women's wishes. However, it is less easy to fulfill the pregnant woman's emotional needs for support, counselling, and care than it is to apply paint to a wall.

Who should provide care in pregnancy?

The sense of security that is so important to pregnant women can only be assured by creating a realistic relationship between care givers and the women who come to them. The ability to form such a relationship is one of the underlying strengths of midwives, in both the hospital and the community. This is sometimes assumed to be because most are women, but it is more likely to be that their working practices make them more available for advice and support than obstetricians. In recent years, however, midwives have failed to build on this strength and have continued with rigid working patterns, such as the 8 h shift, which seriously interfere with continuity of care.

Another factor that interferes with continuity is the traditional medical team system of care in British hospitals, which means that the more senior the doctor, the more wide-ranging are his or her responsibilities. As a result, obstetricians continue to have a heavy commitment to gynecology as well. In the USA and most of Western Europe, continuity of care is only achieved by the presence of many obstetricians and a readily available system of private care. In the UK, achievement of this type of care would require a doubling, at least, of specialist obstetricians and a change in the whole system of remuneration. What is needed is a redistribution of the workload through delegated responsibility. At present, consultant obstetricians are responsible for the care of the great majority of pregnant women in the UK. More than 80 per cent of these women have uncomplicated pregnancies. This and the fact that both maternal and perinatal mortality are so low suggest that midwives could and should provide total antenatal and postnatal care for many more women without any loss of safety.

Midwives have demonstrated their ability to provide safe antenatal and delivery care. In the last century, Semmelweiss (1861) observed that maternal deaths in a large maternity hospital in Vienna were twice as high among women admitted under the care of doctors than among women with exactly the same characteristics who were admitted for care by the midwives. In modern practice, with midwives working alongside obstetricians, there is no problem in referring women who develop a pregnancy complication for a medical opinion. A team approach is undoubtedly the most cost-effective form of care under our present Health Service, but if obstetricians are to preserve it they must be prepared to treat midwives as valued colleagues rather than as nurses without responsibility. A well considered and agreed assignment of responsibility by obstetricians within the health care team is the only way of making best use of the skills of midwives.

Home delivery versus hospital delivery

A longstanding and unresolved issue is whether women are best delivered in hospital or at home. Historically, home delivery was extremely hazardous. Hemorrhage and infection associated with childbirth were the major causes of death in young women in the first 30 years of this century. When blood transfusion, antibiotics, and safe cesarean section became available, it was logical to recommend that delivery occur in hospital. But the 'medicalizing' of maternity care was not without drawbacks. Hospitals are a focus for infection; doctors are prone to intervene at the first sign of a threatening complication and a woman feels more secure and in control in her home.

Nevertheless, while hospitalization may have contributed little to the care of women with normal pregnancies, few would question that it has greatly improved the outcome when life-threatening complications are present. It is unfortunate that debate about whether a woman is best delivered at home or in hospital has become such a political issue, polarizing the power struggle between midwives and obstetricians. A home confinement supervised solely by a midwife is not as safe as delivery in hospital if complications arise and it is not always possible to forecast potential problems correctly. However, it is clearly time to re-evaluate the national policy that hospital is the only place where delivery should take place.

Unfortunately, there are few reliable data to refer to, because it is impossible to compare the outcomes for women with low-risk pregnancies who have planned deliveries at home with outcomes of women at high risk who are delivered in hospital (Campbell *et al.* 1979).

Having a baby at home contributes to a sense of security and well-being for some women. It is important to say 'some' women, because not every woman or every partner is prepared to give up the relative safety of hospital for home. Safety is critical to this discussion, because no woman is prepared to accept any avoidable risk to her baby. Any change in the care which is currently given to women can only be implemented if it can be shown that, at the very least, safety for mother and baby is not diminished. Safety can be improved by reproducing in the home the majority of the services available in hospital. These are 24 h midwifery cover with medical back-up and the facilities for dealing with the occasional emergency such as hemorrhage or a baby that is asphyxiated. In theory, given sufficient staff and good communications, this is possible. In reality, the costs of reproducing emergency facilities in each woman's home may be too high for a health service funded by taxes.

The Parliamentary Health Select Committee (1992) commented that small maternity units are no longer an available option for many pregnant women. It recommended that the policy of closing such units should be reversed, as they provided safe care for healthy women near to their homes. There is much to recommend this type of care, providing that safety remains a priority. Small units are likely to be less cost-effective than large maternity units, but they can be justified by both patient satisfaction and ease of access. The study of general practitioner units around Bath in England, cited by the Parliamentary Health Select Committee (1992), showed that careful selection of women in early pregnancy, the commitment of local general practitioners, a good ambulance service, and the full collaboration of the specialist maternity unit in Bath all contributed to the acceptable level of safety in these units. Undoubtedly, many obstetricians and midwives would prefer this type of care to home delivery.

Finally, women ought to have a strong voice in where they have their babies. Women are accustomed to making up their minds but they need the right information to do so. Informed consumerism is high on the political agenda; client bills of rights have been developed in the USA (Bloom and Fischer 1982) and a Citizen's Charter covering rights in dealing with a number of public sector organizations was published by the UK Government in 1991. Doctors should not over-emphasize safety issues to such an extent as to take away a woman's ability to express her view. Similarly, midwives should not minimize safety issues in their desire to be independent from medical influence. If alternatives to a totally hospital-based practice are to be developed, they should only be introduced after advice from doctors, midwives, and consumers. The feminist movement and consumer lobbies such as the National Childbirth Trust in Britain have rightly begun to question what the medical profession does to pregnant women. It is also important that non-intervention (or 'watchful waiting', as it is often called by doctors who are uncomfortable with the idea of simply doing nothing) be studied as much as intervention. Insisting on a non-interventionist approach is no more appropriate than insisting on total intervention.

Ethical issues

Evaluation of screening tests

All maternity units now use screening tests to identify fetal complications and their results have a major influence on clinical decision-making, including whether to terminate a pregnancy when a fetal anomaly is suspected and whether to deliver a fetus early by induction of labor or cesarean section if it is judged in later pregnancy to be in poor condition. Chalmers *et al*. (1989) have questioned the usefulness of some of these tests and interventions. For example, while biophysical assessments ranging from quantification of fetal movements to continuous fetal heart rate monitoring theoretically provide valuable information on development during pregnancy, their clinical accuracy as predictors of the true condition of the fetus has been disappointing (see Chapter 17).

The issues of whether and when to use screening tests and to what degree monitoring in pregnancy is appropriate are debated heatedly on medical, ethical, and political grounds. How reliable should a screening or monitoring test be at detecting abnormality before it is introduced into clinical practice? The answer must include an assessment of costs and benefits. How should a new test be introduced? No screening test should be introduced as routine unless every woman is informed of the implication of agreeing to have it done. To what extent should the parents be involved in further decision making when the result of the test is known? What is the liability of doctors if they recommend a test of doubtful validity or, conversely, if they fail to recommend a test of proven validity?

Pregnant women are often on the receiving end of interventions which have not been scientifically proved beneficial. Would it be appropriate to abandon a conventional practice which is traditionally accepted by doctors as being good for pregnant women? Would it be appropriate to subject the practice to a proper scientific trial, which will involve random allocation of some women to a group which receives the traditional treatment and some to a group which does not? Established ways of practicing are not easily changed. Some age-old customs have in fact been evaluated in randomized controlled trials. Shaving the perineum (Johnston and Sidall 1922; Kantor *et al*. 1965) and giving enemas at the start of labor (Romney and Gordon 1981) have both been shown to confer no benefit—but both are still in widespread practice.

Screening programs that would benefit individuals directly may not be initiated if the results are not important for the community as a whole. An example of this is screening for toxoplasmosis in pregnancy. The parasite *Toxoplasma gondii* can cause fetal infection resulting in severe and lasting neurological damage when the mother contracts the infection for the first time in pregnancy (see Chapter 20).

Screening programs have existed in France and Austria for some time. An initial blood test is done at booking and, if the mother has not had a previous toxoplasma infection, the test is repeated monthly to ensure that any new infection is detected and treated *in utero* or a termination of pregnancy offered if necessary. About 20–25 per cent of French women need repeat testing (*Lancet* editorial 1990). In Britain, about 25 new cases of congenital toxoplasmosis out of more than 600 000 births are reported each year to the British Paediatric Surveillance Unit. This is about half the expected number estimated from data on acute toxoplasma infection in pregnancy and transmission rates (Lancet 1990). Only 20 per cent of women tested in London had previously had toxoplasmosis (Fleck 1969), so a screening programme in the UK would need to test 680 000 women at the start of pregnancy and 540 000 pregnant women in each month of their pregnancy to detect 25–50 cases each year.

The expense of such a program makes it highly unlikely that toxoplasmosis screening will be introduced in the UK, despite vigorous lobbying by well-informed and highly motivated families who have discovered that their child has been damaged by a potentially detectable and treatable disease. The cost per case discovered, however beneficial to the individual family concerned, is simply too high. Greater benefit to the community as a whole may result from spending the same amount of money on other forms of more cost-effective health care. Health education about minimizing the risks of contracting toxoplasmosis during pregnancy is a more cost-effective way of reducing the incidence (RCOG Multidisciplinary Working Group 1992).

Experience with continuous electronic monitoring of the fetal heart rate in labor is another good example of how complex this issue is. When it is used for monitoring all women in labor, there is a rise in the number of cesarean sections performed but no obvious improvement in the fetal death rate than with the much less sensitive method of counting the heart rate with a fetal stethoscope (auscultation). This finding can be interpreted as evidence that the signs of impending fetal death are so obvious that they can be reliably detected by auscultation. However, the largest study of fetal monitoring in labor (Grant 1989) shows that twice as many babies who were monitored by auscultation developed convulsions after birth compared with those who were monitored by continuous fetal heart rate recording. This is evidence that oxygen lack causing fetal brain damage can be detected at an earlier stage by continuous monitoring than by auscultation.

Electronic monitoring also produces a visible record, which is reassuring evidence for the mother that her baby is in good condition. However, it also provides evidence that can be used in litigation if a baby develops cerebral palsy. Although the majority of cerebral palsy cases are not caused by problems during delivery, judges often prefer to give parents the benefit of doubt if a continuous fetal heart trace looks even slightly abnormal (Nelson 1988).

What happens when parents do not value maternity services?

Parents in the UK have a legal obligation to seek professional help for delivery, but bringing the mother and even her family into decision making raises the difficult question of who should have the final word. Undoubtedly, in most areas of medicine, the patient has an inalienable right—although often not exercised—to decide what is done to him or her. In pregnancy, there is a third party, the fetus, for whom the mother speaks. But can she be allowed to override professional advice in a matter of life or death for the fetus? Does she have the right, having a relatively inexpert opinion, to stand out against clear evidence that, for example, unless the fetus is delivered urgently, it will die? This is almost a metaphorical question because such extreme confrontation rarely arises. However, the ethical and legal implications of the rights of the mother to determine the future of her unborn baby are increasingly becoming a part of many aspects of modern clinical practice.

In a case reported in *The Times* (1992) the parents refused permission, on religious grounds, to perform a cesarean section to save the life of a baby that could not be born vaginally because it was in the wrong position. The obstetrician appealed to the High Court, and 'Permission was given to override the mother's wishes, even though she was competent to decide for herself, on the ground that the baby's life might be saved'. This case illustrates the potential for conflict of interest between the mother and her professional advisers. Clearly it is the duty of those who are caring for a woman to gain her confidence by convincing her of the rationale of the proposed management. But what if this were to prove ineffective? Must the obstetricians stand by until the baby dies? In our present society, they probably do, but is this right? Answer must be found for these questions.

In the future, as women have an increasing voice in their medical care, those who are responsible for their care must create a relationship that ensures mutual respect. Routine care from the early stages of pregnancy must include education about issues of choice and the limits of what is possible. Inevitably, some women will not wish to collaborate and their management will present problems for which no easy solution can be found.

Evaluating maternity services

It has never been more important for clinicians to evaluate their practice and to ensure that maternity services are of value. Antenatal investigations and treatment always involve some degree of risk, however small. Good clinical practice must minimize risks for women and their babies and involve the women in decision making so that they can give truly informed consent to procedures. Medical, social, and financial costs of treatment must be balanced against the theoretical and actual advantages for the patient, so that judgements can be based on facts rather than anecdotes from past experience.

Research

If care is to be evaluated scientifically, women who will be asked to participate in randomized trials need to understand the basis of such studies. Unless women agree to enter a trial in which they may be in a non-treatment (control) group, it may not be possible to determine whether a particular type of treatment is effective. Most patients recognize that although such trials will provide little immediate benefit to them, the studies are important to others in the future and out of altruism most will agree to participate. In pregnancy, however, women are anxious about any adverse effects on the baby of trial procedures and they need clear and convincing reassurance on this point. Unless trials take place soon after the introduction of a new technique or technology, both women and their doctors can be misled by untested claims for the new development. It may also be regarded as almost unethical to subject a new untested treatment to controlled trials if it has already been widely introduced.

In the UK, no person entering a research trial in a hospital should be concerned about the safety of the proposed study. Ethics committees exist in every hospital and it is mandatory that any research study involving human subjects is passed by such a committee before the study can start. In addition, permission must be obtained from anyone asked to take part. Having said this, it is unlikely that the system is perfect and it is sensible for anyone asked to take part in a research study to be fully satisfied that all the proposed procedures are entirely safe.

In a trial to determine whether a new form of treatment is effective, it may be difficult to understand the rationale of being assigned to the non-treatment arm. For example, a new treatment was proposed by Mowbray *et al.* (1985) for women with a history of repeated miscarriages. The only way to test whether it was effective was to assign women randomly to either treatment with the active substance (the experimental group) or to treatment with an inactive substance (the control group). The randomization was designed so that neither the women being treated nor the researchers knew which group the woman had been assigned to. All women who came to the clinic for this condition were asked whether they would like to enter the trial. It was explained to them that at that time there was no information on whether the treatment was effective or not. Interestingly, all but one woman agreed to enter the trial, because they were reassured that if the treatment proved to be successful and they had been assigned to the control group they could subsequently be offered the successful treatment. The result was that 72 per cent of the treated women had a successful pregnancy, while only 34 per cent of the control group did. Subsequently, the women in the control group received the treatment with the same benefit as had been found in the trial.

Audit and clinical practice

In an audit of clinical practice, clinicians set standards for their practice, compare what they do in real life to those agreed standards, and then effect changes to correct discrepancies between what happens and the good practice they want to achieve.

Protocols (agreed ways to deal with common problems) are increasingly being used to set standards in maternity services. For example, high blood pressure in pregnancy may be injurious and occasionally fatal to the mother or the baby.

There are numerous ways to treat this condition, but experience from research and the Confidential Enquiry into Maternal Mortality has shown that certain drugs and procedures are preferable. An additional benefit of using practice protocols is that all those working in a maternity unit become more familiar with (and therefore more effective in) the management of conditions covered by a protocol. It is also easier to determine how effective the agreed practice is, which makes it easier to introduce improvements.

In theory, when some aspect of clinical care has been clearly shown to be of little benefit, all professionals would alter their practice. However, attempts to impose change nationally have not been particularly successful. In Canada, a consensus development conference was held to agree to indications for cesarean section, but it was later found (Lomas *et al.* 1989) that even with intensive circulation to practising clinicians knowledge of the guidelines was poor. Cesarean section rates also failed to fall in the USA after the report of the National Consensus Development Conference in 1980 (Gleicher 1984). These experiences suggest that clinicians need to look at their own practice as well as national guidelines in order to find incentives to change.

Paterson *et al.* (1991) have suggested that a database be compiled on all women delivering in a given health region. Rates would be obtained for, say, induction of labor, cesarean section, and forceps deliveries in low-risk women who would be expected to have low rates for such interventions. The figures for individual units would be compared and presented to all obstetricians and midwives whose units had been assessed. Units with higher than normal rates but without clear benefit from the higher rates would be expected to lower their rates. The process would be repeated annually. While some obstetricians might feel their independence was threatened, on the whole the response has been one of approval.

Recommendations for the future

Audit may well prove the best means of achieving change. Effective audit of care should ensure that there is better use of educated professionals in providing maternity care, with more shared care by interested and effective primary care doctors and midwives in antenatal and intrapartum care for low-risk women. This would leave the more specialized obstetricians more time to spend on the investigation, counseling, and management of high-risk pregnancies. Greater use must also be made of consumer opinions in the audit of local care.

At no time has the safety of the pregnant woman and her baby been so assured as it is now. However, the very success of maternity services could lead to a dangerous sense of complacency. The quality of the woman's experience of pregnancy and the avoidance of damage to babies that live are issues that have surfaced only now that maternal and perinatal deaths are so rare. The immediate challenge lies in finding solutions to these issues and in ensuring that maternity services fulfill the expectations and remain valuable to both women and those providing the care.

References

Bloom, M. and Fischer, J. (1982). *Evaluating practice: guidelines for the accountantable professional*. Prentice Hall, Englewood Cliffs.

Brown, G. W. and Harris, T. (1978). *Social origins of depression: a study of psychiatric disorders in women*. Tavistock Publications, London.

Campbell, R., Davies, I. M., MacFarlane, A., and Beral, V. (1979). Home births in England and Wales, 1976 perinatal mortality according to place of delivery. *British Medical Journal* **289**, 721–4.

Chalmers, I., Enkin, M. W., and Kierse, M. J. N. C. (ed.) (1989). *Effective care in pregnancy and childbirth*. Oxford University Press.

Chown, B., Duff., A., James, J., Nation, E., Ellement, M., Buchanan, D., *et al.* (1969). Prevention of primary Rh immunisation: first report of the Western Canadian trial, 1966–8. *Canadian Medical Association Journal*, **100**, 1021.

Clarke, C., Donohoe, W., McConnell, R., Woodrow, J., Finn, R., Krevans, J., *et al.* (1963). Further experimental studies in the prevention of Rh-haemolytic disease. *British Medical Journal*, **i**, 979.

Fleck, D. G. (1969) Toxoplasmosis. *Public Health*, **83**, 131–5.

Gleicher, N. (1984). Cesarean section rates in the United States. The short term failure of the national consensus development conferences in 1980. *Journal of the American Medical Association*, **252**, 3273–6.

Grant, A. (1989). Monitoring the fetus during labour. *Effective Care in Pregnancy and Childbirth*, Vol. 2, (ed. I. Chalmers, M. W. Enkin, and M. J. N. C. Keirse), pp. 846–82. Oxford University Press.

Infant Mortality Committee (1870). *Transaction of the Obstetricians Society of London*, **II**, (for 1869), 132–49.

Johnston, R. A. and Sidall, R. S. (1922). Is the usual method of preparing patients for delivery beneficial or necessary? *American Journal of Obstetrics and Gynecology*, **4**, 645–50.

Kantor, H. I., Rember, R., Tabio, P., and Buchanon R. (1965). Value of shaving the pudendal-perineal area in delivery preparation. *Obstetrics and Gynecology*, **25**, 509–12.

Lancet editorial (1990). Antenatal screening for toxoplasmosis in the UK. *Lancet*, **ii**, 346–7.

Lomas, J., Anderson, G. M., Domnick-Pierre, K., Vayda, E., Enkin, M. W., and Hannah W. J. (1989). Do practice guidelines guide practice? *New England Journal of Medicine*, **321**, 1306–11.

Mowbray, J. F., Gibbings, C. R., Liddell, H., Reginald, P. W., Underwood, J. L., and Beard, R. W. (1985). Controlled trial of treatment of recurrent spontaneous abortion by immunisation with paternal cells. *Lancet*, **i**, 941–3.

Nelson, K. (1988). What proportion of cerebral palsy is related to birth asphyxia? *Journal of Pediatrics*, **112**, 572–4.

Parliamentary Health Select Committee (1992). *Maternity Services* Second report, Vol. I, Session 1991–92. HMSO, London.

Parliamentary Social Services Select Committee (1980). *Perinatal and neonatal mortality*. Second Report, Vol. 1, Session 1979–80. HMSO, London.

Paterson, C. M., Chapple, J. C., Beard, R. W., Joffe, M., Steer, P. J., and Wright, C. S. W. (1991). Evaluating the quality of maternity services—a discussion paper. *British Journal of Obstetrics and Gynaecology*, **98**, 1073–8.

Peel, J. (1970). *Report of the sub-committee on domiciliary midwifery and maternity needs*.

Standing Maternity and Midwifery Advisory Committee to the Department of Health and Social Security, Welsh Office. HMSO, London.

Pharaoh, P. O. D. (1986). Perspective and Patterns. *British Medical Bulletin*, **42**, 119–26.

RCOG Multidisciplinary Working Group (1992). *Prenatal screening for toxoplasmosis in the UK*. Royal College of Obstetricians and Gynaecologists, London.

Romney, M. L. and Gordon, H. (1981). Is your enema really necessary? *British Medical Journal*, **282**, 1269–71.

Semmelweiss, I. P. (1861). *Die Aetiologie, der Begrieff und die Prophylaxis der Kindbettsiebers*. Pest, Hartleban. *The Times* (1992). 14 October, p. XX.

Wald, N. J., Kennard, A., Densem, J. W., Cuckle, H. S., Chard, T., and Butler, L. (1992). Antenatal Maternal serum screening for Down's Syndrome: results of a demonstration project. *British Medical Journal*, **305 (6850)**, 391–4.

15 Maternal morbidity and mortality

Allan Rosenfield

There have been extraordinary advances in health care in the industrial countries of Europe, North America, and Japan since the turn of the century, with particularly dramatic declines in both infant mortality rates and maternal mortality ratios*. But these advances have been slow to spread to the poorer developing countries of Asia, Latin America, and Africa. This has especially been the case with women's health care generally and with maternity care more specifically. As a result, there is a very significant differential in maternal mortality ratios, even greater than the differential in infant mortality rates, between the developed and developing world. The maternal mortality ratio in rural areas of a poor developing country may be as high as 1000 per 100 000 live births, as compared with ratios in Europe and North America of between eight and 15 per 100 000 live births. What makes this situation so tragic is the fact that the vast majority of pregnancy-related deaths are preventable with relatively inexpensive existing technologies (Rosenfield 1989; Rosenfield and Maine 1985; UNICEF 1989).

Maternal mortality in the developed world, 1700 to the present

Before detailing the situation in the developing world today, it is instructive to review the past in developed countries. Some of the most relevant historical information on maternal mortality comes from Sweden, where mortality levels were reviewed from 1751 to 1980, with a primary focus on changes that took place before 1900 (Hogberg and Wall 1986). In 1751, the estimated maternal mortality was greater than 800 per 100 000 live births, a ratio not very different from that estimated for many developing countries today. According to the notably reliable Swedish data, mortality levels fell dramatically during the period under assessment, particularly in the period from 1861 to 1900, long before modern obstetrical intervention was introduced.

*Maternal mortality ratio is the number of pregnancy-related deaths per 100 000 live births; the term maternal mortality rate, often incorrectly used in place of ratio, refers to pregnancy-related deaths per 100 000 women of reproductive age, 15–45.

Interestingly, the Swedish Board of Health in 1751 stated that '. . . out of 651 women dying in childbirth, at least 400 could have been saved if only there were enough midwives'. By 1861, the ratio is estimated to have fallen to a level of about 567 per 100 000 live births. In the following 40 year period ending in 1900, it fell further to an estimated level of 227 per 100 000 live births.

Two interventions are described as having had the major impact on these falling ratios before the advent of modern obstetrics: the first was the introduction of aseptic techniques and the second was the introduction of trained and licensed midwives.

The introduction of aseptic techniques in the late 1800s had a direct impact in reducing infection rates. This was recognized as being of particular importance because in the new maternity hospitals created in Sweden in the late eighteenth century, the incidence of sepsis was extraordinarily high, often resulting in the deaths of both mother and infant. In 1864–1880, one out of 35 women delivering in the hospital died of sepsis, compared with only one out of 1124 women delivering at home during that time (maternal mortality ratios of 2700 per 100 000 and 89 per 100 000, respectively).

The problems of hospital-related sepsis, seen often during that period, provided some of the most dramatic examples of iatrogenic disease and mortality in medical history. As aseptic techniques were introduced into Swedish hospitals, these rates fell by 1895 to 96 per 100 000. A specific innovation, for example, was introduced in 1881, when a law was passed that required health professionals involved in caring for patients to use carbolic acid to disinfect their hands and instruments. During this same period, mortality due to sepsis also fell in home deliveries to a level of 33 per 100 000, with no apparent reason being noted.

Although Holmes (in 1843) and Semmelweiss (in 1844) are generally credited with introducing the concept of puerperal sepsis, in 1768 a physician named Denman wrote that a disease is carried by a physician or midwife from one parturient to another and White in 1772 wrote that the discharges of septic women were contagious. The most definitive work was by Gordon who, in 1795, wrote that 'this disease seized women only as they were visited by a nurse who had previously attended patients affected with the disease.'

Despite these farsighted writings in the eighteenth century and the work of Holmes and Semmelweiss in the middle of the nineteenth century, not until towards the end of that century did Swedish medicine and law take note of this knowledge. Swedish recognition of the importance of sepsis preceded attention to the issue in the UK and the USA, where maternal mortality rates remained high (427 and 600 per 100 000, respectively) at the turn of the century.

The second intervention contributing to a reduction in mortality rates during this period was the formal training and licensing of midwives, who practiced widely throughout Sweden. By the early 1800s, the midwives were taught to use forceps for delivery and sharp hooks and perforators to remove an already dead baby in cases of severe obstructed labor. Although available data suggests that the midwives did not use these techniques often, in some instances they almost certainly made it possible to save the life of a woman who otherwise would have died.

Records from the late sixteenth century in an English parish suggest maternal mortality ratios as high as 2300 per 100 000 live births (Dobbie 1982). These ratios must be gross estimates; universal reporting of deaths was unlikely, a problem that hinders research in developing countries today. But due to the influence of the clergy and others, unusually complete village-based data systems were established in some parts of England and Europe during the seventeenth and eighteenth centuries. Review of the available data reveals an excess mortality among women aged 15–49 compared with men of the same age group and the difference was related to pregnancy-related deaths. Similar findings have been noted more recently in Bangladesh, India, Pakistan, and Sri Lanka.

What is striking in reviewing the past is that conditions found in much of the developing world today existed in the USA and Europe at the turn of the century. As recently as 1946, Klein and Clahr (1958) described a maternal mortality ratio of 116 per 100 000 live births in New York City, a ratio that fell to 40 per 100 000 over the next 10 years, primarily through reductions in mortality from infection, hemorrhage, heart disease, and anesthesia. Although control of infection played perhaps the single most important role in this decline, as late as 1956 infections remained a leading cause of mortality because of sepsis related to illegal abortions.

Careful studies by the Committee on Maternal Mortality of the Massachusetts Medical Society, initiated in 1941, traced the decline in mortality in Massachusetts from 50 per 100 000 live births in 1954 to 10 per 100 000 live births in 1985. From 1954 to 1957, the leading causes of maternal mortality were infection, cardiac disease, pregnancy-induced hypertension, and hemorrhage. From 1982 to 1985, the leading cause was pulmonary embolus, plus non-pregnancy-related trauma (accidents, homicides, and suicides). The decreases were due to both legislative actions (licensing of maternity services, blood banks, and, probably of greatest importance, the legalization of abortion) and improvements in medical practice (antibiotic therapy, aggressive treatment of toxemia, and prompt replacement of blood in cases of hemorrhage).

One factor taken for granted in the analysis of maternal mortality in the West is that almost 100 per cent of pregnant women either deliver in an institutional setting or have rapid access to such a facility in case of complications in a home delivery. Recent data from Sweden, for example, demonstrate that the declines in maternal mortality ratios during the twentieth century have been even more dramatic than those in the nineteenth century, reaching a level of 6 per 100 000 live births in 1980 (Hogberg and Wall 1986).

Monitoring maternal mortality

The UK has a system to review in detail all maternal deaths. The findings are published in a triennial report entitled, *Confidential inquiries into maternal deaths*. This system was begun in England and Wales in 1952 by the Department of Health and Social Services. The most recent report (1985–1987) for the first time included all cases that occured in England, Wales, Scotland, and Northern Ireland (Hau 1990). The definition of maternal death in the UK is now in line with the international definition in that it includes only deaths that occured within 42 days of the delivery.

The maternal mortality ratio in the UK has fallen from 67.1 per 100 000 births in 1955–1957 to 7.6 per 100 000 births in 1985–1987. Direct deaths (resulting from obstetric complications) were 15 per cent lower in 1985–1987 than in 1982–1984.

The three leading causes for maternal death in the UK were thrombosis and thromboembolism, hypertensive disorders in pregnancy, and early pregnancy deaths including abortions. The importance of the confidential inquiries lies in the detailed recommendations made by the departments of health on each leading cause of maternal death. Not only does the report refer to clinical measures that should be taken, but also issues such as access and organization of the health care system. An example of a clinical recommendation is the prevention of early pregnancy deaths through the widespread availability of highly sensitive pregnancy tests. An example of a policy change is the establishment of expert regional teams capable of advising or accepting the care of any woman with severe preeclampsia or eclampsia.

In the USA there is no equivalent of this confidential inquiry into maternal deaths. Over the years monitoring of maternal deaths has has been accomplished through vital records or state-run maternal mortality committees. Without autopsy results or at least in-depth reviews of medical records, vital records can only provide a very superficial impression of the causes of maternal death. In addition state-run maternal mortality committees have largely disappeared, in part because of the relatively rare occurance of maternal deaths and because of the perception, which may be in error, that information gained by maternal mortality review committees may be used in malpractice litigation.

For a number of reasons a mechanism needs to be established in the USA for monitoring maternal mortality. First we need to understand why there is an almost 4-fold difference in maternal mortality between White and Black women (7.8 vs 20.4 per 100 000 live births in 1985). This difference is even greater than that seen for infant mortality. Understanding it will mean that new public health programs can be set up. Regular review also permits a continued assessment of the impact of any new public health measures introduced. Second, there have been a significant number of new practices introduced into obstetrics, for example, the widespread use of tocolytic agents to treat premature labor and the rise in the number of women electing to try for a vaginal delivery following a prior cesarean section. Both of these examples have risks; tocolytic agents are associated with pulmonary edema and women undergoing trial of labor have a risk of ruptured uteri. As deaths from either cause are probably rare, by collecting cases across the country and reviewing them carefully, safety measures may be introduced. As maternal mortality is usually the tip of a much larger iceberg of maternal morbidity, the implications of any new measures are multipled greatly.

In the USA there are approximately 350 maternal deaths per year. This compares with 265 cases reviewed between 1985 and 1987 in the UK. A detailed review of 1 year in the USA would provide sufficient cases to analyse problems and examine trends. This would only need to be carried out every 3–5 years. With national birth and death-linked vital records registration, there will probably be almost complete ascertainment of cases for later pregnancy-related deaths. Complete ascertainment of first trimester cases, however, may be more difficult even though most states require notification if the woman was pregnant at time of death.

Maternal mortality and morbidity in the developing world

In the past, health professionals working in developing countries devoted most of their attention to eradicating various communicable infectious and parasitic infestations and to improving sanitation and the clean water supply. More recently, a great deal of attention has been given to the 'child survival' movement, which focuses on interventions to reduce the current high rates of infant and childhood mortality. There are as many as 14 million deaths each year among children under the age of 5 from essentially preventable or treatable conditions. Child survival interventions—which include the management of diarrheal disease and immunizations against the most common of the communicable diseases—are all of high priority. Indeed, the World Health Organization (WHO) and the United Nations Children's Fund (UNICEF), together with ministries of health throughout the world, have set a goal of 'Health for all by the year 2000', with an emphasis on delivery of simple primary-care services to under-served children (WHO and UNICEF 1978).

The health status of women of reproductive age in developing countries, however, has until recently been given a notable lack of attention and priority in almost all discussions of health problems in poor countries. This is extraordinary, since it has been recognized for many years that maternal mortality rates are extremely high in most developing countries, not only in rural areas but in urban slums as well. This lack of attention to maternal health is particularly surprising and sad in light of the fact that approximately 500 000 women die world-wide each year from pregnancy-related causes and the vast majority—over 98 per cent—of these deaths take place in developing countries (WHO 1987). Chapter 13 discusses ways in which this is now being addressed.

Recently, the concept of lifetime risk of maternal death has come into use. This results from the risk of death in a pregnancy, multiplied by the number pregnancies a woman has. Whereas infant mortality describes a risk of which the baby is exposed for 1 year only, lifetime risk of maternal death takes into account the fact that a woman's risk of death is repeated each time she becomes pregnant.

The number of maternal deaths each year is significantly greater than the number of annual deaths from AIDS, this century's most tragic epidemic. But unlike AIDS, for which no curative therapy is yet available, the vast majority of pregnancy-related deaths are preventable. The dramatic neglect of the health and well-being of women clearly raises ethical questions. Some feminists have suggested that were there such a preventable cause of death among men, the situation long ago would have received far greater attention and priority.

The world's public health professionals and obsterician–gynecologists have not given priority to this problem until very recently, however. Clinicians in the developing world have been concerned with providing services for the minority of women who present themselves for care, while academicians have focused on subspecialty technological interventions in obstetrics and gynecology. The relatively small number of obstetrician–gynecologists have not had the time or perhaps the interest to investigate the problems posed by the lack of access to maternity care experienced by the majority of women in their countries.

Until recently, the triennial meetings of the International Federation of Gynecologists and Obstetricians (FIGO) gave almost no attention to this issue, other than to review maternal mortality surveillance in developed countries, as exemplified by the outstanding work of the Massachusetts Maternal Mortality Committee (Sachs *et al.* 1987). At the 1985 FIGO meeting in Berlin, only a small number of sessions were devoted to maternal mortality in developing countries and these were poorly attended; the key session drew approximately 150–200 people. At the same meeting, a special lecture on *in vitro* fertilization (IVF) drew thousands of physicians, many of them from developing countries. While IVF is truly an exciting and extraordinary technological advance, the estimated 500 000 deaths of women world-wide per year need attention first. Appropriately, however, at FIGO meetings in Rio de Janeiro and Singapore, the issue of maternal mortality was highlighted.

Since 1987, the World Bank and WHO have given much greater attention than in the past to maternal mortality, initially through sponsorship of the 1987 Safe Motherhood meeting in Nairobi, Kenya (Measham and Herz 1987). Halfdan Mahler, until 1989 the Director General of WHO, gave a keynote address that clearly summarized a history of tragic neglect and stressed the importance of finding ways to lower the rates of mortality (Mahler 1987). At the same conference in Nairobi, a paper by Kwast (1987) of WHO was circulated which presented a series of case reports of recent maternal deaths. To provide a clearer understanding of the many factors that contribute to maternal deaths in developing countries, a few case reports follow here. The names have been changed, but the cases are real ones reported to WHO.

Case reports

Obstructed labor, Nigeria

Bola, aged 17 and her husband were farmers in a remote village in Nigeria. They had no formal education and their house had no electricity, no water supply, and no modern sanitation facilities. Bola was married at the age of 13. Her first child was born dead after 4 days of difficult obstructed labor, with a resultant vesicovaginal fistula. The consequences of this—incontinence of urine and constant odor—almost ended her marriage, but she was fortunate to have reconstructive surgery at a hospital far from her home. Two years later she again became pregnant, but living very far from any maternity care facility she had no prenatal care. After early rupture of her membranes, she eventually went into labor, but did not progress for 3 days. Finally, the family took her the long distance to the nearest hospital, a trip of several hours. The baby had already died and she was febrile and acutely ill with infection and a ruptured uterus. Despite heroic efforts at the hospital, she died.

Postpartum hemorrhage, Yemen

Fatima, who was 27, lived in a remote village on the top of a steep hill. Her husband, Mohammed, worked as a laborer in Saudi Arabia. Fatima had had five girls, whom she had delivered safely in the village and since the nearest health station was a 2 h walk away, she had received no prenatal care. She had a very short sixth labor, delivering in less than a half hour after her membranes had ruptured. The placenta did not deliver as it had in previous pregnancies. Initially, there was little bleeding, but bleeding soon became very heavy and the family became concerned, particularly as Fatima became increasingly weak. Yemen culture required a husband's permission to go to the hospital, but since Mohammed was out of the country another male relative was sought to give permission. However, it took 2 h to find her uncle in a neighboring village. A stretcher was then made and several men began the long trip down the hill and then another 15 km along the road to a main road, where they hoped to flag down a vehicle to take them the last 40 km to the hospital. When they got to the bottom of the hill, they noticed the stretcher covered with blood and Fatima lying very quietly, apparently sleeping. Soon, however, they realized that she had died—the delays were simply too long.

Illegal abortion, Colombia

Esperanza, age 30, had already had five children. Neither she nor her husband wanted another child and they were upset when she again became pregnant. She had received maternal and child health care at a nearby health care center, but they did not offer family planning advice or services and Esperanza did not know about the private family planning clinic in Bogota. She had recently found a job as a house maid in the city and the wages she earned were badly needed by the family. She decided on her own to obtain an illegal abortion. She did not know exactly what the abortionist had done, but it was painful and resulted in much bleeding. After 3 days, the bleeding decreased, but she developed a fever and abdominal pain and began to vomit. Her husband took her to the hospital, where she received antibiotics for 2 days and then was discharged home. The pain returned, but Esperanza was afraid she would lose her job if she took more time off. However, her symptoms worsened and she was readmitted to the hospital where she soon went into irreversible shock. Despite a laparotomy, she died.

These three cases are typical of the pregnancy-related deaths that are tragically common in many parts of the developing world today. The problem is particularly acute in rural areas, because in many countries, most of the physicians, trained midwives, nurses, and hospitals are located in the larger urban areas, with few such resources available in the rural areas (Measham and Herz 1987). In many countries, the capital city has a large, modern, tertiary care hospital which uses an inordinate percentage of the country's total health budget but which is accessible to only a very small percentage of its population. Inequitable distribution of health resources is one of the greatest problems in many developing countries.

Causes of maternal mortality in the developing world

In all the studies from the developing world, the causes of morbidity and mortality are similar, although the ranking may vary. The five major causes of maternal deaths include obstructed labor (complicated by ruptured uterus), postpartum hemorrhage, pregnancy-induced hypertension, postpartum sepsis, and complications from illegal abortion. In addition, certain medical conditions may be exacerbated by pregnancy, such as heart disease, diabetes, hypertension, and certain chronic tropical diseases.

Discussion of the problem of maternal morbidity and mortality in the developing world is hampered by the absence of good data (Rosenfield 1989; Royston 1989). In most developing countries, the vital registration system (for example, birth and death certificates) is poorly developed. Deaths in rural areas are grossly under-reported and when reports are made, the cause of death is often absent since the reports usually originate from untrained villagers. Most published reports about maternal deaths come from hospital studies, but these are limited to data on patients that come to the hospital; it is probable that many women who die in many countries never make it to a hospital, particularly those who live in rural areas. Depending on the country, anywhere from 40 per cent (in many Latin American countries) to over 80 per cent (in sub Saharan Africa and Indian subcontinent countries) live in under-served rural areas and deliver their babies without any modern prenatal care, in their home with a traditional birth attendant, a relative, or in some cases no-one in attendance at the time of delivery.

Royston and Ferguson (1989) of WHO have estimated, from a variety of sources, that close to half of the 128 million infants born in 1983 were born in the home, with the percentage being highest in subSaharan African countries and such Asian countries as Bangladesh, Pakistan, Afghanistan, Nepal, and parts of India.

Kwast *et al.* (1986) conducted a detailed survey of all the women aged 13–49 in 32 215 households in Addis Ababa, Ethiopia to obtain pregnancy outcome data over a 2 year period (1981–1983). There were 45 pregnancy-related deaths among the 9315 pregnancies identified during the 2 year period, for a maternal mortality ratio of 566 per 100 000 live births. Mortality in this urban study was highest among unmarried nullipara, students, and women employed as housemaids. (In contrast, in rural areas it is likely that a majority of pregnancy-related deaths occur among high-parity married women.) The most common cause was complications of illegal abortions (54 per cent), a not uncommon finding in studies of urban populations in the developing world. In a hospital-based study in Lagos, Nigeria, 51 per cent of maternal deaths in a predominantly urban population also were due to abortion complications (Akingba 1977).

In a survey of 60 developing countries conducted by the International

Planned Parenthood Federation in the late 1970s, Rochat *et al.* (1980) found approximately 207 induced abortions per 1000 live births, an unexpectedly high rate considering that abortion is illegal in most of the countries surveyed. From data collected, the authors estimated that in the 60 countries studied, somewhere between 70 000 and 100 000 maternal deaths each year were due to complications of abortion—an extraordinary toll among predominantly poor women desperate not to have another child. More recent estimates from WHO, however, suggest between 60 000 and 100 000 abortion-related deaths annually, although some consider this an underestimate (WHO 1994).

Studies in the relatively developed city of Harare, Zimbabwe suggest that more than 15 per cent of all pregnancies end in incomplete abortions, with varying estimates as to the percentage of these that were induced (Crowther and Verkuyl 1985; Crowther 1986). In a study in Ghana of obstetrical patients who had undergone at least one previous hospital delivery, 20 per cent had had at least one induced abortion (Lamptey *et al.* 1985). At the University Teaching Hospital in Lusaka, Zambia, 26 per cent of 27 maternal deaths were results of induced abortion and ectopic pregnancy (Narone *et al.* 1983). At the same hospital, between 1977 and 1980, 12 096 patients were admitted with the diagnosis of 'spontaneous' abortion; there was no indication of what percentage of these were actually induced. In a report from the major hospital in Nairobi, abortion-related complications accounted for 60 per cent of acute gynecological beds, while in Durban, South Africa, 19 per cent of all maternal deaths were secondary to illegal abortion (Aggarwal and Mati 1982; Melrose 1984). Unpublished reports from the Kenyatta National Hospital in Nairobi suggest that as many as 30–40 induced abortion patients are admitted daily, an extraordinary figure if true.

Rochat *et al.* (1981) conducted interviews in 63 hospitals and 732 non-hospital facilities in Bangladesh during 1978–1979 to investigate maternal and abortion-related deaths. The authors identified 1933 pregnancy-related deaths, of which 26 were secondary to abortion complications. With an overall estimate of 500–600 maternal deaths per 100 000 live births per year, they estimated that there were 21 600 maternal deaths in Bangladesh annually, of which 5573 were secondary to abortion.

Klein and Clahr (1958), in their report on the decline of maternal mortality rates in New York City from 1946 to 1956, concluded that the inability to bring the maternal mortality rate below 40 per 100 000 was largely due to the continuing contribution of abortion, in the era when abortion was still illegal in the USA.

In Latin America, Fortney (1981) reports that septic abortion accounts for a disproportionate share of the funds spent on transfusions and operating room costs, as well as the total bed-nights. It is estimated by many that abortion is the number one cause of maternal mortality in Latin America. In South Africa (Barford and Parker 1977) and India (Lahiri and Konar 1976), approximately 45 per cent of all abortion deaths occur in high-parity women (parity five or more). Anecdotal data from Brazil suggest that between 2.5 and 4 million abortions are performed annually. The number of deaths is unknown, but is thought to be very high.

It is sad commentary that so many women in so many countries where abortion remains illegal still go to great extremes to obtain one, no matter what the risk to their lives. There is evidence, albeit primarily anecdotal, that educated middle-and upper middle-class women generally have access to safe abortions, regardless of the legality, while it is predominantly the poor who resort to highly unsafe illegal procedures.

The issue really is not whether abortions should be legal but whether they will be safe or unsafe. Obstetrician–gynecologists throughout the world have a moral responsibility to initiate a policy change. Women throughout history have attempted to end unwanted pregnancies, often in desperation. Physicians can no longer ignore the fact that when abortions cannot be obtained legally, maternal morbidity and mortality rates from abortions increase dramatically. Physicians have, in general, simply accepted and treated the women who resorted to illegal abortions, ignoring a moral duty to articulate the underlying problems and advocate essential policy changes.

Overall, hospital-based studies on maternal mortality paint a dismal picture (Harrison 1979; Mtimavalye *et al.* 1980; Boerma 1987; Brown 1987). Information from such studies, as well as from studies reported earlier, tends to confirm estimated maternal mortality ratios of between 500 and 1000 per 100 000 live births. And, as data from a number of both developed and developing countries have demonstrated, the reporting systems of most countries under-report maternal deaths by as much as 50 per cent (Maine *et al.* 1987). It appears that in poor countries as many as 21–46 per cent of deaths among women aged 15–49 are pregnancy-related, compared to about 1 per cent in the USA.

In one rural study in Gambia, a mortality rate of over 2000 per 100 000 live births was noted; postpartum hemorrhage and infection were identified as the leading cause of death in this country (Sherton *et al.* 1989). The groups at highest risk were found to be women under 20 and over 40 years old and those who had had multiple pregnancies. In a classic detailed study in Zaria, Nigeria, Harrison (1985) found 219 maternal deaths among 7654 women seen for the first time in labor, compared with 19 deaths among 15 020 women who had prenatal care through the hospital in Zaria; the death rate among the women who had had prenatal care was still high but was dramatically lower than that seen among patients who were 'unbooked'. In a US study of a religious group which refused any modern medical care, a maternal mortality ratio of 872 per 100 000 was noted in the 1980s, a rate lower than the worst seen in the developing world but comparable to overall figures for many developing countries (Kaunitz *et al.* 1984).

Ectopic pregnancies are particularly subject to under-reporting since many rural women never get to a medical facility. From several different studies, Lettenmaier *et al.* (1988) estimate that there can be anywhere between seven and 30 ectopic pregnancies per 1000 deliveries. A study in Benin City in Nigeria concluded that 15 per cent of all gynecological admissions were for ectopic pregnancies (Oronsaye and Odiase 1981). The role of infection varies greatly, but in all studies it is an important factor.

Obstructed labor is of particular importance in African countries, in part because there are so many very young women who are pregnant and also because there is a relatively high incidence of narrow anthropoid pelves (Lawson and Stewart 1967). Harrison (1985), in his Zaria study, suggests that 18–20 per cent of pregnant women had problems secondary to obstructed labor.

Interventions and lessons learned

Overall, as Harrison (1985) and others have written, education of women and general improvements in their status are of key importance in improving women's health. These developmental goals require much higher priority throughout the world. The following discussion, however, will focus on specific interventions that affect maternal health.

A major lesson from the experience of the developed world in the nineteenth and early twentieth century is that aseptic technique plays a key role in reducing maternal mortality. This is important in both hospital and home deliveries (Hogberg and Wall 1986). Traditional birth attendants in many countries have undergone training programs and, clearly, a major focus should be to instill in them an understanding and appreciation of the importance of asepsis. Unfortunately, however, this training has proven to have little impact on maternal mortality rates in most settings because they are able to do little at village level for the major life-threatening complications of pregnancy. Postpartum hemorrhage, obstructed labor, and eclampsia, for example, require emergency obstetrical care in a hospital, as do the more serious complications of a botched abortion. Thus, access to emergency care is essential.

Much greater attention should be given to provision of health education at the community level, so that women and their families have a better understanding of the various warning signs that mean assistance should be sought. In hospital reports on maternal deaths, there are repeated comments on the long delays between the onset of signs of problems and the decision to seek help at a hospital. Unfortunately, the delays may often be more related to distance, difficult access, or fears about costs than to the lack of understanding that a problem exists.

An overwhelming problem in many rural areas is simply the fact that maternity care services are much too far away to be truly accessible to a majority of women. To teach traditional birth attendants or the women themselves the signs that warrant referral, when referral is almost impossible, creates major problems. For example, if a woman of parity greater than five is at high risk of a complication, particularly postpartum hemorrhage, what should she do if she lives 2 or more hours from the nearest hospital or maternity care facility? Once labor has begun, it generally is too late for the woman to move, because higher parity labors are usually shorter than lower parity ones.

In a few countries, there are maternity waiting homes adjacent to a hospital, where a woman can come in the last weeks of her pregnancy to await the onset of labor, assuming that she has been able to arrange for someone else care for her other children (Rosenfield and Maine 1985). The maternity home concept, where facilities and personnel are limited, is attractive, at least for purposes of assessing the effectiveness of such an approach.

Some of the African women at high risk of obstructed labor (for example, those with very short stature or obvious bony pelvic abnormality), who are unlikely to be delivered in an institutional setting, have had symphysiotomies performed in early pregnancy to facilitate a safer home delivery (Lawson and Stewart 1967). This does not appear to be an active practice at present.

In the long run the solution to the problem of maternal deaths lies in the development of networks with the capability of providing blood transfusions and performing emergency cesarean sections. WHO prepared an excellent report on first-level facilities, suggesting the steps needed to increase access to such care WHO 1987). Since the majority of women in many countries today do not have access to such simple facilities, upgrading—while expensive—is of the highest priority so as to increase access. The key to such a plan, however, is not just the building of facilities but the provision of sufficient budgets to pay for the necessary personnel, equipment, and supplies on a continuing basis. Facilities are available in some rural areas, but they have insufficient equipment and supplies, not to mention properly trained personnel. Eventually, all women should be able to deliver in a well-equipped facility, or, at a minimum, have ready access to such a facility. If low-risk women, after appropriate screening, continue to deliver at home, they should be delivered by well-trained personnel.

Another significant problem is that there simply are insufficient physicians, in general and obstetricians, specifically, to staff the first-level referral facilities in rural areas. Nordberg (1984) has estimated that in East Africa, only 10 per cent of women needing a cesarean section for a maternal indication receive one. Most of those not having the procedure suffer from severe morbidity and a high rate of mortality. Where general physicians are available in the absence of surgeons, they should be trained to do simple operations such as appendectomy, herniorrhaphy, and cesarean section. Where there are dramatic shortages of physicians, there have been calls to allow other personnel to be trained in procedures which non-physicians are usually not permitted to perform (Rosenfield 1974; Smith 1984).

White *et al.* (1987) have reported a very important experience from two rural hospitals in Zaire. These hospitals serve as referral centers for the surrounding rural communities and provide obstetrical services for women who often arrive very late for care. In the 1950s, because of severe understaffing of physicians, a pioneer missionary, Dr Wallace Thornbloom, first trained local nurses to serve as emergency surgeons able to perform cesarean sections. In 1984, the role of such trained nurses was expanded to include repair of ruptured uteri, emergency supracervical hysterectomy, laparotomy for ruptured ectopic pregnancy, symphysiotomy, and suction curettage. In an 18 month period in 1985–1986, nurses at the two hospitals performed 310 emergency cesarean sections, primarily for obstructed labor, uterine inertia, previous cesarean section, placenta previa, and in a few cases for fetal distress. There were only three deaths among these 310 women, a remarkable record, particularly given the long delays in arrival at the hospital and the resultant poor condition of many of the women. It is fair to say that without these procedures, a high proportion of these women would have died.

The experience in doing laparotomies for other emergency situations is newer. Three such laparotomies by nurses at one of the hospitals, in which supracervical hysterectomies were performed for ruptured uteri, resulted in one death (from septic shock during surgery); two women survived who otherwise would certainly have died. This experience in Zaire is a dramatic demonstration of what is possible if unconventional approaches are followed when conventional ones are impossible.

Community interventions

In the child survival movement, strategies have been developed for village-level interventions such as immunization programs and provision of oral rehydration fluids (WHO UNICEF 1978). For maternal mortality, such community interventions are more difficult because of the nature of the conditions needing treatment. Nevertheless, in the short run, there are steps that can be taken without having to wait for the establishment of a network of first-level referral facilities (Rosenfield 1989; UNICEF 1989).

One such important community-level intervention is family planning (Rosenfield and Maine 1985). Women at very young ages (less than 17), at older ages (over 35) and, perhaps most importantly, women having their fifth or higher child, are all at increased risk of death during pregnancy. Therefore, effective family planning services, which can be delivered at village level, can have an impact on maternal mortality rates in this group, as well as on the very large numbers of women who have stated in fertility surveys that they do not want any more children than they already have (Cleland *et al.* 1987).

However, in reviewing the five major causes of deaths during pregnancy (obstructed labor and ruptured uterus, postpartum hemorrhage, pregnancy-induced hypertension, postpartum infection, and septic abortion), it becomes apparent that there is not a great deal that can be done for most of these complications other than referral to a first-level facility, if such a facility is readily available. The following are some possible strategies, most of which have not yet been carefully assessed.

At village level, traditional birth attendants and women themselves need to understand the signs of obstructed labor; no matter how far the nearest referral facility, there often is time to get there if the decision to move is taken before 24 h of labor have passed.

Postpartum hemorrhage is most common in high-parity women and unfortunately usually cannot be predicted in advance. When it does occur, the bleeding can quickly become very extensive. This means that very few women in a rural setting will survive a trip to a distant facility. Traditional birth attendants and others can be taught to carry out effective uterine massage and the proper means for removing a retained placenta. While controversial, a case can be made for the provision of ergotrate or oxytocic drugs (which cause uterine contractions) at village level for use with a special checklist. The obvious danger is that oxytoxics might be used during a difficult labor and increase the risk of a ruptured uterus. Making such drugs available would require a well-designed and supervised training program, so that traditional birth attendants would fully understand the risks of using such drugs in all circumstances except as indicated on the check-list. There is little if any experience in the provision of such drugs at village level, and further study is needed.

There is little that can be done for pregnancy-related hypertension at the village level other than to recommend bed-rest and possibly the use of sedatives. Once severe pre-eclampsia or convulsions have occurred, the woman will almost certainly die unless she can be moved to a first-level referral facility.

The use of careful sterile techniques can do much to decrease the incidence of puerperal sepsis and traditional birth attendants in many countries have been so trained. It might be possible to train them to use a broad spectrum antibiotic for women who have had ruptured membranes for longer than 12 or 18 h. The chance of infection rises the longer the membranes are ruptured before delivery, so early introduction of an antibiotic could be beneficial. Provision of antibiotics by traditional birth attendants needs to be studied. Similarly, they should be trained to do as few vaginal examinations as possible during labor and should understand that when such examinations are done, careful asepsis is essential.

Legalization of abortion is the most controversial of all issues within the field of reproductive health. Clearly, the prevention of the need for an abortion through the practice of family planning should be encouraged. However, as the experience of the USA has shown, even widespread availability of contraceptive services does not do away with the demand for abortions. Traditional birth attendants and other untrained practitioners perform abortions in villages as well as in urban slums areas. While politically unacceptable where abortion is illegal, one rational approach is to train illegal abortionists in the safe use of suction equipment. Since it is highly unlikely that this will be possible, a more practical recommendation is that, even where abortion is illegal, first-level referral centers should have suction equipment (together with personnel trained to use it, including midwives or nurses) for managing incomplete abortions, ideally before infection has become established. At the same time, those who are truly concerned about the health of women should advocate that the laws be changed so that abortion is a right to be decided by women themselves, not by legislators or by doctors. And services, once legal, should be accessible to all women.

Conclusion

This chapter has described the current situation in the developing world and suggested some possible interventions for the short- and long-term. The death of a woman in the prime of her life from a pregnancy-related cause is an unmitigated tragedy if it could have been either prevented or treated with simple existing technologies. The fact that some 500 000 women are estimated to die unnecessarily each year from such causes and that these deaths are apparently accepted without an international uproar is extraordinary. It is the responsibility of the obstetrical and public health communities, along with women's groups and others, to protest about this and to work to overcome it. Obstetricians should not allow themselves to become so involved in clinical and academic, often technologically oriented pursuits, as to ignore these tragic deaths. A rededication to the improvement in the health of all women is needed, with particular attention to the poor in rural areas and in urban slums throughout both the developed and developing world.

References

Aggarwal, V. P. and Mati, J. K. G. (1982). Epidemiology of induced abortions in Nairobi, Kenya. *Journal of Obstetrics and Gynecology, East and Central Africa*, **1**, 54–7.

Akingba, J. B. (1977). Abortion, maternity and other health problems in Nigeria. *Nigerian Medical Journal*, **7**, 465–71.

Barford, D. A. and Parker, J. R. (1977). Maternal mortality: a survey of 118 maternal deaths and the avoidable factors involved. *South African Medical Journal*, **51**, 101–5.

Boerma, T. (1987). The magnitude of the maternity mortality problem in sub-Saharan Africa. *Social Science and Medicine*, **24**, 551–8.

Brown, I. (1987). Maternal mortality: a survey of maternal deaths occurring during 1976. *Central African Journal of Medicine*, **24**, 212–14.

Cleland, J., Scott, C., and Whitelegge, D. (1987). *The world fertility survey: an assessment*. Oxford University Press.

Crowther, C. (1986). Maternal deaths at Harare Maternity Hospital during 1983. *South African Medical Journal*, **69**, 180–2.

Crowther, C. and Verkuyl, D. (1985). Characteristics of patients attending Harare Hospital with incomplete abortion. *Central African Journal of Medicine*, **31**, 67–70.

Dobbie, B. M. W. (1982). An attempt to estimate the true rate of maternal mortality, sixteenth to eighteenth centuries. *Medical History*, **26**, 79–90.

Fortney, J. A. (1981). The use of hospital resources to treat incomplete abortions: examples from Latin America. *Public Health Reports*, **96**, 574–9.

Sherton, F. C., Tulloch S., Greenwood, B. M., Bradley, A. K., Williams, K., *et al.* (1987). A perspective survey of the outcome of pregnancy in a rural area of the Gambia. *Bulletin of the WHO*, **65**, 635–43.

Harrison, K. A. (1979). Nigeria. *Lancet*, **ii**, 1229–32.

Harrison, K. (1985). Child-bearing, health and social services priorities: a survey of 22,774 consecutive hospital births in Zaria, Northern Nigeria. *British Journal of Obstetrics and Gynaecology*, **92**, (Suppl. 5), 1–119.

Hau, M. H. (1990). Commentory: confidential enquiry into maternal death. *British Journal of Obstetrics and Gynecology*, **97(8)**, 1752–3.

Hogberg, V., Wau, S., and Brostrom, G. (1986). The impact of early medical technology on maternal mortality in late 19th century Sweden. *Interaction Journal of Gynecology and Obstetrics*, **24 (4)**, 251–61.

Kaunitz, A. M., Spence, C., Danielson, T. S., Rochat, R. W. and Grimes, D. A. (1984). Perinatal and maternal mortality in a religious group avoiding obstetric care. *American Journal of Obstetrics and Gynecology*, **150**, 826–31.

Klein, M. D. and Clahr, J. (1958). Factors in decline of maternal mortality. *Journal of the American Medical Association*, **68**, 237–42.

Kwast, B. E. (1987). Roads to maternal deaths: case histories. Paper prepared for Safe Motherhood conference, Nairobi.

Kwast, B. E., Rochat, R. W., and Kidane-Mariam, W. (1986). Maternal mortality in Addis Ababa, Ethiopia. *Studies in Family Planning*, **17**, 288–301.

Lahiri, D. and Konar, M. (1976). Abortion hazards. *Journal of the Indian Medical Association*, **66**, 288–94.

Lamptey, P., Janowitz, B., Smith, J. B., and Klufio, C. (1985). Abortion experience among obstetric patients at Korle-Bu Hospital, Accra, Ghana,. *Journal of Biosocial Science*, **17**, 195–203.

Lawson, J. B. and Stewart, D. B. (1967). *Obstetrics and Gynaecology in the Tropics and Developing Countries*. Edward Arnold, London.

Lettenmaier, C., Liskin, L., Church, C. A., and Harris, J. A. (1988). Mothers lives matter: maternal health in the community. *Population Reports*, Series L (Issues in World Health), **7**, 1–31.

Mahler, H. (1987). The safe motherhood initiative: a call to action. *Lancet*, **i**, 668–70.

Maine, D., Rosenfield, A., Wallace, M., Kimball, A. M., Papiernik, E., and White. S. (1987). Prevention of maternal deaths in developing countries: program options and practical considerations. Background paper for Safe Motherhood conference; Nairobi.

Measham, A. R. and Herz, B. (1987). The safe motherhood initiative: proposals for action. World Bank background for Safe Motherhood conference, Nairobi.

Melrose, E. B. (1984)., Maternal deaths at King Edward VIII Hospital, Durban: a review of 258 consecutive cases. *South African Medical Journal*, **65**, 161–5.

Mtimavalye, L. A. R., Lisasi, D., and Ntuyabaliwe, W. K. (1980). Maternal mortality in Dar es Salaam, Tanzania 1974–1977. *East African Medical Journal*, **58**, 501–9.

Narone, R. K., Ngulube, T. J., and Narone, J. M. (1983). A study of 'spontaneous' abortions in Zambia. *Journal of Obstetrics and Gynecology, East and Central Africa*, **2**, 150–3.

Nordberg, E. M. (1984). Incidence and estimated need of Caesarean section, inguinal hernia repair and operations for strangulated hernia in rural Africa. *British Medical Journal*, **289**, 92–3.

Oronsaye, A. U. and Odiase, G. I. (1981). Incidence of ectopic pregnancy in Benin City, Nigeria. *Tropical Doctor*, **11**, 160–163.

Rochat, R. W., Kramer, D., Senanayake, G., and Howell, C. (1980). Induced abortion and health problems in developing countries. *Lancet*, **ii**, 284.

Rochat, R. W., Jaheen, S., Rosenberg, M. J., Measham, A. R., Kahn, A. R., Obaidullah, M. *et al.* (1981). Maternal and abortion related death in Bangladesh. *International Journal of Gynecology and Obstetrics*, **19**, 155–64.

Rosenfield, A. (1974). Auxiliaries and family planning. *Lancet*, **i**, 443–5.

Rosenfield, A. (1977)., Modern medicine and the delivery of health care: lessons from the developing world. *Man and Medicine*, **2**, 279–92.

Rosenfield, A. (1989). Maternal mortality in developing countries: an ongoing but neglected 'epidemic'. *Journal of the American Medical Association*, **262**, 376–79.

Rosenfield, A. and Maine, D. (1985). Maternal mortality—a neglected tragedy: where is the M in MCH? *Lancet*, **ii**, 83–5.

Royston, E. and Ferguson, J. (1989). The coverage of maternity care: a critical review of available information. *World Health Statistics Quarterly*, **38**, 267–88.

Sachs, B. P., Brown, A. J., Driscoll, S. G., Schulman, E. Acker, D., Ronsid, B. J., and Jewett, J. F. (1987). Maternal mortality in Massachusetts. *New England Journal of Medicine*, **316**, 667–72.

Smith, S. M. (1984). How might we improve surgical services for rural regulations in developing countries? *British Medical Journal*, **289**, 494–5.

UNICEF (1989). *State of the World's Children*. UNICEF, New York.

White, S. M., Thorpe, R. G., and Maine, D. (1987). Emergency obstetric surgery performed by nurses in Zaire. *Lancet*, **ii**, 612–3.

WHO (1987). *Essential obstetric functions at first referral level to reduce maternal mortality* (Report of a Technical Working Group). WHO, Geneva.

WHO (1987). *Maternal mortality: the dimension of the problem*. Background paper for Safe Motherhood conference, Nairobi.

WHO (1994). *Abortion: A tabulation of available data on the frequency and mortality of unsafe abortion* (2nd edition). WHO, Geneva.

WHO and UNICEF (1978). *Alma Ata, 1978: Primary Health Care*. WHO Geneva.

16 Cesarean section

Thorkild F. Nielsen

History of cesarean section

Cesarean section is an operation of great antiquity. It was practiced by the early Romans, the ancient Hindus, and the ancient Hebrews. These first abdominal deliveries were performed only after the death of the mother, however and it is impossible to ascertain when the operation was first done on a living woman. The first documented cesarean section performed on a living woman in Europe was carried out on 22 April, 1610 by a German surgeon, Jeremias Trautman of Wittenberg. The operation was described in detail by Professor Daniel Sennert who was present during the procedure. The mother died 24 days later; the child survived (Bailer 1982).

In the next two centuries, cesarean section was only performed on living women in rare and desperate cases and the maternal mortality was terrifyingly high. In 1880 Radford reported on 131 cesarean sections; the maternal mortality in this group was 83 per cent. In Paris in the seventeenth and eighteenth centuries, more than 90 per cent of cesarean deliveries were fatal for the patients. The causes of death were primarily hemorrhage and infection. At that time, because of the risk of infection, sutures were not used in the uterine wound because the ends could not be left long for subsequent removal. As a result, the women often died of hemorrhage from the uterine wound. Furthermore, lochia escaped from the uterine cavity into the abdomen, causing severe infections. In 1877, Professor Porro of Padua, Italy advised removal of the uterus after delivery in order to avoid the fatal consequences of hemorrhage and infection originating from the uterus.

The turning point in the evolution of abdominal delivery came in 1882, when Sanger, then an assistant of Crede in the University Clinic of Leipzig, closed the uterine wall for the first time using eight to ten silver wire sutures. The incidence of severe hemorrhage was thereafter reduced.

Also in 1882, Kehrer of Heidelberg described a new type of uterine incision. The traditional method had been to make a longitudinal incision from the upper part of the uterus and down, thus dividing the uterus into two halves. This type of incision is called the classical incision. Kehrer proposed making a transverse incision into the lower uterine segment. In the following decades this techniques became more popular and in 1921 Professor Kerr of Glasgow, Scotland finally recommended this lower segment approach as causing not only less infection, postoperative ileus, and bleeding, but also less uterine rupture and fewer adhesions.

These changes in operative techniques reduced the number of fatalities from hemorrhage, but infection remained an important cause of death. In the early nineteenth century, however, three famous men were born whose work and discoveries greatly influenced obstetric development and eventually brought down the death rate from infection. They were Ignatz Semmelweis (1818–1865), Louis Pasteur (1822–1895), and Joseph Lister (1827–1912). In 1847 Semmelweis, on an empirical basis, proposed methods for preventing puerperal fever: that physicians and nurses wash their hands with soap and a solution of chloride of lime before touching patients' wound and that patients have clean bedclothes. Pasteur was the first to discover bacteria and to demonstrate the importance of bacteria for the processes of infection. In 1867, on the basis of these discoveries, Lister, a professor in Glasgow, began using carbolic acid as an antiseptic agent during operations, thereby reducing mortality and morbidity from postoperative infections.

Rates of cesarean section

The abdominal delivery rate has increased steadily during the last three decades in all Western countries from a rate lower than 1 per cent during the first half of this century. The incidence in Sweden was 0.87 per cent in 1946–1950 and was still only 2–3 per cent in the 1960s. It increased sharply, by at least 3-fold, during the first half of the 1970s in most obstetric departments (Nielsen 1984). There was a similar trend in 19 other Western industrialized countries during a comparable period and the annual rate of increase in these countries seemed to be coverging (Urquhart *et al.* 1987).

The increase in the rate of cesarean section has been most remarkable in the USA. The reported abdominal delivery rate in 1987 was 24.4 per cent and cesarean section is now the most common surgical procedure in North American hospitals (Jonas 1989). The primary cesarean section rate seems to be leveling off. However, because repeat cesarean sections account for 20–30 per cent of all procedures, the total rate will continue to rise for some time. Researchers at the US National Centre for Health Statistics predict that without a change in obstetric delivery trends, the national cesarean section rate could reach 40 per cent by the year 2000 (Taffel *et al.* 1987).

Current indications for cesarean section

The reasons for the rise in the cesarean section rate are numerous and complex. They include liberalization of indications to include quality of life considerations and improved survival of infants with conditions known to be associated with trauma during vaginal delivery. For example, cesarean section has replaced difficult midforceps deliveries in most cases and has become an important tool for improving fetal condition in these deliveries.

Cesarean sections for breech presentation and transverse lie have increased dramatically and are now routine in many practices. Many obstetricians believe that vaginal delivery in these cases results in a higher incidence of fetal injury and asphyxia than delivery by the abdominal route, because the risks are magnified by the relative infrequency of these presentations (Lilford 1990).

In multiple pregnancies, both the fetuses and the mother are at high risk for complications. Use of a liberal abdominal delivery policy in selected cases has lowered fetal morbidity and mortality (Chervenak *et al.* 1985).

During the last several decades, there has been a dramatic increase in the use of electronic fetal heart rate monitoring. It had been hoped that earlier identification of fetal distress during labor and intervention by cesarean delivery would greatly improve fetal survival (Paul *et al.* 1980). However, over the last two decades there is no evidence that there has been a decline in the incidence of cerebral palsy and mental retardation despite the widespread introduction of electronic fetal monitoring and increased cesarean deliveries (See Chapters 17 and 24).

A placental covering of the internal birth canal in late pregnancy is a life-threatening condition for mother and child. Abdominal delivery in these cases is often life-saving for both (Nielsen *et al.* 1989).

Another indication for cesarean delivery is active vaginal herpes infection at the time of labor. Abdominal delivery is essential if the fetus is to be protected from this serious infection. Up to 60 per cent of infected fetuses die and 50 per cent of the survivors have severe, permanent neurologic sequelae (Hankins and Gilstrap 1988).

The great advances in medical care—improved anesthetic techniques, blood products and blood transfusions, wider choice of antibiotics, and better control of maternal diabetes, hypertension, and heart disease—have significantly lowered maternal morbidity and mortality in abdominal deliveries and consequently have made the choice of cesarean birth easier for the obstetrician in many cases. The broadening of indications for cesarean section has certainly produced better results for the fetus (Nielsen 1984).

Yet the range of problems for which cesarean section is indicated is now cause for concern. There is great danger in believing that abdominal delivery is the only way out in every difficult obstetric situation. It is a major operation and may be associated with any severe intraoperative or postoperative complication that besets major surgery, as well as late complications such as secondary infertility and, in subsequent pregnancies and deliveries, uterine scar rupture (Nielsen 1984). Compared with vaginal delivery, cesarean section is associated with higher maternal morbidity and perhaps mortality.

Maternal morbidity and mortality

Intraoperative complications

Surgical complications in association with cesarean section are rarely reported in the literature and then usually as case reports. In one prospective study of 1319 patients, the overall complication rate was 11.6 per cent (Nielsen and Hokegard 1984). Intraoperative complications were divided into two groups. Group A comprised minor complications: intense bleeding necessitating blood transfusions, minor rupture and lacerations in the lower part of the uterus, minor injuries from knife or scissors without sequelae to the child, and difficulty in delivering the child. Group B comprised major complications: injury to the urinary bladder, tears into the cervix and vagina, severe life-threatening bleeding from the uterine arteries, severe lacerations involving most of the uterus, complicated by heavy bleeding, intestinal surgical trauma, and injury to the child with sequelae. It must be acknowledged that cesarean section can be complicated by severe intraoperative difficulties that necessitate great surgical skill. In this study, 2.5 years of regular operative obstetric training was necessary before the surgical complication rate for the young obstetrician had declined to an acceptable level.

Postoperative complications

Infections are the most common postoperative complications associated with cesarean delivery, with an incidence between 13 and 65 per cent in different studies (Nielsen 1984). The most common infectious complications are infection of the uterus (endometritis), urinary tract infection, wound infection, severe intra-abdominal infections, and generalized whole body infection (sepsis). The fact that the rate of infection following abdominal delivery varies widely suggests that the risk depends on a variety of predisposing factors such as duration of labor, rupture of membranes, low hematocrit, socio-economic status, maternal age, lack of prenatal care, parity, experience of the surgeon, and type of anesthesia. Cesarean section is complicated by a much higher incidence of maternal postpartum infection than delivery by the vaginal route; in one study, a 7-fold increase was found (Sweet and Ledger 1973). Reasons for the higher rate of infection include impairment of the local blood supply resulting from trauma to the blood vessels in the uterus, presence of foreign bodies (i.e. suture), destruction of tissue by surgical manipulation, and lacerations and blood clot formation. Bacteria from the vagina may enter damaged sites in the uterus and produce infections. In patients at high risk for infection, however, morbidity can be significantly reduced by pretreatment with prophylactic antibiotics (Ledger 1983).

Late sequelae

Few studies have attempted to describe late complications of cesarean section. Kirchoff speculated that there is an increased incidence of spontaneous abortion and extrauterine pregnancy (Kirchoff 1977). Postoperative complications may also put the woman's reproductive future at risk: severe postcesarean intra-abdominal infections, although rarely seen, result in infertility in more than half of cases (Hurry *et al.* 1984).

Placenta Previa

Bender (1954) suggested that the uterine scar itself predisposes to placental complications in subsequent pregnancies. Cesarean section damages the uterine wall, predisposing to low placental implantation and consequently to a higher risk of placenta previa. Other studies have confirmed that abdominal delivery significantly increases the risk of placenta previa during later pregnancies (Clarck *et al.* 1985; Nielsen *et al.* 1989). In fact, the risk of this severe complication in a patient with a previous cesarean section is about five times as high as in patients with an unscarred uterus.

Uterine scar rupture

Rupture of the uterus during pregnancy and labor is considered one of the major hazards in obstetrics. Since 1916, when Edward Cragin pronounced his now-famous dictum 'Once a cesarean section, always a cesarean section', previous cesarean section has been considered to be the most important predisposing factor for uterine rupture (Beacham *et al* 1970). Between 1980 and 1983, repeat cesarean section accounted for 55 per cent of the cesarean deliveries in the USA (National Centre for Health Statistics 1985). However, whereas scars from classical cesarean incisions are at high risk for uterine rupture (Lavin *et al.* 1982), scars from transverse segment incisions rarely rupture during succeeding pregnancies and labors. Data from many studies on the safety of a trial of labor after previous abdominal birth show that in selected cases, vaginal delivery after previous cesarean section is safe and there is no increased incidence of maternal or perinatal morbidity. Lavin reviewed 30 years of literature on vaginal delivery after previous abdominal birth (Lavin *et al.* 1982) and found and that it is associated with a 0.7 per cent incidence of uterine rupture and no maternal deaths. Vaginal delivery should be considered the safest route of delivery in most of these patients (Nielsen *et al.* 1989).

Maternal mortality

With improvements in anesthesia and supportive care, cesarean section has evolved from an operation of last resort to an elective procedure and maternal mortality has become a less significant factor.

In the eighteenth century, the mortality associated with cesarean section was 80–90 per cent. This rate fell to 4–10 per cent in the first half of this century in most Western industrialized countries. After the introduction of antibacterial therapy and hospital blood banks in the early 1940s, maternal mortality associated with abdominal delivery fell to less than 1 per cent (Nielsen 1984).

A report on maternal deaths in England and Wales (Department of Health

1989) noted a continued decline in mortality over a 15 year period, despite the increasing number of cesarean sections. In 1970–1972, the cesarean rate was 5.2 per cent and the maternal fatality rate 99 per 100 000 live births in 1982–1984, the maternal fatality rate fell to 37 per 100 000 while the cesarean section rate climbed to 10.1 per cent. The decline in maternal deaths was attributed to better patient selection, better anesthesia, and better surgical technique.

In conclusion, the overall picture is one of greatly improved safety for the mother delivered by the abdominal route and even further improvement in these figures can and should be expected. The fact cannot be overlooked, however, that maternal cesarean mor tality is still estimated to be 10–20 times higher than mortality in women giving birth by the vaginal route (Moldin *et al.* 1984;), although some of the increase can be ascribed to the high-risk factors of many of the women who require abdominal delivery.

Perinatal morbidity and mortality

Many physicians have cited concern for infants' health as justification for the sharply rising rate of cesarean sections, claiming that the increasing cesarean birth rate correlates with improved perinatal mortality and morbidity.

The question of whether such a correlation really exists has been examined by O'Driscoll and Foley (1983), who compared statistics from the USA and Dublin, Republic of Ireland. In the USA, cesarean birth rates increased from 5 per cent in 1965 to more than 15 per cent in 1980. During the same period in Dublin, the cesarean section rate remained virtually unchanged (4.2 per cent in 1965 and 4.8 per cent in 1980) and the perinatal mortality fell from 42.1 to 16.8 per 1000 infants born at 500 g or more. The decrease in perinatal mortality in the USA during the same time was not greater than that in Dublin. Obviously, perinatal results from medical centers on different continents must be compared with caution; it does seem possible, however, to draw conclusions from simple trends in two specific items (cesarean section rates and perinatal mortality) which lend themselves to accurate definition and which start from the same baseline.

O'Driscoll's results are supported by a study of all the obstetric departments in Sweden (Nielsen *et al.* 1986), which found that while the incidence of abdominal delivery varied from 8 to 19 per cent between different obstetric departments, there were no significant differences in perinatal mortality or in the number of infants who were depressed at birth (Apgar score less than 7 at 5 minutes).

A concern has been raised that babies born by cesarean section have a higher risk of respiratory distress (Nielsen 1984). Although the route of delivery may be a factor in some cases, prematurity (iatrogenic or planned) may be the underlying cause in others.

Ethical, demographic, and legal issues

Ethical concerns

Few medical interventions in Western societies are performed with as much emotion and expectation as a cesarean section. The ethical principles associated with this operation are generally not specific to this procedure and correspond well to established patterns governing the doctor–patient relationship. Implicit in the relationship is the doctor's traditional commitment to the patient's best interests and his or her respect for the patient's right to make decisions concerning her health.

Particularly in an era when people are having fewer children, parents have high expectations for healthy babies and many are convinced that the abdominal birth route is the safest. Therefore, women's expectations and their demands on the physician undoubtedly influence the decision for or against operative delivery. For an obstetrician, it may be more convenient to comply with the patient's request for cesarean delivery than to try to convince her that the vaginal route is preferable. Furthermore, the malpractice climate in many countries has led many obstetricians to practice more defensive medicine, which certainly lowers their threshold for resorting to cesarean section. However, the physician is bound by medical ethics to offer advice to the patient that is based solely on sound medical experience and principle. Before the final decision concerning operative intervention, every obstetrician must consider whether all the issues have been adequately addressed.

Demographic issues

The most controversial feature of modern obstetrics is the rapidly increasing incidence of cesarean section. Factors independent of medical indication may play an important role in this development. In a study by Gould *et al.* (1989) the primary cesarean birth rate was shown to vary directly with socio-economic status. Women with an annual family income of more than $30 000 had a primary cesarean section rate of 22.9 per cent—nearly double that of women with a family income of less than $11 000 (13.2 per cent). This difference could not be explained by differences in maternal age, parity, birth weight, ethnic group, or complications of pregnancy or childbirth.

One of the single most important factors contributing to election of cesarean section seems to be the obstetrician's personal attitude to the procedure. To investigate this influence, Goyert *et al.* (1989) studied 1533 women at low risk of obstetric complications. The mean rate of cesarean delivery was 26.9 per cent, but the individual rates for the 11 obstetricians who cared for them ranged from 19.1 per cent to 42.3 per cent. A stepwise logistic-regression model of the determinants of cesarean section, including the obstetrician involved, parity, birthweight, and maternal age, showed that only nulliparity was more important than the identity of the physician in influencing the rate of abdominal delivery.

The influence of malpractice litigation

Obstetricians' fear of malpractice suits plays an increasingly important role in the rising cesarean section rate. In the USA and other countries, malpractice suits can be brought directly against an obstetrician by a patient. The threat of a malpractice suit has become an integral part of obstetric care and obstetricians increasingly report that it is of prime influence in their decisions to perform abdominal delivery. In the USA, the average number of claims per 100 physicians tripled over five years (1980–1985) and it is estimated that more than 70 per cent of the fellows of the American College of Obstetricians and Gynecologists have been sued at least once (ACOG 1990). Furthermore, the rise in malpractice claims has been accompanied by a 2300 per cent increase in the number of awards of more than $1 million.

The risk of a malpractice suit varies by country. Suits are often brought when neurologically impaired infants are born (for example, infants with cerebral palsy). Yet Freeman and Nelson and other authors writing in this book have concluded that the cause of cerebral palsy is usually unknown and that when a presumed cause can be identified, it more often occurred before the onset of labor (see Chapter 24). On the basis of present knowledge, it can be concluded that intrapartum events account for no more than 10 per cent of cases of cerebral palsy (Nelson 1988).

The view that cerebral palsy is not the result of birth trauma but is probably caused sometime during pregnancy or after delivery is gaining wider acceptance. If this new view is accepted by parents, health authorities, and obstetricians, the incidence of malpractice claims may be reduced. Such a reduction could result in a no-fault compensation scheme involving a comprehensive disability allowance to support both parents and infants.

Cost—benefit analysis

The medical cost of delivery by cesarean section is generally higher than that of vaginal delivery.

Myers and Gleicher (1988) found that the abdominal delivery rate could be substantially reduced—without adverse effects on the outcome for mother or infant—with a program that included setting objective criteria for the four most common indications for cesarean section, a detailed review of all cases, and a stringent requirement for a second opinion. However, it was also found that revenues decreased for both the staff and hospital as a direct result of the initiative to reduce the cesarean section rate. The hospital's reimbursement for vaginal delivery was approximately $3 000 lower than for cesarean section. Also, the individual physician's fee was usually $250–500 lower for vaginal delivery.

The components of the costs associated with abdominal delivery include higher physician fees, an average of 3 extra days of hospitalization, and the cost for treatment of associated complications (Danforth 1985;). There may also be non-medical costs: the longer period of convalescence may necessitate time off work for the husband and the cost of caring for the newborn as well as for other children in the household may increase for the same reason.

Finally, Gleicher (1984) estimated that every 1 per cent increase in the cesarean section rate in the USA would raise health costs by $63 million each year. In light of this, the goal must be to avoid unnecessary operations that increase medical costs for both the patient and the community.

Reducing cesarean section rates

Is it possible to reduce the cesarean rate in Western industrialized societies? Certain obstetric departments have developed successful programs to lower cesarean rates without adverse effects on outcome for mother or infant, although there are no reports of the same development on a nationwide basis.

In Sweden, medical birth registration began in 1973. A birth registration form is completed for all newborn babies, living or stillborn. Recorded variables include maternal age, parity, obstetric history, pregnancy complications, intra- and postpartum complications, mode of delivery (with indication for cesarean section, if necessary), fetal presentation, birthweight, perinatal mortality, Apgar score at 1, 5, and 10 min, and pediatric morbidity. Figures from this database show a significant decline in the cesarean section rate in Sweden during the last 10 years. The rate rose from 5.25 per cent in 1973 to 12.30 per cent in 1983 but then stabilized at around 12 per cent. In 1989, the last year for which figures are available, there was a significant decline to 10.99 per cent. The number of operations fell by almost 3000 a year. During the same period, perinatal mortality declined from 0.66 per cent (1983) to 0.61 per cent (1989), while the number of depressed infants at birth (Apgar score less than 7 at 5 minutes) has been consistently low. A review of the literature during the last decade shows that this is without parallel in any other country with reliable statistics. Closer examination of the findings in Sweden could become a model for similar developments in other countries.

The cesarean section rates between 1983 and 1989 for placenta previas, placental abruptions, cephalopelvic disproportion, and dysfunctional labor have virtually remained the same. These indications have been well defined for many years and one would not expect any major changes in these indications for medical reasons.

For malpresentation, the incidence significantly decreased, from 1.89 per cent in 1983 to 1.37 per cent in 1989. Cesarean section was routinely performed for breech presentation in many countries in the 1970s after studies showed an increase in neurological abnormalities after vaginal delivery compared with abdominal delivery (Westgren and Ingemarsson 1988). However, recent studies with long-term follow-up of infants born in breech presentation indicate that outcome after vaginal delivery is comparable to that after cesarean section (Svenningsen *et al.* 1985). Strict criteria are necessary to select cases for a trial of vaginal delivery, including anticipated normal fetal weight, normal pelvic dimensions, and obstetricians with sufficient experience and manual skill to manage complications associated with vaginal breech deliveries. The macrosomic infant is excluded.

Electronic monitoring of fetal heart rate became routine in the early to mid-1970s (Nielsen 1984). Adoption of this new technology, however, was not preceded by critical evaluation of its implications and the obstetric profession was not prepared for nor educated in the interpretation of fetal monitoring. Today, routine use of fetal monitoring during labor might be considered injudicious, because one of the main factors responsible for the overall increase in the cesarean section rate seems to be unnecessary interventions due to fetal heart rate changes that are not specific for fetal hypoxia, but cause medical anxiety (Prentice and Lind 1987). Inappropriate action based on misinterpretation of suspicious or abnormal fetal heart rate changes may lead to litigation; fear of such litigation may contribute to the number of unnecessary interventions. In Sweden during the past decade, training programs in the use of monitors and scalp sampling for fetal acid–base status have been instituted in most maternity units. These programs seem to have been very successful; the cesarean section rate for fetal distress declined from 31.9 per cent in 1983 to 18.0 per cent in 1989. Thus, the expertise with which information from fetal monitoring is interpreted seems to be the single most important factor in reducing the abdominal delivery rate overall.

Cesarean section has been proposed when the presentation of twins is other than vertex and particularly when gestation is less than 34 weeks (Cetrulo 1986). However, published studies have failed to show any correlation between cesarean delivery and improved prognosis for low-birth weight twins (less than 2500 g), even if their presentation is taken into account (Rydstrom *et al.* 1990). Thus, the case with twins seems to be parallel to breech presentation: indiscriminate use of abdominal delivery will hardly improve the fetal outcome.

The dictum of Cragin (1916) has been followed in most obstetric departments and repeat cesarean sections make a large contribution to the increasing abdominal delivery rate. As discussed above, however, many studies on the safety of a trial of labor after previous abdominal birth have been performed and data from the great majority show that, in selected cases, vaginal delivery after previous cesarean section is safe and there is no increased incidence of maternal or perinatal morbidity. Thus, it must be concluded that vaginal delivery is the safest route of delivery in most patients with previous abdominal delivery.

In Sweden, the indication of 'psychologic and/or bad obstetric history' significantly increased in incidence from 1983 to 1989, perhaps in part because of malpractice litigation in the USA. The increased threat to obstetricians has become a prime factor in their decision to perform cesarean section and seems to be the most difficult problem for the obstetric community in the future. Facing this problem, it is necessary to recognize the importance of frequent national obstetric meetings, postgraduate courses in obstetrics, and research into the nature of economic incentives for or against cesarean delivery, combined with legal and ethical concern, on a nation-wide basis.

Conclusion

Cesarean section has become an integral and essential part of modern obstetrics in most Western countries. As safety has increased, so too have the range of problems that cesarean section is employed to address, to a degree that raises medical concern. There is little evidence that a high cesarean section rate can be justified on the grounds of outcome for the mother or baby, or both. This discrepancy between clinical practice and evidence from controlled clinical trials is probably unparalled in medicine. Aggressive measures to combat the tide of cesareans should be one of the major challenges undertaken by the obstetric community in the nineties.

References

Bailer, P. (1982). History of cesarean section. *Obstetrics and Gynecology*, **59(2)**, 135–48.

Beacham, W., Beacham, D., Webster, H., and Fielding, S. (1970). Rupture of the uterus at New Orleans Charity Hospital. *American Journal of Obstetrics and Gynecology*, **106**, 1083–7.

Bender, S. (1954). Placenta previa and previous LSCS. *Surgery, Gynecology and Obstetrics* **98**, 625–27.

Cetrulo, C. L., Ingardia, C. J., and Sbarra, A. J. (1980). Management of multiple gestation. *Clinical Obstetrics and Gynecology*, **23(2)**, 533–48.

Chervenak, F. A., Johnson, R. E., Youcha, S., Hobbins, J. C., and Berkowitz, R. L. (1985). Intrapartum management of twin gestation. *Obstetrics and Gynecology*, **65(1)**, 119–24.

Clarck, S. L., Koonings, P. P., Phelan, J. P. (1985). Placenta previa/accreta and prior cesarean section. *Obstetrices Gynecology* **66**. 89–92.

Danforth, D. N. (1985) Cesarean section. *Journal of the American Medical Association*, **253(6)**, 811–18.

Gleicher, N. (1984). Cesarean section rates in the United States. The short-term failure of the National Consensus development Conference in 1980. *Journal of the American Medical Association*, **252(23)**, 3273–6.

Gould, J. B., Davey, B., and Stafford, R. S. (1989). Socioeconomic differences in rates of cesarean section. *New England Journal of Medicine*, **321(11)**, 233–9.

Goyert, G. L., Bottoms, S. F., Treadwell, M. C., and Nehra, P. C. (1989). The physician factor in cesarean birth rates. *New England Journal of Medicine*, **320(11)**, 706–9.

Hankins, G. D. V., Gilstrap, L. C. (1988). Additional maternal and fetal indications. In *Cesarean delivery* (ed. Phelan, J. P. & Clarck, S. L.) pp. 541–55, Elsevier, New York, Amsterdam, London.

Hurry, D. J., Larsen, B., and Charles, D. (1984). Effects of postcesarean section febrile morbidity on subsequent fertility. *Obstetrics and Gynecology*, **64(2)**, 256–60.

Jonas, H. S., and Dooley, S. L. (1989). The search for a lower cesarean rate goes on. *Journal of American Medical Association*, **262(11)**, 1512–13.

Kirchoff, H. (1977). Birgt die berechtigte Intensivierung der prospektiven Geburtsleitungen zum Nutzen des Kindes fur die Mutter eine gehöte Gefar? *Geburtshilfe und Frauenheilkunde* **37**, 103–9.

Lavin, J., Stephens, R., Miodovnik, M., and Barden, T. (1982). Vaginal delivery in patients with a prior cesarean section. *Obstetrics and Gynecology*, **59**, 135–48.

Ledger, W. J. (1983). Prophylactic antibiotics. *Clinical Obstetrics and Gynaecology*, **10(1)**, 23–36.

Lilford, R. J., van Coeverden de Grott, H. A., Morre, P. J., and Bingham, P. (1990). The relative risks of caesarean section (intrapartum and elective) and vaginal delivery: a detailed analysis to exclude the effects of medical disorders and other acute pre-existing physiological disturbances. *British Journal of Obstetrics and Gynaecology*, **97(10)**, 883–92.

Moldin, R., Hokegard, K. H., and Nielsen, T. F. (1984). Cesarean section and maternal mortality in Sweden. Acta Obstetricia Gynelogcia Scandanaviea, **63(1)**, 7–11.

Myers, S. A., and Gleicher, N. (1988). A successful program to lower cesarean-section rates. *New England Journal of Medicine*, **319(23)**, 1511–16.

Nelson, K. (1988). What proportion of cerebral palsy is related to birth asphyxia? *Journal of Pediatrics*, **112**, 572–5.

Nielsen, T. F. (1984). Cesarean section. A clinical study on the incidence and type of complications associated with abdominal delivery. *Thesis*, Department of Obstetrics and Gynecology, Central Hospital Borås and the Department of Obstetrics and Gynecology, University of Gothenburg, Sweden.

Nielsen, T. F., Hagberg, H., and Ljungblad, U. (1989). Placenta previa and antepartum hemorrhage after previous cesarean section. *Gynecology and Obstetrics Investigation*, **27(2)**, 88–90.

Nielsen, T. F., and Hokegard, K. H. (1984). Cesarean section and intraoperative surgical complications. *Acta Obstetrics and Gynecology Scandanavia*, **63(2)**, 103–8.

Nielsen, T. F., Hokegard, K. H., and Ericson, A. (1986). Indications for Cesarean section in Sweden in 1983. (Indikationer for kejsarsnitt i Sverige 1983). *Lakartidningen*, **83(41)**, 3417, 3419–20. S.

Nielson, T. F., Ljungblad, U., and Hagberg, H. (1989). Rupture and dehiscence of cesarean section scar during pregnancy and delivery. *American Journal of Obstetric and Gynecology*, **160(3)**, 569–73.

O'Driscoll, K. and Foley, M. (1983). Correlation of decrease in perinatal mortality and increase in cesarean section rates. *Obstetrics and Gynecology*, **61(1)**, 1–5.

Paul, R. H., Gauthier, R. J., and Quilligan, E. J. (1980). Clinical fetal monitoring. The usage and relationship to trends in cesarean delivery and perinatal mortality. *Acta Obstetrics and Gynecology Scandanavia*, **59(4)**, 289–95.

Prentice, A. and Lind, T. (1987). Fetal heart rate monitoring during labour—too frequent intervention, too little benefit? *Lancet*, **2(8572)**, 1375–7.

ACOG (American College of Obstetricians and Gynecologists) (1990). *Professional liability insurance and its effects: report of a 1990 survey of ACOG's membership. American College of Obstetricians and Gynecologists*, Washington, DC.

Rydhstrom, H., Ingemarsson, I., and Ohrlander, S. (1990). Lack of correlation between a high caesarean section rate and improved prognosis for low-birthweight twins (less than 2500g). *British Journal of Obstetrics and Gynaecology*, **97(3)**, 229–33.

Svenningsen, N. W., Westgren, M., Ingemarsson, I. (1985). Modern strategy for term breech delivery—a study with 4-year follow-up of the infants. *Journal of Perinatal Medicine* **13**, 117–26.

Sweet, R. L., and Ledger, W. J. (1973). Puerperal infectious morbidity: a two-year review. *American Journal of Obstetrics and Gynecology*, **117(8)**, 1093–100.

Taffel, S. M., Placek, P. J., and Liss, T. (1987). Trends in the United States cesarean section rate and reasons for the 1980–85 rise. *American Journal of Public Health*, **77(8)**, 955–9.

Urquhard, D. R., Grieve, R. M., and Geals, M. F. (1987). The rising caesarean section rate—a year's audit to assess the trend. *Health Bulletin*, **45(6)**, 316–28.

Westgren, M., and Ingemarsson, I. (1988). Breech delivery and mental handicap. *Clinical Obstetrics and Gynecology* Vol. **2**, 187–94.

IV Pregnancy and Prevention of Adverse Infant Outcomes

17 Evaluation of monitoring techniques in pregnancy

Roger K. Freeman

Introduction

With the advances in technology emanating primarily from the space, biochemical, and electronics industries, there has been an understandable desire to apply this new knowledge to health care. Medical researchers have been aiming to use new scientific methods to develop new strategies that can improve outcomes for many previously devastating diseases. In obstetrics, there certainly have been great benefits seen from the introduction of antibiotics, the understanding, treatment and prevention of rhesus disease, amniocentesis and the ability to prevent the birth of children with Down syndrome, and the use of blood and blood products to replace substances necessary for the sustenance of life.

Beginning in the 1960s, scientific advances in biochemistry offered the ability for obstetricians to begin to measure various substances emanating from the previously inaccessible fetus *in utero*. Thus were born expectations that these monitoring techniques would allow the clinician to develop interventional strategies that could improve fetal outcome. The ability to measure estriol, human placental lactogen, and heat stable alkaline phosphatase gave high expectations that it would be possible to measure placental function and identify causes of intrauterine death, fetal growth retardation, and perhaps even the embryopathy affecting infants of diabetic mothers.

A large number of scientific papers examined the correlations of abnormalities in levels of these substances with fetal problems, and indeed it appeared that outcome could be improved with such programs of fetal surveillance. Biophysical methods which allowed for a quicker answer soon began to replace biochemical surveillance and today techniques involving fetal heart rate monitoring and ultrasonic modalities have completely replaced biochemical tests. I would like to trace the development of three of these biophysical technologies, especially the initial hopes and their subsequent adoption as standards of practice on the basis of non-randomized trials. It is hoped that we can learn some lessons from this piece of modern medical history as we are deluged with multitudes of new technologies.

Electronic intrapartum fetal heart rate monitoring

Before intrapartum electronic fetal heart rate monitoring the cesarean section rate was low, intrapartum fetal death and asphyxia neonatorum were usually unexpected and these events were largely considered to be unavoidable acts of God. When I trained in the 1960s, cesarean birth was still vividly remembered by my teachers as a dangerous procedure that was to be avoided if at all possible and the fetal/neonatal outcome was not the primary concern. All primary cesarean sections were discussed in detail at morning rounds and we were frequently criticized by the more experienced practitioners for not having persisted further with forceps or oxytocin or both. Success was considered a vaginal delivery and birth trauma suffered by the fetus and mother were usually accepted as a small price to pay for avoiding a cesarean section. While there had been references to a relationship between intrapartum events and subsequent cerebral palsy (Eastman and De Leon 1955; Lilienfield and Pasamanick 1955), there were no prevention strategies during this era of mechanical obstetrics, when the discipline was dominated by maternal advocates.

Electronic fetal monitoring, more than any other aspect of modern obstetrics, has changed the focus from the mother to the fetus. The contributions of Edward Hon in the USA and Caldeyro-Barcia from Uruguay and Hammacher from Germany gave insight into fetal oxygenation during labor. In the late 1960s and 1970s there were large numbers of reports comparing outcome with fetal monitoring and auscultation, using historical or non-randomized concurrent controls, which appeared to show enormous benefits of electronic monitoring during labor (Shenker *et al.* 1975; Lee and Baggish 1976; Amato 1977; Paul *et al.* 1977). The classic paper by Benson *et al.* (1968) from collaborative study data concluded that, except at the extreme, auscultation did not predict fetal outcome. Certainly, it was believed that having access to all the fetal heart rate data must be better than sampling only a few per cent of the heartbeats by intermittent auscultation.

Since the chance of being pronounced dead on the day of birth exceeded the risk for the next 40 years of life combined, the birth process must be extremely treacherous. Any method that would allow us to predict fetal acidosis, death, low Apgar scores, and poor performance in the nursery must therefore be of great value. After all, uterine contractions, while necessary for successful vaginal delivery, cause intermittent oxygen deprivation, so labor itself must contribute to this newly recognized preventable intrapartum asphyxia. While intrauterine resuscitation was discovered by observing improvement in ominous fetal heart rate patterns by stopping oxytocin, changing mother from the supine to lateral position, increasing intravascular volume, and administering oxygen, all too often cesarean section was the only solution available for a 'non-reassuring fetal heart rate pattern'.

Ultimately, the belief (based on large amounts of correlative data) became prevalent that most fetal injury was due to intrapartum asphyxia, trauma, or both. To prevent such disastrous events, we believed that a low threshold for cesarean section, and avoiding difficult forceps deliveries, would serve our patients and their fetuses well. Furthermore a perceived standard of care evolved which implied that a ill baby was due to intrapartum negligence until proven otherwise. This concept has led to a huge medico-legal problem for obstetricians.

The first randomized controlled trial of electronic fetal monitoring was done by Haverkamp *et al.* (1976). Patients were managed with either continuous electronic fetal heart rate monitoring (the study group) or intermittent auscultation with a dedicated 'one-on-one' nurse (the control group). The study was criticized by many because the numbers were small, but more importantly because the results, which showed no benefit to electronic monitoring over auscultation, did not fit the previous correlative results from non-randomized reports. By this time most academicians had accepted that fetal monitoring was of great benefit and so these results just did not make sense to them.

A second study by the same investigators included another group managed by both fetal scalp blood sampling and electronic monitoring. This also showed that auscultation gave similar results to electronic monitoring in terms of fetal outcome. The previously noted higher cesarean section rate in the electronically monitored group persisted although with the addition of fetal scalp blood sampling there were fewer than with electronic monitoring alone (Haverkamp 1979). Interestingly the higher cesarean section rate in the electronically monitored group was not due to those done for fetal distress but rather was primarily attributed to failed progress, a finding that has never been completely explained.

Since these initial studies, there have been six more randomized trials, none of which has found clear benefit for electronic fetal monitoring (Renou *et al.* 1976; Kelso *et al.* 1981; Neldham *et al.* 1981; Wood *et al.* 1981; McDonald *et al.* 1985; Leveno *et al.* 1986). There were significantly less neonatal seizures in the electronically monitored groups than in the intermittent auscultation groups when results of all the randomized trials were combined. This difference was largely due to the Dublin study results, but at 4 years of age there was no difference in neurological outcome between the two groups (Grant *et al.* 1989). The long-term follow-up of Haverkamp's original series also failed to show any difference in neurological outcome (Langendoerfer *et al.* 1980).

Many of the critics who originally said that the numbers were insufficient to show the benefit of electronic fetal monitoring have had to agree that, with some 17 500 prospectively randomized patients now studied, if there were even a small demonstrable benefit to monitoring there would at least be a trend in the combined data. There is no such trend.

Until the study by Luthy *et al.* (1987), which randomized patients in premature labor, it was generally felt that results would support observations by Martin *et al.* (1974) and Hobel *et al.* (1972) suggesting that electronic fetal monitoring was beneficial in premature labor. In fact, Luthy *et al.* (1987) showed no benefit in short-term outcome and a recent report of long-term follow-up of these premature neonates (Shy *et al.* 1990) confirmed that monitoring had no demonstrable benefit (Freeman 1990). The study was flawed, however, in that the results actually showed an excess of cerebral palsy among electronically monitored infants who weighed under 1750 g. Scrutiny of the study design showed that an abnormal fetal scalp blood pH was required before intervention for fetal distress in the monitored group, which was not required in the intermittent auscultation group. This resulted in about 1 h longer interval between recognition of the abnormal fetal heart rate pattern in the electronically monitored group and delivery than occurred in the intermittent auscultation group. Unfortunately, the lay press picked this up and suggested that electronic fetal monitoring actually caused cerebral palsy, but infact the data only indicated no protective effect over intermittent auscultation.

We are now left with the problem of trying to explain why a technique that clearly does identify hypoxic fetuses even at an early stage, that does correlate with Apgar scores, fetal scalp, and umbilical cord pH, and that can be reproduced in hypoxic animal models (Meyers 1972) does not appear to offer information that can allow the clinician to deliver better babies than with such a crude technique as intermittent auscultation. Perhaps we have to question the role that labor plays in fetal compromise and even whether the intrapartum period really is the dangerous journey that we have been taught is a major cause of death and long-term neurological morbidity (Nelson and Ellenberg 1986). It appears that there are at least three possible explanations:

1. Most hypoxic deaths and morbidity occur before the intrapartum period. While electronic monitoring can identify a fetus that enters labor with hypoxic compromise, it is usually too late to offer an opportunity for rescue.

2. It is now well known that fetuses with neurological abnormalities of a non-hypoxic nature, such as trisomy 13 or 18 or anencephaly, have heart rate patterns indistinguishable from hypoxic fetuses with neurological dysfunction. Furthermore, they are very prone to intrapartum asphyxia, probably caused by the abnormality rather than the reverse. It is possible therefore, that fetuses with neurological abnormalities from any cause may develop intrapartum asphyxia that is secondary to their neurological problem. Our perspective in the past has been to attribute the cause as the asphyxia and the effect as the neurological abnormality.

3. Certainly there are acute intrapartum hypoxic events such as abruptio placenta, prolapsed cord, ruptured uterus, bleeding vasa previa, and maternal cardiovascular collapse that give rise to sudden acute total asphyxia and can result in fetal death or damage to the neonate. However, these will usually be obvious and the profound fetal heart rate changes can be appreciated by auscultation. There is probably a very narrow window in these cases between normal outcome and fetal death or neurological damage, giving little opportunity for the more precise information from electronic fetal monitoring to have a demonstrated advantage.

What then shall we do about intrapartum fetal surveillance? The American College of Obstetrics and Gynecology (ACOG) has recommended either continuous electronic monitoring, or intermittent auscultation every 15 min in the first stage, increasing to every 5 min in the second stage for high-risk patients only. This is based on the protocol used in the randomized controlled trials. It should be pointed out that in the trials, there was usually a dedicated nurse with each patient in the intermittent auscultation group. It appears that, on most labor and delivery services, continuous electronic monitoring will provide greater likelihood of meeting the ACOG recommendation for intrapartum surveillance and a $10 000 fetal monitor works 24 h a day, 7 days a week. The question of patient choice in surveillance technique is often raised. This decision must be left to the individual hospital, physician, and patient to decide. It would be ideal to have a guaranteed personal nurse for all laboring patients, but current hospital budgets make that unlikely.

Finally I would like to point out that we really do not know how much benefit there is to intrapartum fetal surveillance since there have been no studies comparing either method to no surveillance. For this reason we will continue to be required to provide surveillance either by electronic monitoring or appropriate intermittent auscultation.

Home uterine activity monitoring

Preterm birth continues to be the greatest problem faced by obstetricians and neonatologists, accounting for the great majority of perinatal deaths. Although intrapartum hypoxia has not proved to be a major cause of developmental abnormalities as was initially believed, there is no doubt that preterm birth is the single major cause of long-term developmental problems resulting in long-term disability and tremendous costs to society. In spite of this relationship, there has been no decline in the preterm birth rate in the USA (Vital Statistics of the United States 1977, 1987), and preterm birth accounts for the USA's high infant mortality compared with other developed nations (Committee to study Prevention of Low Birthweight 1985).

The approach advocated by Herron *et al.* (1982), involving intense education of providers and patients coupled with frequent cervical examination, was initially hopeful in that there was a marked decline in the preterm birth rate compared with historical controls in the same system. However, when this technique was subjected to randomized prospective trials in patients at high risk for preterm birth, the benefit could not be seen (R. Creasy, personal communication). In spite of these disappointing results, such techniques have been instituted in many public health programs.

There have been numerous studies correlating increasing uterine activity with the onset of labor whether at term or before term (Main *et al.* 1982; Nageotte *et al.* 1988). Other studies have shown that pregnant women are unable to feel a large percentage of the contractions measured by a home uterine activity monitoring device (Newman *et al.* 1986; Brustman *et al.* 1988).

Early non-randomized controlled trials by Katz *et al.* (1986) involved giving patients at high risk for preterm birth a monitoring device to use at home. Uterine activity measurements were transmitted to the hospital by telephone and a professional spoke to each patient every day. This system detected preterm labor much earlier than was the case for standard prenatal care and tocolytic intervention was more successful. Perhaps because of the disappointment about results of randomized trials of electronic fetal heart rate monitoring, this technique was subjected to randomized trials even before it was accepted in practice.

The first randomized trial by Morrison *et al.* (1987) showed that, in a very high-risk group with over 60 per cent preterm labor, the use of a home monitor and a daily phone call from an educated nurse markedly reduced the preterm birth rate compared with no monitoring or nurse-initiated phone contact. These exciting results were later questioned and three randomized controlled trials comparing home monitoring with daily provider-initiated phone contact showed no advantage for monitoring (Iams *et al.* 1987; Scioscia *et al.* 1988; Dyson *et al.* 1991). Another study of monitor use with daily phone contact showed the same outcome whether or not the monitor data was looked at (Porto *et al.* 1987). But, again, standard prenatal care given to a third group was associated with a higher preterm birth rate than in either group with provider-initiated phone contact and use of the home monitor. A recent analysis of home uterine activity monitoring by the American Medical Association panel on diagnostic and therapeutic technology assessment (DATTA) concluded that nursing contact is the major contributor to the system's success, and that further study is necessary (Cole 1989).

It would appear therefore that while the device does detect uterine activity more accurately than the patient and uterine activity does herald the onset of preterm labor, the truly significant contractions appear to be detectable by the patient who has frequent provider-initiated phone contact. The benefits of home monitoring programs seem to derive from a heightened awareness of high-risk patients coupled with a solicitous attitude on the part of the provider that breaks down the usual barriers to early evaluation, detection, and treatment of preterm labor. The device alone does not appear to offer any independent benefits. A recent analysis of the randomized controlled trials by Grimes and Schultz (1992) concluded that, until the efficacy of home monitoring has been established, this proceedure should not be used clinically, and Sachs *et al.* (1992) also concluded that current data does not support the value of the home monitoring device and the cost of such programs is high.

The US Food and Drug Administration (FDA) has been unwilling to allow the manufacturers of home uterine activity monitors to claim on labels that they prevent preterm birth and ACOG continues to classify home monitoring as experimental. In spite of the evidence, and the FDA and ACOG opposition, there has been tremendous commercial pressure to promote the home monitors, for which charges often exceed $100 per day or $5000 per pregnancy. Insurance companies are anxious to limit their losses related to premature birth and some have agreed to pay these high prices in the belief that monitoring is cost-effective. The industry has been estimated to have potential revenues in excess of a billion dollars annually. There has been a proliferation of companies producing these devices, with the leading company having registered spectacular profits and growth. Recently, the FDA approved the product of one company as an aid to diagnosis of preterm labor at an earlier cervical dilatation, even though the study on which this approval was based showed no decrease in preterm birth attributable to the device (Mou *et al.* 1991). The company was immediately purchased for more than $30 000 000 on the basis of this approval. Home uterine activity monitoring programs are now being heavily marketed to obstetricians, obstetric nurses, and insurance companies, often with the implication that the device is required by the medico-legal standard of care.

What should the practitioner do? Since there is evidence that frequent provider-initiated phone contact may decrease the preterm birth rate in high-risk women, third-party payers should be encouraged to pay for this service which could be done by existing office or hospital staff nurses at a fraction of the cost of the home monitoring programs being marketed. There is some progress being made in this area. If home uterine activity monitoring becomes accepted as the standard of care in the same way as was electronic fetal monitoring, the cost to society will be very high, the medico-legal effect will be chilling, and ultimately the patient will pay for it.

Umbilical doppler velocimetry

Doppler velocimetry is a technique that uses ultrasound to measure the speed of blood moving through the umbilical cord. The velocity patterns are then analyzed in various ways, to give the systolic to diastolic ratio, the resistance index, the pulsatility index, and the absence of or direction of flow during diastole. It is believed that these results allow the clinician to have a measure of impedance to flow in the umbilical vessels, which ultimately relates to placental flow, and such clinical entities as intrauterine growth retardation.

There has been a great deal of literature on this new technology in fetal evaluation, but its exact role has yet to be established. There are those who believe that it should be the gold standard for evaluation of the fetus *in utero*, but others believe that it adds nothing to current biophysical methods of fetal evaluation. Results of randomized trials that allow a comparison between umbilical Doppler velocimetry and antepartum fetal heart rate testing have only recently appeared. The results of metanalysis (Neilson 1991) of four randomized trials (Trudinger *et al.* 1987; Pearce and McFarland 1988; Omtzigt 1990; Newnham *et al.* 1991) indicated that umbilical Doppler velocimetry had no effect on rates of hospital admission, elective delivery, fetal distress, cesarean section for fetal distress, or neonatal condition. The analysis did show, however, a significant fall in perinatal mortality of normally formed babies who had Doppler antepartum fetal surveillance. It should be pointed out that the corrected perinatal mortality in the combined Doppler groups was 18 per 1000 and in the combined control groups was 35 per 1000—both significantly higher than usually reported with conventional methods of antepartum surveillance. The ACOG committee on obstetrical practice recently reviewed Doppler velocimetry for fetal surveillance and concluded that it should remain investigational.

Unfortunately, the control groups in these trials had primarily non-stress testing for fetal surveillance which was shown in four previous randomized trials to have no beneficial effect on perinatal mortality (Brown *et al.* 1982; Flynn *et al.* 1982; Lumley *et al.* 1983; Kidd *et al.* 1985). It was also not possible to determine the exact protocols for fetal surveillance in either the Doppler or control groups. We therefore currently need a randomized controlled trial of umbilical Doppler velocimetry vs either contraction stress testing or full or modified biophysical profile testing. While there are no randomized trials comparing the latter two techniques with non-stress testing, there is some evidence that the antenatal death rate is much less with these methods than with non-stress testing for primary surveillance (Freeman *et al.* 1982; Manning *et al.* 1987; Clark *et al.* 1989). It is doubtful at this point, however, that umbilical Doppler velocimetry surveillance of high-risk pregnancies improves perinatal survival compared with populations being surveyed by non-stress testing only.

As with other new forms of technology, Doppler umbilical velocimetry carries a risk of increased expense due to the technology itself, but more importantly to the high cost of intervention and the cascade of testing by other methods which may begin when the Doppler results are a little abnormal.

Discussion

Currently in the USA the FDA is responsible for approving new measuring devices. Traditionally they saw the scope of their charge as extending only to approval of safety and accuracy of the claimed measurements. Recently they have extended their charge to approving devices only with demonstrated clinical efficacy. For example, the home uterine monitoring devices were originally approved only for monitoring term labor based on the fact that intrapartum fetal monitors contained similar technology and were already approved. When asked for approval for use in preterm birth prevention, they withheld approval initially. When they recently approved the device, it was as an aid in preterm labor diagnosis, since there are no studies that show that use of the device itself decreases preterm birth rates. Even though the FDA has been appropriately unwilling to give such approval, the devices have become widely used as a result of the facts that approval is in place for term labor monitoring and that a physician may prescribe the approved device for an unapproved indication.

This example illustrates the need to develop a mechanism of consensus among clinical organizations to determine when and if a new technology becomes appropriate for generalized clinical application. Unfortunately, at the moment the FDA is the regulator of practice and the mechanism of using approved devices for unapproved indications has completely undermined their well-meaning attempts to limit the use of such new technologies until clinical efficacy is established. It is my opinion that there needs to be a mechanism whereby the FDA approves only the safety and accuracy of such diagnostic devices and the appropriate practice organizations such as the ACOG and or the AMA should determine their role in clinical practice. It is important to separate the research funding by manufacturers and researchers to avoid the obvious conflicts of interest that can occur. Ideally, the manufacturers would provide funding for research designed and supervised by a consortium of such organizations as the FDA, NIH, and ACOG. Recently ACOG has committed to a technology assessment group that will help the practice committees evaluate the research and determine the appropriate role, if any, for new technologies.

We have lived through an age of technology explosion in medicine, much of which has been greatly beneficial. However, with limited resources for health care, unproved new technologies are competitors for dollars that may be more appropriately allocated to other uses. The lessons we have learned from the acceptance of technology before proven efficacy should be used to establish criteria that must be met before new technologies are allowed to become established practice standards.

References

Amato, J. C. (1977). Fetal monitoring in a community hospital: a statistical analysis. *Obstetrics and Gynecology*, **50**, 269–74.

Benson, R., Shubeck, F., Deutschberger, J., Weiss, W., Bererdes, H. *et al.* (1968). Fetal heart rate as a predictor of fetal distress. Obstetrics and Gynecology, **32**, 259–66.

Brown, V., Sawers, S., Parsons, R., Duncan, L., and Cooke, I. (1982). The value of antenatal cardiotocography in the management of high risk pregnancy: a randomized controlled trial. *British Journal of Obstetrics and Gynaecology* **et al.** 716–722.

Brustman, L. Anyaegbunam, A., Belle, C., Ingrasin, J., and Langer, O. (1988). Uterine activity: Perception vs electronic recording. In *abstracts of the eighth annual meeting of the Society of Perinatal Obstetricians*, Abstract 67.

Clark, S. L., Sabey, P., and Jolley, K. (1989). Nonstress testing with acoustic stimulation and amniotic fluid volume assessment: 5973 tests without unexpected fetal death. *American Journal of Obstetrics and Gynecology*, **160**, 694–7.

Cole, H. M. (ed.) (1989). Home monitoring of uterine activity. *Journal of the American Medical Association*, **261**, 3027.

Committee to Study Prevention of Low Birthweight, Institute of Medicine (1985). *Preventing low birthweight*. National Academy Press, Washington DC.

Dyson, D. C., Crites, Y. M., Ray, D. M., and Armstrong, M. A. (1991). Prevention of preerm birth in high-risk patients. The role of education and provider contact versus home uterine monitoring. **164**, 756–762.

Eastman, N. J., and De Leon, M. (1955). The etiology of cerebral palsy. *American Journal of Obstetrics and Gynecology*, **70**, 93.

Flynn, A., Kelly, J., Mansfield, H., Needham, P., O'Connor, M., and Viegas, O. (1982). A randomized controlled trial of non-stress antepartum cardiotocography. *British Journal of Obstetrics and Gynaecology*, **89**, 427–33.

Freeman, R. K. (1990). Intrapartum fetal monitoring—a disappointing story. *New England Journal of Medicine*, **322**, 624–626.

Freeman, R., Anderson, G., and Dorchester W. (1982). A prospective multi-institutional study of antepartum fetal heart rate monitoring, II. Contraction stress test vs non-stress test for primary surveillance. *American Journal of Obstetrics and Gynecology*, **143**, 778–81.

Grant, A., Obrien, N., Joy, M. T., Hennessy, E., and MacDonald, D. (1989). Cerebral palsy among children born during the Dublin randomized trial of intrapartum monitoring. *Lancet*, **ii**, 1233–6.

Grimes, D., and Schultz, K. (1992). Randomized controlled trials of home uterine activity monitoring: a review and critique. *Obstetrics and Gynecology*, **79**, 137–42.

Haverkamp, A. D., Thompson, H. E., McFee, J. G., Murphy, J., Thompson, H. G. *et al.* (1976). The evaluation of continuous fetal heart rate monitoring in high risk pregnancy. **125**, 310.

Haverkamp, A. D., Orleans, M., Langendoerfer, S., Murphy, J. Thompson, H. E. *et al.* (1979). A controlled trial of the differential effects of intrapartum fetal monitoring. **134**, 399–412.

Herron, M. A., Katz, M., and Creasey, R. K. (1982). Evaluation of a preterm birth prevention program: a preliminary report. *Obstetrics and Gynecology*, **59**, 452–6.

Hobel, C. J., Hyvarinen, M., Oh, W. (1972). Abnormal fetal heart rate patterns and fetal acid base balance in low birth weight infants in relation to respiratory distress syndrome. *Obstetrics and Gynecology*, **39**, 83–88.

Iams, J. D, Johnson, F. F., O'Shaughnessy, R. W., and West, L. C. (1987). A prospective randomized trial of uterine activity monitoring in pregnancies at increased risk of preterm labor. *American Journal of Obstetrics and Gynecology*, **157**, 638–43.

Katz, M., Gill, P., and Newman, R. (1986). Detection of preterm labor by ambulatory monitoring of uterine activity for management of oral tocolysis. *American Journal of Obstetrics and Gynecology*, **154**, 1253–6.

Kelso, I. M., Pasons, R. J., Lawrence, G. F., Arora, S. S., Edmonds, D. K., Cooke, I. D. *et al.* (1981). An assessment of continuous fetal heart rate monitoring in labor: a randomized trial. *American Journal of Obstetrics and Gynecology*, **141**, 526–32.

Kidd, L. C., Patel, N., and Smith, R. (1985). Non-stress antenatal cardiotocography—a prospective randomized clinical trial. *British Journal of Obstetrics and Gynaecology*, **92**, 1156–9.

Langendoerfer, S., Haverkamp, A. D., Murphy, J., *et al.* (1980). Pediatric follow-up of a randomized controlled trial of intrapartum monitoring techniques. *Journal of Pediatrics*, **97**, 103–7.

Lee, W. K. and Baggish, M. S. (1976). The effect of unselected intrapartum fetal monitoring. *Obstetrics and Gynecology*, **47**, 516–20.

Leveno, K. J., Cunningham, F. G., Nelson, S., Roark, M., Williams, M. L., Gujick, D. *et al.* (1986). A prospective comparison of selective and universal electronic fetal monitoring in 34, 995 pregnancies. *New England Journal of Medicine*, **315**, 615–19.

Lilienfield, A. M., and Pasamanick, B. (1955). The association of maternal and fetal factors with the development of cerebral palsy and epilepsy. *American Journal of Obstetrics and Gynecology*, **70**, 93.

Lumley, J., Lester, A., Anderson, I., Renou, P., and Wood, C. (1983). A randomized trial of weekly cardiotocography in high risk obstetrical patients. *British Journal of Obstetrics and Gynaecology*, **90**, 1018–26.

Luthy, D. A., Shy, K. K., Van Belle, G. (1987). A randomized trial of electronic fetal monitoring in preterm labor. *Obstetrics and Gynecology*, **69**, 687–95.

Main, D. M., Katz, M., Chiu, G., Campion, S., and Gabbe, S. G. (1988). Intermittent weekly contraction monitoring to predict preterm labor in low risk women: a blinded study. *Obstetrics and Gynecology*, **72(2)**, 757–61.

Manning, F., Morrison, I., Harman, C., Lange, I., and Menticoglou, S. (1987). Fetal assessment based on biophysical profile scoring: experience with 19, 221 referred high-risk pregnancies. *American Journal of Obstetrics and Gynecology*, **157**, 880–4.

Martin, C. B., Siassi, B., and Hon, E. H. (1974). Fetal heart rate patterns and neonatal death in low birthweight infants. *Obstetrics and Gynecology*, **44**, 503–510.

MacDonald, D., Grant, A., Sheridan-Pereira, M., Boylon, P., Chalmers, I. *et al.* (1985).

The Dublin randomized controlled trial of intrapartum fetal heart rate monitoring. *American Journal of Obstetrics and Gynecology*, **152**, 524–39.

Meyers, R. E. (1972). Two patterns of perinatal brain damage and their conditions of occurrence. *American Journal of Obstetrics and Gynecology*, **112**, 246–76.

Morrison, J. C., Martin, J. N., Martin, R. W., Goodkin, K. S., and Wiser, W. L. (1987). Prevention of preterm birth by ambulatory assessment of uterine activity: a randomized study. *American Journal of Obstetrics and Gynecology*, **156**, 536–40.

Mou, S. M., Shirazali, G. S., Gall, S., *et al.* (1991). Multicenter randomized clinical trial of home uterine activity monitoring: for detection of preterm labor. *American Journal of Obstetrics and Gynecology*, **158**, 858–66.

Nageotte, M. P., Dorchester, W., Porto, M., Keegan, K. A., and Freeman, R. (1988). Quantitation of uterine activity preceding preterm, term and postterm labor. *American Journal of Obstetrics and Gynecology*, **72**, 757–60.

Neilson, J. P. (1991). Doppler ultrasound study of umbilical artery waveforms in high risk pregnancies. In *Oxford database of perinatal trials*, (ed. I. Chalmers), Version 1.2, Disk Issue 6, Record 3889.

Neldam, S., Osler, M., Harsen, P. K., Nim, J., Smith, S. F., and Herter, J. (1986). Intrapartum fetal heart rate monitory is a combined low and high-risk population *European Journal of Obstetrics and Gynecology*, **23(1–2)**, 1–11.

Nelson, K. B., and Ellenberg, J. H. (1986). Antecedents of cerebral palsy: multivariate analysis of risk. (1977). *New England Journal of Medicine*, **315**, 81–6.

Newman, R. B., Gill, P. J., Wittreich, P., and Katz, M. (1986). Maternal perception of prelabor activity. *Obstetrics and Gynecology*, **68**, 765–9.

Newnham, J. P., O'Dea, M. R., Reid, K. P., and Diepeveen, D. A. (1991). Doppler flow velocity waveform analysis in high risk pregnancies: a randomized trial. *British Journal of Obstetrics and Gynaecology*, **98**, 956–63.

Omtzigt, A. W. J. (1990). *Clinical value of umbilical Doppler velocimetry*, MD thesis. University of Utrecht.

Paul, R. H., Huey, J. R., and Yaeger, C. F. (1977). Clinical fetal monitoring—its effect on cesarean section rate and perinatal mortality: five year trends. *Postgraduate Medicine*, **61**, 160–6.

Pearce, J. M., and McFarland, P. (1988). Doppler blood flow in pregnancy. *Placenta*, **9**, 427–50.

Porto, M., Nageotte, M. P., Hill, O., Keegan, K. A., and Freeman, R. K. (1987). The role of home uterine activity monitoring in the prevention of preterm birth. In *Abstracts of the seventh annual meeting of the Society of Perinatal Obstetricians*, Abstract 7.

Renou, P., Chang, A., Anderson, I., Wood, C. (1976). Controlled trial of fetal intensive care. *American Journal of Obstetrics and Gynecology*, **126**, 470.

Sachs, B. P., Hellerstein, S., Freeman, R., Frigeletto, F., and Hauth, J. (1991). Home monitoring of uterine activity: does it prevent prematurity? New *England Journal of Medicine*, **325**, 1374–7.

Scioscia, A., Nickless, N., Hodgson, P., Belanger, K., and Hobbins, J. (1988). A randomized clinical trial of outpatient monitoring of uterine contactions in women at risk for preterm delivery: self palpation vs tocodynamometer. *In Abstracts of the eighth meeting of the Society of Perinatal Obstetricians.*

Shenker, L., Post, R. C., and Seiler, J. S. (1975). Routine electronic monitoring of fetal heart rate and uterine activity during labor. *Obstetrics and Gynecology*, **46**, 185–9.

Shy, K. K., Luthy, D. A., Benett, F. C., Whitfield, M., Lerson, E. B., Van Belle, G. *et al.* (1990). Effects of electronic fetal heart rate monitoring as compared with periodic auscultation on the neurologic development of premature infants. *New England Journal of Medicine*, **322**, 588–93.

Trudinger, B. J., Cook, C. M., Giles, W. B., Connely, A. J., and Thompson, R. S. (1987). Umbilical artery flow velocity waveforms in high risk pregnancy: randomized controlled trial. *Lancet*, **i**, 188–90.

Vital Statistics of the United States. (1977). *New England Journal of Medicine, Natality*, vol. 1, pp. 1–22.7. US Department of Health and Human Services, Rockville.

Vital Statistics of the United States. (1987). *Natality*, pp. 1–255. US Department of Health and Human Services, Rockville.

Wood, C., Renou, P., Oates, J., Farreu, E., Beisoner, N., Anderson, I. *et al.* (1981). A controlled trial of fetal heart rate monitoring in a low-risk population. *American Journal of Obstetrics and Gynecology* **141**, 527–534.

18 Substance abuse in pregnancy

Wendy Chavkin

Introduction

In recent years illicit drug use by pregnant women has garnered an unprecedented level of medical and popular concern. In part this is a direct result of a dramatic increase in their drug use. It also results from heightened medical sophistication. Advances in perinatology and epidemiological research have led to recognition of a wider range of consequences of *in utero* exposure to drugs.

Since 1982, crack has been the most commonly used form of cocaine. It is a heated mixture consisting of pure cocaine and baking soda that forms into 'rocks'. Ingestion of the substance is usually accomplished by smoking the rocks in a pipe or cigarette. Because it is so accessible and inexpensive, many first-time users begin their cocaine experiences with crack and this shortens to weeks the lag from the onset of use to the development of addiction. In 1985, the US National Institute for Drug Abuse (NIDA) estimated that 5.8 million Americans were currently using cocaine, of whom 15–20 per cent were seriously dependent on the drug—more than five times the number reported to be addicted to heroin. By 1987, 20 million people in the USA had tried cocaine at least once, with 5 million regular users among all racial and socio-economic groups. The New York State Department of Substance Abuse Services (DSAS) reports that women make up a larger percentage of people addicted to crack than to any other drug. An estimated 30–40 per cent are women. On the national level, a NIDA survey in 1987 revealed that 30 per cent of women between 18 and 24 used illicit drugs in the previous year.

In 1980, in New York City, maternal illicit drug use was mentioned on the birth certificate in 6.7 cases per thousand live births. By 1988, this rate had risen to 20.3 per thousand—an increase of more than three times since 1980 (Habel *et al.* 1988). Individual hospital incidence rates in New York City ranged from 1 to 27 per cent (Chavkin 1990).

New York City statistics mirror a national trend. Based on a survey of 36 hospitals across the country, the National Association for Perinatal Addiction Research and Education (NAPARE) estimated that 11 per cent of women used illicit drugs during pregnancy, resulting in the births of 375 000 drug-exposed infants annually. Because many private patients deliver in the hospitals surveyed in this study, the authors inferred that prenatal drug use was not restricted to any one socio-economic class, although, in fact, only public patients were systematically surveyed.

The House Select Committee on Children, Youth, and Families surveyed 18 hospitals nationally in 1989 and reported that 15 of them (14 public and one private) experienced a 3–4-fold increase in births of drug-exposed infants between 1985 and 1988.

Associated risks

The compulsive pursuit of illegal drugs for women has been linked with traditional prostitution and the immediate exchange of sex for drugs, as well as sex with male drug users. In US inner cities this has resulted in close association between drug use and the acquisition of sexually transmitted diseases and HIV infection. Minkoff *et al.* (1990) reported that 18.7 per cent of parturient women in one hospital, whose newborns had positive toxicology results for cocaine derivatives, were infected with syphilis and 7.6 per cent with HIV—increased risks of approximately 7- and 5-fold, respectively. In a study done in 1987–1989, New York City birth certificate data revealed that women infected with syphilis were 3.9 times more likely to be cocaine users than those not infected (Greenberg 1991).

Nationally, the increase in drug use by young women paralleled rises in syphilis (20 per 100 000) and congenital syphilis (10.5 per 100 000), both of which skyrocketed during the 1980s (MMWR 1988, 1991). In New York City, the incidence of female primary and secondary syphilis rose by 240 per cent between 1986 and 1988. Congenital syphilis jumped to 147 cases in 1987, after holding steady at about 60 reported cases annually for many years. In 1988, the incidence increased yet another 2.4 times to 357 cases or 2.7 per thousand live births. This pattern has also been associated with trends in HIV infection. New York State Department of Health data from 1989 indicated that one of every 61 babies born in New York City was born to a mother who was seropositive. The HIV prevalence among newborns was 0.66 per cent in the state overall and 1.25 per cent in New York City. The rate of seropositivity was almost three times higher in zip code areas with high rates of drug use in New York City (Novick *et al.* 1989).

Prenatal care

The data also indicates that women who abuse cocaine are more likely than others to be covered by Medicaid or to be uninsured. Maternal cocaine users were seven times more likely than non-users to have received no prenatal care. Birth certificate data from 1978–1986 indicates that only 61 per cent of methadone users and only 49 per cent of cocaine users obtained any prenatal care, compared with 87 per cent of all mothers. They were also much more likely to have used cigarettes, alcohol, heroin, methadone, or marijuana during their pregnancies. Of the cocaine-positive mothers in one study, 48.3 per cent had received no prenatal care, compared with 20.6 per cent of other mothers (Habel *et al.* 1988).

Consequences for the fetus and infant

Illicit drugs: crack/cocaine and opiates

Knowledge of the effects of prenatal crack/cocaine exposure on the fetus remains rudimentary. Studies have not yet rigorously evaluated the possible relationship between dosage, the time of exposure during gestation, and the mode of administration with known morphologic, physiologic, and behavioral outcomes. However, clinicians concur that preterm delivery, placental abruption, low birth weight, increased pregnancy loss, and other sequelae consistent with the known vasoconstrictive action of cocaine are all increased in crack-using mothers and their infants.

Various clinical investigators have reported 2–10-fold higher rates of placental abruption among cocaine-using women than among opiate users and drug-free women (Bingol *et al.* 1987; MacGregor *et al.* 1987; Handler *et al.* 1991; Finnegan *et al.* 1992). The association between maternal cocaine use and depressed birth weight is derived from case series, controlled studies, and birth certificate data, and appears to be one of the most consistently reported findings (MacGregor *et al.* 1987; Keith *et al.* 1989; Handler *et al.* 1991; Finnegan *et al.* 1992). However, despite statistical efforts to control for confounding variables, researchers currently reserve judgement as to whether reductions in birth weight and length of gestation are directly attributable to crack/cocaine use or to the many related life-style factors known to independently and synergistically depress birth weight.

The research on the consequences of opiate use during pregnancy, while similarly plagued by associated life-style confounders, predates the era of multiple drug use. Heroin has been significantly associated with retard fetal growth. Methadone has been associated with higher birth weight, although some postulate that this reflects the benefits of participating in a treatment program and reducing the hazards of the illicit drug using life-style (Kandall *et al.* 1976).

It is difficult to disentangle whether specific drugs adversely affect maternal or infant mortality directly or through their association with a host of risk factors. In a review of medical examiner records in New York City for 1983–84, drug use was recognized for the first time to be a cause of maternal death (Allen *et al.* 1990). HIV infection is also a newly recognized cause of maternal death, although data are conflicting as to whether pregnancy aggravates or ameliorates the course of the syndrome (Selwyn *et al.* 1984).

Large databases, such as vital statistics, confirm elevated infant mortality rates among offspring whose mothers used cocaine or opiates during pregnancy. This appears to be mediated via birth weight. The race-adjusted infant mortality rate for drug-exposed infants born between 1978 and 1985 was 38.8 per 100 000, or 2.6 times higher than for infants in New York City in general (Habel *et al.* 1988).

There is a well-described neonatal abstinence syndrome following *in utero* exposure to opioids, which includes central and autonomic nervous system signs, and gastrointestinal and respiratory abnormalities and can be successfully medically managed with non-specific supportive measures, substitute opiates (paregoric), or CNS depressants (phenobarbital). Although most opiate abstinence becomes apparent after birth, 5–10 per cent of methadone-exposed newborns have a delayed abstinence syndrome beginning at 7–14 days (Kandall and Gartner 1974).

There is no true abstinence syndrome amongst cocaine-exposed newborns; a self-limited mild neurologic dysfunction characterized by irritability, poor interactive behavior, and poor organizational response to stimuli has been described, although not yet rigorously documented. This pattern appears to be transitory and does not generally require medical treatment (Doberczak *et al.* 1988).

Neither heroin nor methadone have been reported to cause an increase in congenital malformations. There have, however, been case reports of increases in genitourinary, cardiac, and limb reduction anomalies among cocaine-exposed newborns. While other studies have not documented this, some investigators have postulated a biologically coherent model of vascular disruption to explain these varied findings (Finnegan *et al.* 1992).

The long-term consequences of cocaine or opiate exposure are far from clearly understood. Despite long clinical experience with opiate exposure during pregnancy, follow-up studies of the children are still fragmentary and generally have not revealed consistent neurobehavioral abnormalities (Mayes *et al.* 1992). In general, cognitive function in children born following *in utero* opiate exposure appears to be similar to their (socio-economically deprived) peers.

Cocaine-exposed children have been popularly characterized as severely neurodevelopmentally impaired, despite a lack of methodologically sound scientific evidence. Single studies have reported structural changes in the brain (echodensities and echolucencies) (Dixon and Bejar 1989) and long-term cognitive and emotional impairment (Howard 1989). However, short-term studies have not confirmed these findings in infants, and long-term longitudinal studies have rarely been performed. These studies are confounded by multiple drug use, as well as by a host of factors which are often the result of the chaotic parental life-style associated with substance abuse.

Alcohol

Fetal alcohol syndrome was recognized in the 1970s as a constellation of birth defects encompassing intrauterine growth retardation, specific cranial dysmorphology, and CNS dysfunction. In the Western world, fetal alcohol syndrome is considered to be the leading cause of mental retardation (Waldman 1989). A dose–response relationship has yet to be clearly defined. There appears to be a demonstrably higher risk for heavy drinkers, who drink the equivalent of five or more drinks per day at least twice a month, or an average of three drinks a day during pregnancy. The evidence that light or moderate drinking (less than two drinks per day) during pregnancy has deleterious effects on the fetus is scant and inconclusive (Alpert and Zuckerman 1991; Ernhardt 1991).

At another point on the continuum of alcohol-mediated problems are 'fetal alcohol effects', the manifestations of which are often subjectively interpreted. The term has been applied to various neurobehavioral disorders, which are present at birth or develop later in life. These effects have not yet been studied rigorously and therefore remain ill defined (Ernhardt 1991; Smith and Eckhardt 1991).

Smoking effects on pregnancy and reproductive health

Cigarette smoking is associated with a range of adverse pregnancy outcomes and appears to have a negative impact on reproductive health through a variety of mechanisms. Approximately 26 per cent of US women of reproductive age (18–44 years old) smoke, an average of almost one pack (18 cigarettes) per day. The number of adolescent women smokers appears to be growing, although the highest prevalence is among older women, Black women, and women with less than a high school education (Hellerstein and Sachs 1992).

The major chemical components thought to be responsible for the effects of smoking on reproductive health are carbon monoxide, nicotine, and tar. Many chemical components have not yet been adequately evaluated (Surgeon General 1990). Carbon monoxide absorbed through the placenta results in oxygen depletion for which the fetus cannot compensate (Longo 1977). Nicotine acts to increase the levels of norepinephrine, epinephrine, and acetylcholine, ultimately raising fetal blood pressure (Surgeon General 1989).

In men, smoking impairs sperm concentration, motility, and morphology (Rosenberg 1987). Passive smoking also involves the inhalation of smoke and systemic absorption, so smoking by male partners may constitute an exposure for a pregnant woman.

Smoking appears to reduce fecundity by a factor of 1.3–1.6 (Gindoff and Tidey 1989). Fertility may be impaired as a result of disorders of oocyte depletion, ovulatory function, tubal function, implantation, and early pregnancy loss (Hellerstein *et al.* 1992). Smoking also appears to shorten a women's reproductive life-span. According to a review by the Surgeon General (1990) women smokers reach menopause 1–2 years earlier than non-smokers.

The risk of ectopic pregnancy in smokers has been shown in several studies to be 2.2–4 times greater than for non-smokers (Campbell and Gray 1987). The mechanism is not yet understood, although nicotine has been found to alter tubal motility in animals.

A clear link between smoking and perinatal loss has been consistently demonstrated. Placenta previa, abruptio placentae, and premature rupture of membranes are the leading causes of perinatal loss associated with smoking (Surgeon General 1990). In a population-based study where 30 per cent of the pregnant women smoked, there was a 25 per cent increase in total fetal and infant mortality among primiparous smoking women and a 56 per cent increase in multiparous women (Kleinman *et al.* 1988), although the study did not control for alcohol or drug abuse. However, a study by the office of the Surgeon General (1990), which did control for these variables, found strong, dose-dependent associations between smoking and perinatal loss.

There is overwhelming evidence of a relationship between smoking and low birth weight. More than 100 epidemiological studies have shown that birth weights of smokers' infants are 170–120 grams less than the infants of non-smokers. Smokers have 3.5–4.0-fold increased risk of delivering small for gestational age babies (Hellerstein *et al.* 1992). Proposed mechanisms affecting birth weight include: hypoxia due to carbon monoxide, placental vascular problems due to nicotine, decreased transfer of amino acids across the placentas of smokers, and the limited availability of zinc (Hellerstein *et al.* 1992).

More recently, a strong association has been established between smoking and sudden infant death syndrome (SIDS). Perinatal exposure increases the risk of SIDS by 2–6-fold and among women who smoke nine or more cigarettes a day the risk increases with the number of cigarettes smoked (Haglund and Cnattingius 1990; Li and Daling 1991; Mitchell *et al.* 1991; Nilsen and Laederdal 1991; Heilerstein *et al.* 1992). According to Kandall and Gaines (1991), the association between perinatal exposure to smoking and SIDS is stronger than that for opiates, cocaine, or alcohol, for which the association ranges from weak (for opiates) to non-existent (for alcohol).

As with other substance abuse problems, pregnancy appears to provide strong motivation for cessation. One-fifth of women report that they gave up smoking by the time they make their first prenatal visit (Surgeon General 1990). Some have advocated use of the nicotine patch during pregnancy for heavy smokers if non-pharmacological methods have failed, despite its FDA classification in Category D (positive evidence of human fetal risk) (Benowitz 1991; Fiore *et al.* 1992). A low level of serum nicotine appears to reduce craving and other unpleasant withdrawal symptoms of smoking. However, smoking cessation programs have rarely been linked with prenatal care.

Causes of addiction

There are a host of theories about the etiology and mechanism of addiction. Dissension surfaces initially at the point of definition. Most concur that addiction is a disorder characterized by initial gratification with use, followed by delayed negative effects with loss of control over use, which causes interference in any major life function, such as health, job, family, friends, and obeying the law. However, competing models vary as to how they explain the high relapse rates which typically mark efforts to moderate or abstain from use of the chemical. (The term chemical dependency covers compulsive use of all psychoactive agents, including alcohol and nicotine.) Classically, this has been explained in terms of physiological dependence, with increased tolerance, cellular adaptation, and withdrawal symptoms. The fact that agents reversing withdrawal symptoms have only limited efficacy in resolution of addiction and that cocaine is not associated with physiological withdrawal symptoms led proponents of the physiologic model to refine their model. They now consider chemical interaction between drugs and the brain to produce further neurochemical pathology, which in turn, drives the addiction. Opiod addiction has been demonstrated to be related to norepinephrine and beta-endorphins, cocaine addiction involves nor epinephrine and dopamine, addiction to sedative hypnotics is considered to involve gamma-aminobutyric acid (GABA) depletion, and GABA depletion and abnormalities of G protein are implicated in alcohol addiction (Gawin *et al*. 1988).

Some proponents of this disease or physiologic model emphasize genetic predisposition. Studies have been most developed in regard to alcohol and various EEG patterns and enzyme levels have been described as characterizing genetic subgroups with higher susceptibility to the development of alcoholism.

Others ascribe the clusters of addicted people in different generations of a family to psychopathologic factors. The more biologically oriented version of this model places emphasis on underlying hereditary psychiatric disorder, a psychodynamic version focuses on ego and personality deficits resulting from (addicted) parental dysfunction, and a more cognitively–behaviorally oriented version stresses learned behaviors and conditioning.

While these psychopathological models emphasize the importance of factors specific to the person to explain drug use, they concur that environmental factors also play key roles. These factors include family and peer behaviors and values, community norms and options, and socio-economic status, and associated exposures and expectations. They also comprise more macro-level phenomena such as poverty, social despair, availability and price of specific drugs, advertising and public education, and the cohort phenomenon in which there is widespread exposure of a particular age group to a specific drug. Examples of this are the use of hallucinogens in the 1960s among White middle-class adolescents and young adults and crack use in the urban ghettos in the 1980s.

Obviously, these competing models affect inferences made about treatment and about public policy. Methadone maintenance is a treatment based on a medical disease model, drug-free therapeutic communities concentrate on personality restructuring, the 12-step fellowships (derived from the original Alcoholics Anonymous model) combine a disease model (progressive disorder which can be arrested but not cured, requiring lifetime abstinence) with a non-medical therapy, and the psychopathologic model underlies both psychodynamically oriented counseling and psychopharmalogical treatment aimed at psychiatric disorder.

Lately, these models have begun to be considered as complementary, rather than competing. The World Health Organization straddled the physiological–psychological divide with use of the term neuroadaptation. The American Psychiatric Association is using behavioral, rather than solely physiological criteria to define drug dependence. Gawin and Kleber (1988) have hypothesized that prolonged high-dose cocaine use generates sustained neurophysiological changes whose chemical manifestations appear solely psychological. The classic public health triangle of host, agent, and environment. finds no difficulty in comprising these many models simultaneously, with each considered a possible contributory component at certain times.

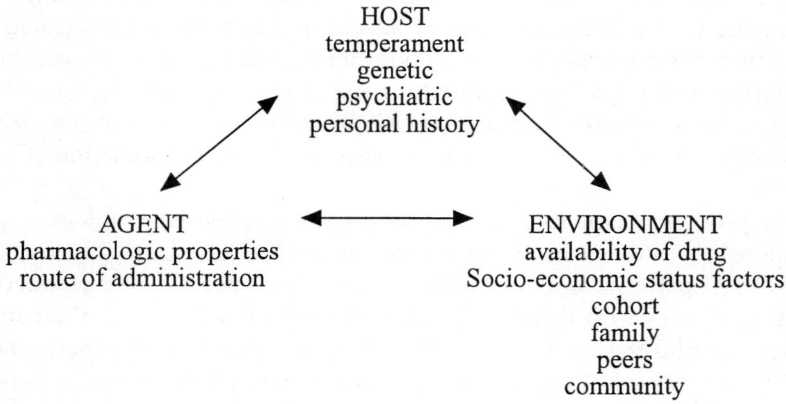

The public policy debate in the USA in the twentieth century has centered on the question of willful criminal behavior versus medical disease. In the early part of the century the criminal model prevailed and physicians were prosecuted for prescribing drugs to addicts. Organized medicine initially colluded in condemning any treatment which placed opiates in the hands of addicts for self-administration. However, this view was reversed by the 1950s when the American Medical Association (AMA) urged decriminalization of addicted status and the development of comprehensive medical and social treatment. Indeed, psychoactive substance dependency disorder currently occupies a place in the *Diagnostic and statistical manual of mental disorders* (Chavkin 1990).

In addition to these competing attempts to explain addiction generically, several other factors have been considered to explain the explosion of drug use by reproductive age women in the USA in the 1980s. These include the feminization of poverty and the rise of homelessness, particularly involving women with young children. The profile of poor families has changed dramatically over the past 30 years. In 1959, 23 per cent of all poor families were headed by women; by 1989 this proportion had risen to 51.7 per cent. Currently, nearly 40 per cent of the poor in the USA are children, more than half of whom live in families headed by women (Sidel 1992).

In addition to whatever contribution social decay and hopelessness may make to subcultures of drug use, the welfare hotels and other congregate domiciles provided by the state for the homeless became recruiting grounds for the initiation of young mothers into drug use (Kozol 1988). This transpired either through direct coercion by drug dealers, security guards, and landlords on the clientele or through massive exposure and peer pressure in these highly straitened circumstances.

Recent research has underscored associations between personal histories of sexual assault and drug use. An interview study of 150 crack-using mothers in New York City demonstrated a significant association between past sexual assault and level of drug use, involvement with an abusive man, and the exchange of sex for drugs. The younger the age at the time of the assault, the more pronounced the association (Paone *et al.* 1992).

Legal implications

The federal emphasis on interdiction and deterrence evinces an implied belief in an environmental contribution to drug use, although not one that considers drug users' economic or socio-political circumstances. Critics have postulated that women are in fact deterred from seeking treatment for their substance abuse because this punitive approach instills fear. In seeking prenatal care a woman may be vulnerable to civil or criminal prosecution resulting in a possible jail sentence or loss of custody of her child. Women may also be discouraged from giving accurate drug histories to prenatal care providers.

The vision of addiction as a medical or criminal matter is a critical one, not only for the obvious policy implications regarding resource allocation to sanction or therapy, but also for the logical consistency of the criminal justice system itself. The imposition of criminal punishment presupposes the capacity of the defendant to voluntarily conform her conduct to the requirements of the law. If a psychoactive substance dependency is acknowledged to be a compulsive medical disorder, then it would appear logical that criminal sanctions alone cannot deter it. The US Supreme Court recognized addiction to be a disease as early as 1925 in the Linder decision 'addicts . . . are diseased and proper subjects for such (medical) treatments'. The court held in Robinson vs California (1962) that criminal conviction for being addicted to the use of narcotics violated the eighth and Fourteenth Amendments, and explicitly stated that drug addiction constituted a disease status:

> It is unlikely that any state at this moment in history would attempt to make it a criminal offense for a person to be mentally ill or a leper, or to be afflicted with a venereal disease . . . in light of contemporary human knowledge, a law which made a criminal offense of such a disease would doubtless be universally thought to be an infliction of cruel and unusual punishment in violation of the Eighth and Fourteenth Amendments . . . the prosecution is aimed at penalizing an illness, rather than at providing medical care for it. We would forget the teaching of the eighth amendment if we allowed sicknesses to be made a crime and permitted sick people to be punished for being sick.

In the case of addiction during pregnancy, another heated political controversy converges with the medical vs criminal debate, that is whether a pregnant woman and her fetus should be viewed separately, with discrete and even competing interests. Fueled by the debate over abortion and the corollary arguments over maternal autonomy, maternal obligation to the fetus, and fetal status, many attempts have been made to prosecute women for illicit drug use during pregnancy. Currently, nine states in the USA define drug use in pregnancy as child abuse and 20 states have attempted to criminally prosecute drug-using pregnant women. Of these 20 states, only nine have treatment and prevention programs and only two give priority to pregnant substance-using women seeking treatment.

Many efforts at prosecution have foundered on a question of non-recognition of fetal personhood by the law. In Florida prosecutors attempted to circumvent the question of fetal status by charging women with delivery of controlled substances to minors via the umbilical cord (a charge usually reserved for dealers).

Opponents of these policies have objected to the construction of a new crime—drug use while pregnant—which does not fit the extant legal models relating to illicit drugs. They have also documented discriminatory application. Approximately two-thirds of women prosecuted for drug use during pregnancy were from a minority group and all were poor (Congressional Record 1989). In Florida, positive urine toxicology tests from pregnant Black women were reported to health authorities at approximately 10 times the rate for White women (Chasnoff *et al.* 1990).

Both the American College of Obstetricians and Gynecologists and the American Medical Association have rejected the route of punishment or coercion because of respect for the pregnant woman's right of privacy, autonomy, and bodily integrity and because of a concern about adverse consequences for the physician–patient relationship.

Although the criminal prosecutions have captured public attention, many more women and infants have been affected by interpretation of maternal prenatal drug use as presumptive risk of child neglect. Grounds for suspicion of maternal drug use vary and can include clinical symptomalogy in mother or newborn, or maternal characteristics such as public patient status, inadequate prenatal care or unregistered status at delivery, age less than 20, or residence in neighborhoods where drug use is widespread.

Even states that did not construct the special category of 'prenatal child abuse' have applied child protective laws on the basis of maternal drug use during pregnancy. In New York, for example, positive neonatal urine toxicology screens for illicit drugs were interpreted in the 1980s as evidence of chronic maternal drug use and impaired parental function. The child protective service agency was obliged to conduct an investigation and make a determination regarding parental fitness. If the parent was deemed neglectful then the agency staff devised a plan which could include supervision or foster care placement for the child. According to the New York State Welfare Reform Act, preventive or rehabilitative services were to be provided in such cases, as the 'state's first obligation is to help the family with services to prevent its break-up or to reunite it if the child has already left home' (Temporary Commission on Child Welfare 1980).

The reality was, however, that resources to assist these families were often not provided, because of budgetary constraints. The increasing numbers of these cases meant that the investigations were sometimes perfunctory, sometimes prolonged, and often accompanied by disruption of maternal custody pending the case disposition. In New York City in the 1980s, for example, when case volume was high and there was a shortage of certified foster care homes, many babies boarded in hospitals or congregate care facilities (group facilities that were run by the city's Human Resources Administration where between six and 24 infants were cared for together). In 1987, substance abuse was the primary reason for boarder baby status in New York City, accounting for 40 per cent of the more than 300 cases per day (Driver *et al.* 1987). In 1988, maternal drug use and homelessness were the two primary reasons; more than 300 babies boarded in New York City hospitals each day and another 130 per day in congregate care (Office of Policy Management 1989).

Because of this state of affairs, New York State changed its policy in 1992 and now permits continuation of custody during investigation of maternal fitness, although a positive newborn toxicology screen is still considered grounds for initiating an investigation. New York City has also initiated services to aid the maintenance of families: the establishment of a network of social workers with limited case loads offering support, frequent contact, and referral services to women in need of treatment for drug use, other types of health care, and social services.

Treatment

Obviously treatment approaches vary according to theories of etiology and sometimes with substance of abuse. No one treatment modality has been clearly demonstrated to be better than others. The efficacy of treatment appears to be predicted by a combination of the treatment modality, substance(s) used, time in treatment, and aftercare. Methadone maintenance, drug-free (out-patient), and therapeutic community approaches all consistently have similar moderate rates of success: an estimated 15–50 per cent of program participants appear to overcome their substance abuse problem. Across modalities, time in treatment is the most important factor affecting its efficacy. Detoxification is therefore reported to be the least successful of the four major approaches. The availability of aftercare—a post-treatment plan for clients' maintenance of sobriety—appears to be critical as well (Price *et al.* 1991; Tim *et al.* 1991). This may reflect the lack of data resulting from the difficulties in performing long-term follow-up on drug users and the methodological limitations of the existing research, as much as the limited efficacy of the treatment models.

Critics have also described ways in which drug treatment programs inadequately meet the specific needs of women. In the early 1970s the National Institute of Drug Abuse (NIDA) began to sponsor research and program development which specifically addressed women addicts. Surveys of drug treatment staff and addicted women indicated that the male staff and participants were often hostile to women clients, employed a confrontational 'therapeutic' style uncomfortable for women, and directed them into gender-stereotyped tasks and training which offered minimal compensation or chance for success after completion of the program. Moreover, programs did not address the environment of sexual exploitation and violence in which female addicts often lived, they made no provision for care of the addicted women's children and thus effectively limited or precluded their participation in treatment, and they did not provide contraceptive or prenatal medical services.

In 1979, after a decade and a half of encouraging treatment programs to recognize the specific needs of addicted women, NIDA surveyed those which described themselves as specifically geared towards female addicts. Only 25 could be found nationally and more than half of the women treated in these reported that they did not receive gynecologic care and three-quarters did not receive contraceptive counseling. Unfortunately, this lack of hospitality to addicted women developed into outright discrimination against pregnant women. A 1989 survey in New York City revealed that 54 per cent of treatment programs categorically excluded pregnant women. Effective availability was further limited by restrictions on method of payment or specific substance of abuse. Sixty-seven per cent of the programs rejected pregnant Medicaid patients and only 13 per cent accepted pregnant Medicaid patients addicted to crack (Chavkin 1989). The justification for the exclusion of pregnant women has been medical uncertainty over optimal medical management during pregnancy, set against the current backdrop of fear of obstetric liability.

Medical management and uncertainty

Initially the medical debate about treatment during pregnancy centered on the use of methadone for detoxification or maintenance for pregnant heroin addicts. In the early 1970s, the Food and Drug Administration (FDA) first recommended 21 day methadone detoxification during pregnancy and then withdrew the recommendation. Accounts appeared in the obstetric and pediatric literature of fetal compromise and death associated with maternal withdrawal from narcotics. Obstetricians voiced concern about detoxification during pregnancy unless biochemical monitoring of fetal status could be assured. Clinicians then disagreed about the optimal dosage for methadone maintenance. Several investigators reported a correlation between maternal methadone dose and the severity of neonatal withdrawal symptoms and concluded that maternal methadone use should be decreased to less than 20 mg per day as early in gestation as possible. Other investigators, however, did not confirm a straightforward relationship between maternal dose and neonatal abstinence syndrome. Some argued that the dose must be sufficiently high to prevent relapse and the use of additional illicit drugs and to accommodate the volume expansion and hemodilution of pregnancy. Kandall *et al.* (1976) reported a positive relationship between maternal methadone dose and neonatal birth weight and head circumference. They speculated that higher doses in the first trimester might promote fetal growth and still allow time for tapering the dose later in gestation in order to minimize neonatal abstinence symptoms.

Currently, there are not enough data on non-opioid drugs to substantiate whether the detoxification approach should be abrupt, graduated, or involve substitution, or other medication. Drug treatment options for women have recently been expanded, although the need for such services still far outdistances available treatment opportunities. In New York State in 1990, for example, it was estimated that only 42 000 treatment slots were available for an estimated 500 000 drug abusers of both sexes.

Interdisciplinary approach

Comprehensive preventive and therapeutic programs that provide a wide range of supports and resources for families with substance abuse problems are currently expanding. In a recent study, 150 addicted women and 50 experts in drug treatment described what they felt would constitute an effective drug treatment program (Chavkin *et al.* 1993). The following features were considered essential for success:

(1) a continuum of addiction services (for example, residential, out-patient, and home based);

(2) multiple counseling modalities (for example, individual, group, and family);

(3) counseling on other issues (for example, history of sexual abuse and domestic violence);

(4) services for children (day care, play therapy, child development, child development monitoring, and parent training);

(5) concrete services, including food, housing, and transportation;

(6) Program orientation (for example, long-term, community-based, and individualized care);

(7) comprehensive health care, including prenatal care, family planning, and HIV prevention;

(8) services related to women's educational needs (for example, job training and high school equivalency);

(9) appropriate staffing, including female staff, with non confrontational and culturally and racially sensitive attitudes;

(10) an advocacy role with, for example, child protective services and welfare;

(11) Aftercare (for example, 12 step, transitional housing, or individual counselling after completion of the intensive treatment program), as the recovering woman attempts reintegration into sober life.

In identifying the specific needs of women, the experts accentuated the differences between chemically dependent women and men and concurred on the importance of providing gender-specific treatment. Imperatives for programs include efforts to assist women in maintaining relationships with their children, in strengthening relationships with their partners and families, and developing extended support networks. This emphasis on relationships represents a departure from previous treatment ideology, which has advocated severance from drug-using associates and not addressed the addicted woman's responsibilities towards dependents.

The study's findings highlight the desirability of an approach that combines treatment for drug addiction with medical and therapeutic services for mother and child, education and job training, assistance with concrete needs such as day care and housing, and long-term after-care focused on relapse prevention and management. While the approach is not new—it has formed the basis for model programs established in New York, Philadelphia, Chicago, Detroit, Boston, and elsewhere over the past 20 years—it still is not widespread.

Research needs

The varied political controversies centering around drug use in pregnancy have obscured the research agenda. Outcomes of interest can be as divergent as maternal blood pressure, birth weight, urine toxicology results, and assessment of parental function by clinical or governmental authorities. Specification of outcomes of interest is obviously required in order to define the research agenda. Some key topics include

(1) interaction between drug-and alcohol-mediated changes and the physiologic changes of pregnancy, and between these and associated conditions such as syphilis;

(2) timing and dosage of specific agents and consequences for maternal and fetal health;

(3) medical management of detoxification during pregnancy and specification of maternal and fetal outcomes of interest and parameters to monitor;

(4) efficacy of treatment, defined according to maternal, newborn, and childhood behavioral and physiologic parameters;

(5) efficacy of related interventions, to improve maternal level of function in job holding, maintenance of permanent housing, resistance to abuse, parenting abilities, etc, and cognitive and affective development;

(6) length of follow-up—since chemical dependency is understood to be a chronic relapsing condition, length of follow-up and definition of recovery are essential for judging efficacy of interventions.

Much remains to be learned regarding the behavioral, physiologic, and treatment aspects of chemical dependency in pregnancy. The impact on the mother, fetus, and infant requires elucidation. Thoughtful delineation of outcome, agent, locus, timing, and mechanism is required for progress in this area.

Conclusion

The medical and public health communities generally concur in emphasizing prevention and treatment of chemical dependency, rather than interdiction and punishment. Remediation efforts with women and children who may have been multiply traumatized offer the most promising routes for breaking the intergenerational cycle of chemical dependency and improving quality of life and function. While such preventive and remedial efforts may be complicated, costly, and time-consuming, they appear to be essential. The link between drug use and HIV infection and the impact on children of familial dysfunction and disruption of parental custody lend urgency to the situation. Experimentation with treatment approaches, evaluation of efficacy, and widespread replication of promising models represent our best hope.

References

Allen, M. H., Chavkin, W., and Marinoff J. (1991). Ascertainment of maternal deaths in New York City. *American Journal of Public Health*, **81**, 380–2.

Alpert, J. and Zuckerman, B. (1991). Alcohol use during pregnancy: what is the risk? *Pediatrics in Review*, **12**, 375–9.

Benowitz, N. L. (1991). Nicotine replacement therapy during pregnancy. *Journal of the American Medical Association*, **266**, 3174–7.

Bingol, N., Fuchs, M., Diaz V., Stone R., and Gromisch D. (1987). Teratogenicity of cocaine in humans. *Journal of Pediatrics*, **110**, 93–6.

Campbell, O. and Gray, R. (1987). *Smoking and Reproductive Health*. PSG Publishing, Littleton.

Chasnoff, I., Landress, H., and Barrett, M. (1990). The prevalence of illicit drug or alcohol use during pregnancy and discrepancies in mandatory reporting in Pinellas county, Florida. *New England Journal of Medicine* **322**, 1202–6.

Chavkin, W. (1989). Help, don't jail, addicted women. *New York Times*, 18 July, p. A21.

Chavkin, W. (1990). Drug addiction and pregnancy: policy crossroads. *American Journal of Public Health*, **80**, 483–7.

Chavkin, W., Paone, D., Friedmann, P., and Wilets, I. (1993). Reforming the debate: towards effective treatment for inner city drug abusing mothers. *Bulletin of the New York Academy of Medicine*, **70(1)**, 50–68.

Congressional Record (1989). National Drug Control Strategy. *congressional Record*, 6 September, S10603.

Dixon, S. D., and Bejar, R. (1989). Echoencephalographic findings in neonates associated with maternal cocaine and methamphetamine use: incidence and clinical correlates. *Journal of Pediatrics*, **115**, 770–8.

Doberczak, T. M., Shanzer, S., Senie, R. T., and Kandall S. (1988). Neonatal neurologic and electroencephalographic effects of intrauterine cocaine exposure. *Journal of Pediatrics*, **113**, 354–8.

Driver, C., Chavkin, W., and Higginson, G. (1987). *Survey of infants awaiting placement in voluntary hospitals 1986–87*. New York City Department of Health.

Ernhardt, C. B. (1991). Clinical correlations between ethanol intake and fetal alcohol syndrome. *Recent Developments in Alcoholism*, **9**, 127–50.

Finnegan, L., Mellott, J., Williams, L., and Wapner R. (1992). Perinatal exposure to cocaine: human studies. In *Cocaine: Pharmacology, Physiology and clinical Strategies* (ed. J. Lakoski, M. Galloway, and F. White), pp. 391–409. CRC Press, Boca Raton.

Fiore, M. C., Jorenby, D. E., Baker, T. B., and Kenford, S. L. (1992). Tobacco dependence and the nicotine patch. *Journal of the American Medical Association*, **268**, 2687–94.

Gawin, F. H. and Kleber, H. D. (1988). Evolving conceptions of cocaine dependence. *Yale Journal of Biology and Medicine*, **61**, 123–6.

Gindoff, P. and Tidey, G. (1989). Effects of smoking on female fecundity and early pregnancy outcome. *Seminars in Reproductive Endocrinology*, **7**, 305–13.

Greenberg, M. Z., Singh, T., Htoo, M., and Schultz, S. (1991). The association between congenital syphilis and cocaine/crack use in New York City: a case control study. *American Journal of Public Health*, **81**, 1316–8.

Habel, L., Kaye, K., Lee, J., and Grossi, M. T. (1988). Trends in reporting of maternal substance abuse in New York City 1978–1987. Presented at the American Public Health Annual Meeting, Boston.

Haglund, B. and Cnattingius, S. (1990). Cigarette smoking as a risk factor for sudden infant death syndrome: a population based study. *American Journal of Public Health*, **80**, 29–32.

Handler, A., Kristin, N., Davis, F., and Ferre, C. (1991). Cocaine use during pregnancy: perinatal outcomes. *American Journal of Epidemiology*, **133**, 818–25.

Hellerstein, S. and Sachs, B. P. (1993). Smoking in pregnancy. *ACOG Technical Bulletin*, v **180**.

Howard, J. (1989). Cocaine and its effects on the newborn. *Developmental Medicine and Child Neurology*, **31**, 255–7.

Kandall, S. and Gaines, J. (1991). Maternal substance use and subsequent sudden infant death syndrome (SIDS) in offspring. *Neurotoxicology and Teratology*, **13**, 235–40.

Kandall, S. and Gartner, L. M. (1974). Late presentation of drug withdrawal symptoms in newborns. *American Journal of the Diseased Child*, **127**, 58–61.

Kandall, S. R., Albin, S., Lewison, J., Bearle, B., Eidelman, A., and Gartner, L. (1976). Differential effects of maternal heroin and methadone use on birth weight. *Pediatrics*, **58**, 681–5.

Keith, L. G., MacGregor, S., Freidell, S., Rosner, M., Chasnoff, I., and Sciarra, J. J. (1989). Substance abuse in pregnant women: recent experience at the perinatal center for chemical dependence of Northwestern Memorial Hospital. *Obstetrics and Gynecology*, **73**, 715–20.

Kleinman, J., Pierre, M., Madans, J., Land, G., and Schramm W. (1988). The effects of maternal smoking on fetal and infant mortality. *The American Journal of Epidemiology*, **127**, 274–82.

Kozol, J. (1988). *Rachel and Her Children*, p. 111. Crown Publishers, New York.

Li, D. K. and Daling, J. R. (1991). Maternal smoking, low birth weight, and ethnicity in relation to sudden infant death syndrome. *American Journal of Epidemiology*, **143**, 958–64.

Longo, L. (1977). The biological effects of carbon monoxide on the pregnant women, and newborn infant. *The American Journal of Obstetrics and Gynecology*, **129**, 69–103.

MacGregor, S., Keith, L., Chasnoff, I., Rosner, M., Chisum, G., Shaw, P. *et al.* (1987). Cocaine use during pregnancy: adverse perinatal outcome. *American Journal of Obstetrics and Gynocology*, **156**, 686–90.

Mayes, L. C., Granger, R., Bornstein, M., and Zuckerman, B. (1992). The problem of prenatal cocaine exposure: a rush to judgement. *Journal of the American Medical Association*, **267**, 406–8.

Minkoff, H. L., McCalla, S., Delke, I., Stevens, R., Salwen, M., and Feldman, J. (1990). The relationship of cocaine use to syphilis and human immunodeficiency virus infections among inner city parturient women. *American Journal of Obstetrics Gynecology*, **163**, 521–6.

Mitchell, E. A., Scragg, R., Stewart, A. W., Becroft, D. M., Taylor, B. J., Ford, R. P.

et al. (1991). Results from the first year of the New Zealand cot death study. *New Zealand Medical Journal*, **104**, 191.

MMWR (1988). Syphilis and congenital syphilis—United States, 1985–1988. *Morbidity and Mortality Weekly Report*, **37**, 486–9.

MMWR (1991). Primary and secondary syphilis—United States, 1981–90. *Morbidity and Mortality Weekly Report*, **40** 314–5.

Nilsen, S. T. and Laederdal, A. (1991). Crib death and smoking during pregnancy (Krybbedod or royking i svangerskapet). *Tidsskr-Nor-Laegeforen*, **111**, 3493–5.

Novick, L. F., Berns, D., Stricof, R., Stevens, R., Pass, K., and Wethers, J. (1989). HIV seroprevalence in newborns in New York State. *Journal of the American Medical Association*, **261**, 1745–50.

Office of Policy Management. (1989). *Whatever happened to the boarder babies*? Office of the Comptroller, city of New York.

Paone, D., Chavkin, W., Wilets, I., Friedmann, P., and Des Jarlais, D. (1992). The impact of sexual abuse: implications for drug treatment. *Journal of Women's Health*, **1**, 149–53.

Price, R. H., Burke, A. C., D'Aunno, T., Klingel, D. M., McCaughrin, W., Rafferty, J. A., and Vaughn, T. E. (1991). Outpatient drug abuse treatment services, 1988: results of a national survey. *National Institute of Drug Addiction NIDA* **106**, 63–92.

Robinson vs California (1962). 370 US 660, 8 L ed 2d 758, 82 S Ct 1417 [No 554].

Rosenberg, M. J. (1987). *Smoking and Reproductive Health*, PSG Publishing, Littleton.

Rush, D., Andrews, J., and Kristal, A. (1990). Maternal cigarette smoking during pregnancy, adiposity, social class, and perinatal outcome in Cardiff, Wales 1965–1977. *American Journal of Perinatology*, **7**, 319–26.

Selwyn, P. A., Schoenbaum, E. C., Davenny, K., and Robertson, V. J. (1984). Prospective study of human immunodeficiency virus infection and pregnancy outcomes in intravenous drug using women. *Journal of the American Medical Association*, **261**, 1289–94.

Sidel, R. (1992). Women and children first: towards a US family policy. *American Journal of Public Health*, **82**, 664–5.

Smith, K. J. and Eckhardt, M. J. (1991). The effects of prenatal alcohol on the central nervous system. *Recent Developments in Alcoholism*. **9**, 151–64.

Temporary Commission on Child Welfare (1980). *The Children of the State III*. New York City and Albany.

Tim, F. M., Fletcher, B., and Hubbard, R. L. (1991). Treatment outcomes for drug abuse clients. *National Institute of Drug Addiction*, **106**, 93–112.

Surgeon General (1989). *Reducing the health consequences of smoking: a 25 year progress report: a report of the Surgeon General*. US Department of Health and Human Services Publication no. (CDC) 89–8411, 75–85, Washington DC.

Surgeon General (1991). *The health benefits of smoking cessation: a report of the Surgeon general*. US Department of Health and Human Services, Publication no. (CDC) 90–8416, Washington DC.

Waldman, H. (1989). Fetal alcohol syndrome and the realities of our time. *ASDC Journal of Dentistry for Children*, **56**, 435–7.

19 Prevention of preterm birth in France

Emile Papiernik

Definition of preterm delivery

A fetus is considered mature when the pregnancy has lasted 37 weeks since the first day of the last menstrual period (LMP). Preterm birth is defined as a birth before the fetus has reached maturity.

The severity of a preterm birth is measured by the risk of death, the need for artificial ventilation, the need for prolonged intensive care, and the risk of developmental delay and handicaps. These risks are proportional to the gestational age and to birth weight.

Traditionally, the risk to the baby was described only with reference to birth weight, as pediatricians thought this measure was easier to establish and not subject to inexact estimates of gestation duration. The weight of a baby can be correlated with gestation duration: a normal growing baby born at 28 weeks will weigh 1100–1200 g, at 32 weeks, the baby will weigh 1400–1600 g, and at 37 weeks, it will weigh 2400–2600 g.

But estimating the degree of prematurity only on the basis of the baby's weight does not differentiate between short gestation (real preterm birth), and a second condition, low birth weight (less than 2500 g at birth) in a full-term infant, which can result from growth retardation. These conditions may be associated. This chapter, however, will deal only with true preterm birth resulting from shortened gestation.

The risks of being born too early

A baby born preterm is not able to adapt to the outside world—specifically, to breathing air. The major complication of preterm birth is immaturity of the lungs: they are unable to extract oxygen from air and to release carbon dioxide. The ensuing respiratory distress can lead to asphyxia and death. It is usually necessary to transfer the baby to a neonatal intensive care unit and to place it on mechanical ventilation.

Immaturity of the lung and asphyxia can have dramatic effects, particularly on the brain. The immature brain of the preterm neonate is extremely fragile. If the baby suffers asphyxia, the veins of the choroid plexus inside the lateral ventricle of the brain may become dilated and rupture. The walls of these blood vessels are only one cell thick, so rupture is seen frequently. If the bleeding is limited to the ventricle, there may not be any associated complications. However, if the bleeding damages important neurological tissue (the pyramidal pathways in the brain) this is manifested later in motor disabilities. These bleeding episodes are the reason why so many preterm babies who do survive suffer developmental impairments and motor handicaps.

Other organ systems also suffer from immaturity in the preterm baby. Jaundice occurs, although it is the least severe of the immaturity related diseases and occurs even in babies born very close to term. The therapies for some of the complications of immaturity can themselves cause adverse effects: high oxygen levels can result in blindness and mechanical ventilation can produce bronchopulmonary dysplasia.

The degrees of lung and brain immaturity and the severity of their consequences are closely related to the age of the fetus (the duration of pregnancy). For very short gestations (less than 28 weeks since LMP), organ immaturity is so extreme that many babies will not survive. As gestation lengthens, the risk of death decreases rapidly (it is reduced by half by every week of gestation duration). This is confirmed by the findings of a study of more than 3000 babies admitted to five tertiary care centers in the United States from 1983 to 1986. Duration of stay, severity of pulmonary disease and severity of bleeding in the cerebral ventricles were all related to length of gestation (Robertson *et al.* 1992).

Very few babies die who are born after 34 weeks since LMP (7.5 months of gestation). The risk of death beyond that point has been greatly reduced by innovations in technology—but other factors have also been important in improving survival of preterm babies during the past 20 years. Regionalization of care is one (McCormick *et al.* 1985). In the USA, for example, mothers at high risk for early preterm births are transported before the birth to tertiary care hospitals with neonatal intensive care units. This has made it possible to offer each preterm baby the best chances of survival.

Today, the major problem for the baby born too early and for his or her parents is the risk of developmental disability. While remarkable progress in neonatal intensive care has greatly lowered the preterm baby's risk of death, the risk of handicap or impairment among survivors has remained stable or has not decreased significantly. This means that with more survivors, the number of handicapped children from preterm births has increased.

A distinction must be made between impairments, disabilities, and handicaps. According to World Health Organization (1980) definitions, an impairment is any loss or abnormality of psychological, physiological, or anatomical structure or function. A disability is any restriction or lack of ability (resulting from impairment) to perform an activity in the manner or within the range considered normal for a human being. A handicap is a disadvantage for a given individual resulting from an impairment or a disability that limits or prevents the fulfillment of a role that is normal (depending on age, sex, and social or cultural factors) for an individual.

A large population-based study in The Netherlands measured the risks of impairment, disability, and handicap for babies born before 32 weeks. The babies were followed for up to 5 years. Of 966 such babies born in 1983, 73 per cent were normal, 13 per cent were disabled, and 14 per cent were handicapped (Veen *et al.* 1991).

The Parisian regional study of 539 preterm babies (Dehan *et al.* 1990) also described handicaps related to duration of pregnancy; survivors were followed to age 2. With increased survival of very tiny babies, more sequelae have been observed: in particular, more blindness due to adverse effects of oxygen therapy (Gibson *et al.* 1989) and more chronic respiratory disease related to the mechanical ventilation needed after birth (Zuspan *et al.* 1991). Severe bronchopulmonary dysplasia has become a major medical problem in neonatal intensive care nurseries, costing thousands of dollars per patient, many hours of care by physicians and nurses, and incalculable pain and grief to parents (Stahlman 1989).

McCormick *et al.* (1982) followed babies who needed intensive care after birth, but did not include preterm infants who did not need intensive care. The study is nevertheless of interest because of its long follow-up period. At ages 8–10, children born too soon or too small were evaluated both for severe handicaps and for less severe disabilities that affected their ability to learn. Among the babies who weighed less than 1500 g at birth, a significant proportion suffered later from severe neurological impairments with handicaps. A much larger proportion suffered from less severe developmental delays related to health problems due to being born too early or too small.

Supported by advances in technology and by aggressive obstetric and neonatal therapies and encouraged by popular support for the 'right of life', physicians who care for these tiny babies have been able to stretch the limits of viability beyond any previous expectations. Their achievements have raised a controversial question: How small is too small? (Hack and Fanaroff 1988). The answers have major financial implications (US Congress Office of Technology Assessment 1987).

The problems of medical intervention

New medical technologies have allowed babies to survive after very short gestations. Twenty years ago, most preterm babies would have died. But the very high proportion of handicapped children among these survivors opens a major discussion of the limits of our actions. Do we need to define a minimum gestational age, below which no action would be allowed? Or must we give each child its best chance of survival, no matter what the risk of impairment?

Are there limits to the actions that can be taken during neonatal care? Should pediatricians be allowed to stop their interventions if there is a very high risk of handicap? Pediatric teams around the world have begun to deal with these major questions.

Many pediatricians are aware of the dramatically increasing costs of care as technology allows infants of lower and lower gestational age or weight to survive. Despite the high levels of mortality, morbidity, and sequelae for these tiny babies, the success in allowing some to survive to normal childhood and adulthood sometimes seems enough to justify all the costs and handicaps (Hernandez *et al.* 1986). There will not be easy answers to these questions. For the mother, the father, the society, and the child, the best answer is to prevent preterm birth in the first place. Later in this chapter, I explain how, between 1971 and 1988, a prevention policy in France reduced the rate of preterm births by more than one-third and the rate of very early preterm births by more than two-thirds.

Social factors in preterm deliveries

To propose methods of prevention, however, it is necessary to understand how this accident occurs. Such understanding has not come easily. Preterm birth is a common outcome of a combination of medical and social factors. In fact, it may be said to be a social disease: it happens much more frequently if the mother is poor, less educated, without social links, single, or too young.

Preterm birth is highly influenced by the social class to which the patient belongs. Most authors have agreed on this correlation between preterm birth and social class, regardless of the population studied. National data are unequivocal on this major point; for example, preterm birth is closely related to social class in the UK (Butler and Alberman 1969; Chamberlain *et al.* 1975). This is also true in the USA (Garn *et al.* 1977) and in France, both on a nation-wide scale (Rumeau-Rouquette *et al.* 1978) and in hospital populations (Rumeau-Rouquette *et al.* 1979). Rumeau-Rouquette's results were for 12 000 pregnancies followed from the first trimester during the late 1960s in public hospitals in Paris. Similar results were seen in a prospective study of a population in Haguenau, France (Mamelle *et al.* 1984). The social differences are even more obvious for gestations of less than 33 weeks; for these, the ratio of privileged to underprivileged women for a preterm delivery is 1 : 3.3 (Mamelle *et al.* 1981, 1984).

Social class seems at first not to be amenable to any measures or policy because the clinician cannot change the social class to which a pregnant woman belongs. Such a resigned approach, however, is an inappropriate response to the problem. There has been insufficient research into why social class is such a basic cause of preterm birth. In 1969, we hypothesized that social class is not a simple factor but is made up of several different, complex components which must be distinguished in order to focus the preventive actions (Papiernik 1969). Four essential factors that vary according to social class were considered:

(1) physical work;

(2) access to information;
(3) choice of care channels;
(4) other social factors.

Physical work

One of the first clues to risk factors for preterm births was given by Adolphe Pinard, a French obstetrician in the last years of the last century (Pinard 1895). He showed that one of the reasons for the social distribution of preterm deliveries was hard physical effort at work. He discovered a very high risk of preterm births among the women who worked in the laundry factories in the district of Vaugirard in Paris. He tested his hypothesis by making it possible for these women to avoid hard work during the last weeks of their pregnancy. As a result, the women delivered at term, like 'bourgeoises' who did not work. These findings were confirmed by Debre *et al.* (1934) and by Stewart (1955), who showed that physical overexertion, as a result of either salaried or domestic work, was related to preterm delivery.

Modern studies in France have shown more precisely the relationship between preterm births and hard work. Paid work *per se* does not increase the risk of preterm labor. On the contrary, women doing paid work have fewer preterm births than women who work at home. The paradox is only apparent when results are analyzed in relation to their social context. Obviously, groups of working and non-working women do not have the same social composition or equivalent levels of education. In France, women having no paid work are of a lower social rank, have received less education, and, as a group, have a higher rate of preterm births (Rumeau-Rouquette *et al.* 1979; Mamelle *et al.* 1981). Furthermore, women working outside the home are better informed about pregnancy and make better use of medical resources (Rumeau-Rouquette *et al.* 1979).

Table 19.1 Professional fatigue index

Item contributing to fatigue	Index is 'high' if:
Posture	Standing more than 3 h per day
Machine	Assembly line work on an industrial machine
	Independent work on industrial machine with high degree of exertion or vibrations
Physical stress	Strong physical effort in 'fits and starts'
	Carrying loads of more than 10 kg
Mental stress	Recurrent tasks
	Variable tasks requiring little attention and without stimulation
Environnment	At least two of the following: high sound level, cold temperature, and very wet atmosphere
	Handling of chemicals

Table 19.2 Preterm delivery rate by low or high professional fatigue index

Professional fatigue index	Per cent of women		Preterm delivery rate		
	Low	High	Low	High	
Posture	59	41	4.6	7.5	$p < 0.01$
Machine	85	15	5.3	8.5	$p < 0.05$
Physical stress	70	30	4.8	8.1	$p < 0.01$
Mental stress	53	47	4.0	7.8	$p < 0.001$
Environment	80	20	4.9	9.4	$p < 0.001$

Mamelle *et al.* (1981) collected data on posture at work, use of machines, mental stress, and environmental noise; indexes were developed for each of these factor (Table 19.1). A relationship existed between the number of positive indexes of tiring conditions at work and the rate of preterm births (Tables 19.2, 19.3). When there was no positive index, the preterm birth rate was 2.3 per cent, with one positive index, it was 5.1 per cent, with two indexes, 6.2 per cent, with three, 9.4 per cent, and with four, 11.1 per cent. A second, independent relationship was shown between the number of working hours per week and the preterm birth rate: 3.6 per cent among women who worked less than 40 h a week, 5.6 per cent among those who worked 40 h, 7.0 per cent for 41–45 h, and 10.0 per cent for more than 45 h a week. Physical work and stress were unequally distributed within each social group. The Mamelle *et al.* (1981) study took account of social class and access to information and found that the relationship between physical effort and preterm birth was independent of social class. Some of the most adverse work conditions were found among self-employed women or saleswomen. Important knowledge gained in the last 10 years confirms Mamelle's early studies (McDonald *et al.* 1988; Ahlborg *et al.* 1990; Homer *et al.* 1990; Saurel-Cubizolles *et al.* 1991).

When women are questioned during their pregnancy, some know that specific physical effort can induce uterine activity. They may mention fast walking, domestic work in a bent position, or lifting infants in their arms. Some other physical activities may be an immediate trigger to preterm labor. Women who have preterm labor have often been on a long car journey, or packed a household

Table 19.3 Preterm delivery rate by low or high domestic fatigue index

Item contributing to fatigue	Per cent of women		Preterm delivery rate		
	Low	High	Low	High	
Housing	39	61	6.4	8.5	$p < 0.05$
Amenities	38	62	6.0	8.0	NS
Laundry	75	25	5.9	11.4	$p < 0.001$
Children	77	23	7.1	7.8	NS

for moving within the few days before labor. Long daily commuting time, an hour or more in a public transport system, is another adverse factor (Papiernik and Kaminski 1974). A similar effect of travelling has not been quoted as a risk factor in small towns.

An important study in the USA eliminated the effect of social class by studying female medical residents (who are assumed to work harder than most other women), and comparing the outcomes of their pregnancies (n = 984) with the outcomes of pregnancies of wives of male residents (n = 1218). The female physicians did not have more preterm deliveries, but they did have twice the rate of preterm labor as the non-physicians: 11.3 versus 6.0 per cent (Klebanof *et al.* 1990). Women in residency programs also had pre-eclampsia or eclampsia more frequently: 8.8 versus 3.5 per cent.

The strong relationship between preterm birth and hard work a standing-up position has also been demonstrated in Guatemala City, in a study of 15 786 women (Laumier *et al.* 1990).

Work can also be dangerous for reasons other than physical exertion. Psychologic stress—defined as high psychologic demands and limited control over the response to these demands—may be harmful (Homer *et al.* 1990). In a study in Sweden, after the physical exertion entailed in a given job was accounted for, occupational stress as measured by job title alone was not associated with preterm birth. But for women who did not want to remain in the work-force, work-related stress did increase the risk of preterm delivery (Ahlborg *et al.* 1990).

Information

Pregnant women's access to information seems to be of major importance. In studies, it is difficult, if not impossible, to measure precisely each woman's level of information; however, two observations are of value: preterm birth is significantly related to the mother's educational level, as measured by the number of years at school and the preterm birth rate is higher in nulliparous women. The close relationship between preterm birth and schooling is well known and has been frequently reported (Garn *et al.* 1977). When making comparisons within a given socio-economic group, the preterm birth rate is lowest in women spending the longest time at school. Teachers, for example, have the lowest rate of preterm birth. Among Black women in the USA, educational level is the most distinctive factor associated with the rate of preterm birth. Among the women in France, we were surprised to find a very effective information system—characteristic of the village communication system that has almost disappeared in our cities—in a community of immigrant women who had recently moved from Morocco (Berardi *et al.* 1988). We expected to find a very high rate of preterm birth in this particular group, due to poverty and immigrant status. In fact, the preterm birth rate was lower than that of the nearest indigenous population. There was clear evidence of an information system among these immigrant women which spread specific knowledge and advice to pregnant women in a manner similar to the dissemination of traditional knowledge of folk medicine.

Care channels

In France, the choice of a care provider is up to the patient herself and depends on her information, education, and social level. We have shown that patients actively choosing to attend the department of obstetrics and gynaecology at Clamart had outcomes unrelated to their social status or years of schooling. Outcomes depended on antecedent factors such as infertility or a previous perinatal death. Our analysis was based on single pregnancies and took account of the place of residence, distance from the hospital, social and cultural levels, and time of booking. Among these women, social level was not more related to rate of preterm delivery; all social groups had a rate of preterm birth of 4 per cent.

The social roots of preterm birth can also be analyzed in light of other predictive factors, including characteristics of the patient, single status or adolescence, and race.

Single status and adolescence

The high rate of premature delivery among single women, particularly adolescent single women, illustrates the importance of social aspects in preterm birth. These women are often isolated, in terms of social and family integration and have the lowest access to help, information, and protection; such factors may explain the high rate of preterm birth. In addition, single women often feel some uncertainty about their desire for the pregnancy and often want to keep their pregnancy hidden from their immediate social contacts. They do not obtain regular prenatal care and may have a poor diet. Many reports have shown that adolescent pregnancies are prone to deliver too soon with very small infants (Douglas 1950; Donnely *et al.* 1964; Fedrick and Anderson 1976; Clewell 1979). This is specially true for very young women with no social or family support who conceal their pregnancies.

Social isolation is probably the major factor influencing the high rate of preterm birth in adolescent girls; this explains the positive effect of a maternity shelter seen in a study involving 112 teenage girls in New York (La Guardia *et al.* 1989). On the other hand, for adolescents who refuse an abortion and show a real desire to remain pregnant, the prognosis may be entirely different. When they can be protected from moral and social isolation and if the pregnancies are correctly monitored, the rates of preterm birth may not be very different from those in a normal population (Papiernik and Tresmontant 1984).

Race

Race may be an important factor in preterm births. In the USA, for example, African American women are reported to have twice the rate of preterm births (Niswander and Gordon 1972). It is difficult to identify factors that could be responsible for such a difference. Social factors play a large role: Black women in the USA are frequently unmarried, are of a lower level of education, and are more likely to endure hard physical work. Such points must be considered when defining a preventive policy to counteract those factors, but the possibility of ethnic differences in duration of gestation cannot be excluded. It would be possible to determine this only if other elements were controlled (Alexander *et al.* 1985; Papiernik *et al.* 1986*a*).

Living conditions

Finally, it may be possible to control risks for pregnant women that are related to their everyday living conditions. Low socio-economic status, for example, cannot be accepted as a real explanation for preterm deliveries; there is no adverse physiological mechanism related to poverty or ignorance. Yet the social bases for preterm birth are often forgotten by physicians, who prefer to deal with 'medical causes' with which they are familiar. Later in this chapter, I will discuss ways to address the social reasons for preterm births. Some, such as age, marital status, or social isolation, cannot be changed. Others are more amenable to action; for instance, access to information. If one cannot change during pregnancy the years of school attendance a woman has had, one can nevertheless find other ways by which information can reach the less-educated woman.

But one preventive action is simple, at least in principle: avoid exposing a pregnant woman to hard work. The ease with which this can be implemented depends on the society in which the woman lives and whether it decides to protect her during pregnancy. This strategy has long been a major intervention in Europe. More specific action has been undertaken in France since 1970, with a focus on helping pregnant women exposed to hard work to avoid that work. The statistical relationship between hard work and preterm delivery may be weakened if preventive measures related to workload are adopted. This has happened in Finland (Hartikainen-Sorri and Sorri 1989), in Sweden (Ahlborg *et al.* 1990), and in France, where progressive reduction of exertion in work reduced its predictive value at the same time as preterm birth rate decreased (Saurel-Cubizolles *et al.* 1991).

The social factors responsible for preterm birth have not disappeared, but their role has been diminished in all countries successful in providing modern prenatal care, with free access to care, a high number of prenatal visits, social protection against hard work, help in case of isolation, and shelter for very exposed women, single women, and teenagers. The low rates of preterm births in Scandinavian countries are a modern phenomenon, observed 70 years after a good prenatal protective system was first established. The results in countries such as France, where a reduction in the preterm birth rate has been achieved by social intervention, are also convincing.

A high prevalence of premature births is the major cause of infant mortality in the USA. The analysis of all infant deaths in North Carolina from 1980 to 1984 shows prematurity as the major cause, accounting for 1883 of a total of 5624 deaths. There was an overrepresentation of non-White, unmarried, young teenage mothers, and mothers with less than adequate prenatal care (Dollfus *et al.* 1990). As long as an organized prenatal system is not available in the USA, the best medical journals will continue to publish papers from pediatricians desperate in their fight against the consequences of preterm birth and clamoring for prevention (Stahlman 1989).

Prematurity is in many instances the result of a variety of social problems in which the medical condition of the mother or the fetus is of secondary importance. Most premature infants are born to the socially disadvantaged of the USA—the poor, the unemployed, the welfare recipients, the undereducated, the school dropouts, the medically underserved, the teenage mothers, the unloved children, the poorly fed, the inadequately housed, and all those for whom the stress of day to day living and survival is of paramount concern (Stahlman 1989).

Medical reasons for preterm deliveries

There are a great number of medical reasons for preterm births, but most of them cannot be changed—at least, not during a given pregnancy. They can be classified into three main categories.

The first category is abnormal opening of the uterus, often called cervical incompetence. This is rare. It is often the cause of repeated preterm births or of repeated losses with spontaneous miscarriage in the second trimester. It is more frequent in women who have had two or more induced abortions.

Very similar to this abnormal opening of the uterine cervix are cases in which the cervix has been altered by surgery for precancerous disease (consization) (Jones *et al.* 1979) or in which the uterus was impaired by prenatal exposure to the artificial estrogen diethylstilbestrol (Herbst *et al.* 1980; Stillman 1982).

The second group of medical causes of preterm births are those related to abnormalities of the placenta or fetal membrances. A low-lying placenta leads to bleeding in the second trimester or early in the third trimester, and often very preterm birth results. In addition, sudden augmentation of amniotic fluid (hydramnios), in which the normal association of the placenta to the uterine wall is disrupted by bleeding, can lead to a preterm birth.

The third group is related to impaired growth of the fetus in the last weeks of intrauterine life. The consequence of such impaired growth can be a spontaneous beginning of labor. More and more frequently, however, growth impairment can be recognized by clinical signs or by ultrasound scans, leading to a medical decision to induce preterm birth. The first objective is to avoid fetal death, which would result if no action were taken. A second major objective is to avoid the birth of a baby with severe impairments, by avoiding the cerebral destruction that ensues if the fetus is maintained for too long *in utero* with a reduced blood volume, reduced cardiac flow, and reduced arterial flow to the brain. Methods that are effective at preventing preterm birth of normal, growing babies are not effective when a baby's growth is impaired *in utero* (Bouyer *et al.* 1989).

In developed countries, intrauterine growth retardation is seldom related to a lack of food; this is only observed in countries with a chronic famine or inadequate nutrition. In developed countries, growth retardation is more often

Table 19.4 Spontaneous and induced preterm births, by gestation duration: Haguenau longitudinal study 1971–1982

	1971–1974	1975–1978	1979–1982	*p*-value
<32 weeks induced	19	18	18	
Total preterm	97	60	47	
per cent induced	19.6	30.0	38.3	<0.05
33–34 weeks induced	8	12	14	
Total preterm	63	44	45	
35–36 weeks induced	20	17	30	
Per cent induced	12.6	27.2	31.1	<0.05
Total preterm	168	106	144	
per cent induced	11.9	16	20.8	<0.05

related to severe malformation of the fetus or to maternal disease, such as a vascular abnormality such as might be obvious from high blood pressure or a more discrete flow problem affecting the uterine vessels.

Uteroplacental conditions are common reasons for preterm deliveries in countries such as Finland, where control of social factors has been successful (Hartikainen-Sorri and Sorri 1989).

In France, preterm births related to a medical complication of pregnancy accounted for about 2 per cent of deliveries in the longitudinal study of women followed in the city of Haguenau (Huel *et al.* 1989; Mamelle *et al.* 1989) and many of these deliveries were induced by the medical team (Table 19.5).

Multiple pregnancies deserve mention, particulary because the number of multiple pregnancies has been rising since 1974, when new drugs were introduced for induction of ovulation in infertile women. It has long been known that

Table 19.5 Preterm births among live births, by gestation duration: Hagueneau longitudinal study 1971–1982

	1971–1974	1975–1978	1979–1982	*p*-value
Preterm births				
<37 weeks	299	192	210	
Total births	5548	4787	5811	0.01
Per cent preterm	5.4	4.0	3.6	
<32 weeks	81	51	29	0.001
%	1.5	1.0	0.5	
33–34 weeks	59	39	39	0.05
%	1.1	0.8	0.7	
35–36 weeks	159	102	142	NS
%	2.9	2.1	2.4	

twinning is a very important risk factor for preterm deliveries. Twins occur naturally in about 1 per cent of all pregnancies; the proportion of twins born preterm is between 40 and 50 per cent in all published series. Even more worrisome, twins are at very high risk (10 per cent) for being born before 32 weeks gestation and of miscarriage in the second trimester.

For a triplet pregnancy, the risk of preterm delivery is 95 per cent, the risk of birth before 32 weeks gestation is 25 per cent. For quadruplets, all known births have been preterm and the risk of being born before 32 weeks is 50 per cent.

These statistics raise the question of whether the use of ovulation-induction drugs for infertile women is justified, considering that triplet and quadruplet pregnancies have a risk of preterm birth more than ten times greater than in single pregnancies. The justification of assisted fertilization techniques can also be questioned in certain circumstances, since the higher the number of transfered embryos, the higher the risk of triple or quadruple pregnancies. Guidelines for good practice (as proposed in Chapter 11) should be accepted by infertile couples and by the medical teams caring for them.

What can be done?

In Western countries, the rate of live births before 37 weeks is between 5 and 9 per cent. The rate of early preterm births (gestation less than 33 weeks) is about 1 per cent. In most countries, these rates have not changed in 20 years in spite of new medical interventions. The rates are lower in Scandinavian countries (4–5 per cent) and in France, where there has been a sharp decrease in preterm births in the last 20 years. The French experience is described here (Table 19.4).

In 1971, the French Ministry of Health and Social Welfare defined a new perinatal policy. Its goal was to reduce the incidence of perinatal deaths and handicaps of perinatal origin, first by improving the quality of all deliveries, and second by reducing the incidence of preterm births (Papiernik 1969). The policy for prevention of preterm births was designed with several components:

(1) free prenatal care for all women;

(2) provision of information that would convince women to change their life-styles;

(3) appropriate use of maternity work-leave;

(4) recognition, during prenatal care, of the risk of preterm birth;

(5) reduction of physical activity as a means for prevention of preterm birth.

Free prenatal care for all women

Free care for all women is an important component of the European concept of protection of the pregnant woman and child. The Scandinavian countries were the first to implement a free, generalized prenatal care system, with a high number of prenatal visits (12–15) for every woman as its first goal. In particular, women who were uninsured, single, or extremely young were urged to seek early care and be followed; so too were women with children at home, who might find it difficult to come for a prenatal visit. The medical care was headed by an obstetrician; midwives oversaw most prenatal visits. Women were given incentives to seek early care.

Soon after the the Swedish system was established in 1935, Norway, Denmark, and Finland built similar systems. In Norway, rates for fetal and early neonatal deaths did not change greatly between 1876 and 1930 but then fell sharply between 1930 and 1951 (Bakketeig and Oakley 1986), in response to the initiation in that country of free generalized prenatal care in the 1930s.

The Netherlands developed a free prenatal care system soon after and after the second World War the UK, Germany, and France also began similar programs. The original program in France was not as well designed and not as generous as the program in Scandinavian countries. For example, in France the number of free prenatal visits was limited to three. Also, rather than being centralized under a specialized team of an obstetrician and midwives, care could be offered by any general practitioner.

The system in France was improved with great effort in 1971 (Vignier *et al.* 1971, Chapelain 1978). The rebuilt system was designed to follow the Scandinavian model more closely, with prenatal care delivered at prenatal clinics by obstetricians and midwives and as often as possible by the team that would actually be in charge of delivery. It was not enough, however, merely to propose a new system of prenatal care; the women had to be convinced to change their habits, and this took several years.

During the first 4 years of the new system (1971–74) the number of prenatal visits to maternity clinic made by different women varied widely; the crucial criteria was education. Women with 13 or more years of schooling had already decided to take advantage of the new offer and seek early care at the out-patient maternity clinic; 47.5 per cent were followed at the clinic from the first trimester. It was 4 years before the women with 10–12 years of education did the same. Eight years after a rebuilt system was in place, women with 9 years or less of education still were not using the system to this extent, although all women eventually did change their habits and came earlier and more often (Papiernik *et al.* 1986*b*).

Provision of information to pregnant women

Prevention cannot be imposed on anybody. Pregnant women must be given information that will convince them to participate in these risk-reduction programs. Specifically, information must be given on risk factors over which the woman has control. In France, for example, women were taught to recognize a uterine contraction and to determine whether the contraction was related to a specific type of exertion. In addition, they were given information on shortening of the uterine cervix and the related risk of preterm labor. The pregnant women were extremely interested in sharing this information, as they became aware of their abilities to modify the risk of preterm labor for themselves and to improve the outcome for themselves and their babies.

The appropriate use of maternity leave

When the issue of maternity work-leave became a political problem in several European countries in the 1920s, a major scientific study contributed to the success of the idea. The Office of Hygiene of the League of Nations sponsored a multinational scientific study in Europe on the causes of fetal and infant deaths (Debre *et al.* 1934). The study showed that preterm delivery was a major cause of infant death in the first week of life. It identified social factors that contributed to preterm birth, but also made clear the relationship of preterm delivery to hard work, both inside and outside the home. One of the study's conclusions was to propose a systematic maternity leave program for pregnant women with the aim of preventing preterm births.

Sweden began granting such leave in 1935 and other Scandinavian countries soon followed suit. Women who went on leave received financial compensation and job protection. Maternity leave was mandated by law for all women and, along with free prenatal care, was an important part of the European 'System for Protection of Mother and Child'.

Presently, all European countries have maternity leave for the specific purpose of preventing preterm birth. Leave begins during the last 6–8 weeks of pregnancy in Belgium, France, Germany, Ireland, Italy, and The Netherlands, 10 weeks prenatally in Sweden, and 12 weeks prenatally in Norway and the UK. All countries provide sick leave in addition to maternity leave, for as long as necessary during the pregnancy, although the proportion of salary compensation for sick leave is less than that given for maternity leave. In Belgium, Bulgaria, Germany, The Netherlands and Poland, salaries are compensated at 100 per cent during maternity leave. In Czechoslovakia, Denmark, and Sweden, salaries are compensated at 90 per cent. In Italy and Greece, the compensation rate is about two-thirds (Ierodiaconon 1986).

The recognition of warning signs during prenatal care

The goal of prenatal care is to discover signs of abnormalities during pregnancy, because the timely recognition of such abnormalities could permit intervention against severe complications. In the last years of the last century, an important goal was to recognize the warning signs of breech presentation (Pinard 1895). In the 1930s, the new goal became the prevention of toxemia of pregnancy by monitoring weight gain, testing for protein in urine, and measuring blood pressure. In the 1960s, the new goal was the prevention of preterm birth—which proved to be extremely difficult.

The first method of screening for risk of preterm delivery was proposed by Wood *et al.* (1965). They proposed watching for two major clinical signs: uterine contractions, which can be recognized by the woman early during pregnancy and which can lead to preterm delivery and the length of the opening of the uterine cervix, which can be measured by vaginal examination. A prospective study of 8303 pregnant women clearly demonstrated the value of these clinical signs in measuring the risk for a preterm delivery (Table 19.6; Bouyer *et al.* 1986, Bouyer and Papiernik 1989). Wood's use of early shortening and opening of the cervix as a clinical indicator is based on Bishop's proposal of clinical signs for assessing the maturity of the uterus for induction of labor at term (Bishop 1964).

Physiologic studies have since shown that cervix distensibility is a good predictor for preterm labor because a distended cervix prematurely reaches the low resistance normally observed at term (Cabrol 1991). Shortening of the uterine cervix can be reliably measured at the out-patient clinic. The predictive value of vaginal examination has been tested in different prenatal clinics in studies of 2943 women examined between 29 and 31 weeks (Blondel *et al.* 1991). The same clinical signs are valuable for predicting preterm birth in twin pregnancies (Neilson *et al.* 1988).

Obstetricians, midwives, and nurse practitioners must take the time to be attentive to the observations and claims of their patients. When questioned carefully, pregnant women describe precisely the circumstances of daily life that induce uterine contractions. For some, it is a fast walk, for others, it is

Table 19.6 Attributable risks factors of preterm delivery by type of sign (permanent or changeable) by parity (nulliparas vs multiparas) pregnancy phase 25–28 weeks gestation

		Nulliparas (%)	Multiparas (%)
CHANGEABLE SIGNS	Bleeding	5.0	12.6
	High blood pressure	0.2	7.6
	Short cervix	17.6	14.5
	Dilated internal os	11.3	15.7
	Low presenting part	9.0	9.6
	Expanded lower segment	9.7	5.7
	Uterine contractions	15.9	14.6
	At least one of the five signs of uterine maturity	27.9	35.1
PERMANENT SIGNS	Maternal profession blue collar	8.2	1.7
	Young[a]	6.3	1.1
	Age >35	7.7	8.2
	Primary education	14.4	17.0
	Prior stillbirth	–	2.3
	Prior preterm delivery	–	16.7

[a]Less than 20 years for primiparas; less than 22 years for multiparas.

carrying an older child in her arms, and for others, it is the way their work is demanding in bearing heavy loads or in climbing stairs (this may be true even in modern offices). Women can be questioned on the effect of coitus on the appearance and frequency of uterine contractions. Physiological studies have shown that coitus is followed for several hours by more uterine contractions, and this effect has been measured by home monitoring in high-risk women (Brustman *et al.* 1989). However, coitus has not been demonstrated as a dangerous activity during pregnancy.

Infection of the fetus and of the placenta are extremely frequent in preterm deliveries and particularly in very early preterm deliveries. It is known also to be frequently associated with miscarriages in the second timester. Infection is a secondary mechanism of premature birth, however, meaning that bacteria are very seldom the first trigger of preterm delivery, except in very rare cases such as infection by *Listeria* species. Usually, infection of the fetus and placenta are observed in women who carry abnormal bacterial flora (*Streptococcus* or *Colibacillus*) in their vagina (Chambers *et al.* 1990). But even in these women, infection of fetus and placenta does not occur when the uterine cervix—the normal barrier against infection—is closed. When the uterine cervix is shortened and opened, however, bacteria in the vagina can colonize the placental membranes, the placenta and the fetus and precipitate preterm delivery.

Reduction of physical activity

In 1969, I proposed reducing preterm deliveries by reducing the pregnant woman's work-load (Papiernik 1969). It had become obvious in the 1960s that, while maternity leave starting at 35 weeks (in France) could prevent preterm births among women whose pregnancies lasted to at least 35 weeks, the worst preterm cases were born long before 35 weeks. Thus, a means for earlier intervention had to be proposed.

My theory was based on information collected by Stewart (1955) showing that hard work was dangerous during pregnancy, even before the beginning of maternity work-leave. I also observed that nurses who worked in standing positions were prone to preterm births, particularly if they worked in very demanding jobs in the neonatal intensive care unit.

Obviously, such a major intervention as work-load reduction could not be proposed for all women. The cost would be enormous and many women would not accept it. It was necessary to define an intervention and a specific group of women for whom it would be effective and acceptable.

The point of the intervention was to reduce physical effort in daily life for those women with a risk factor identified at the prenatal visit (either a complaint of uterine contractions or evidence of uterine cervix shortening, softening, or opening). In some cases, the reduction of physical efforts could be achieved by a simple change in behavior, with less fast walking, not bearing an older child in the arms, not shopping for long periods, or avoiding long-distance travel by car. If the effort was related to work, such as long hours in a standing-up position, bearing heavy weights, or commuting 2 h or more, then simply changing domestic

Table 19.7 Sickness work-leave prescriptions during pregnancy: national studies among women working outside their home (Rumeau-Rouquette *et al.* 1985)

	1972		1976		1981	
	N	%	*N*	%	*N*	%
N	5727		2463		2955	
Work-leave prescription						
First trimester	682	12.5	430	18.3	646	23.2
Second trimester	996	18.4	622	26.6	923	33.3
Third trimester	1301	24.0	843	36.4	1104	40.8
p-value		0.001		0.001		

habits could not reduce physical exertion. In these situations, the only way to modify the physical load was to propose leave from work. At the time, French law did not permit maternity leave to begin earlier than 35 weeks. (The law was changed in 1976 to permit 2 weeks maternity leave before 35 weeks.) The only solution was sickness leave. I was able to convince the physicians in the social security system responsible for approving sickness leave that during pregnancy this should be considered a preventive intervention.

The use of sickness leave was monitored on representative samples of all French women having a baby in 1972, 1976, and 1981. Hardness of work and work in a standing-up position was also monitored. The hardness of work has decreased with years ($p < 0.001$, comparing 1972 with 1976, with 1981) (Rumeau-Rouquette *et al.* 1985). Leave prescribed by medical doctors—general practitioners or obstetricians—was carefully analysed, and their distribution by trimester is shown in Table 19.7 (Rumeau-Rouquette *et al.* 1985). Leave for sickness during pregnancy had certainly been used before, but since my work in this area, it has been prescribed more often in each of the three trimesters of pregnancy: it was prescribed for 24.0 per cent of women in the third trimester in 1972 and 40.8 per cent in 1981. This represents a major change in the working habits of pregnant women in France. The costs of this change were high, as we will discuss later by comparing them with the expected result—a reduction in preterm births.

Medical interventions

During the past 20 years, new drugs to reduce the risk of preterm deliveries have been used extensively in all developed countries. Accumulated experience shows that they are effective in preterm labor, when preterm delivery is close. But these new drugs have not reduced the rate of preterm births.

Oral beta-mimetics are efficient for maintenance after preterm labor or recurrence of preterm labor, but the number of available controlled trials is small (Keirse *et al.* 1989). Other drugs, such as indomethacin, may be effective for the treatment of preterm labor, but each drug is associated with specific dangers and should be used only in very particular circumstances.

For many years, cervical cerclage was considered useful for prevention of preterm deliveries in women at risk because of cervical incompetence. It became obvious, however, that this surgical intervention itself introduced a risk for hospitalization and for cesarean section (Lazar *et al.* 1989). In precisely defined high-risk cases (loss of two previous pregnancies by preterm delivery or second trimester loss), this intervention was effective at preventing further loss by preterm delivery (MRC–RCOG working Party 1988; Grant 1989). When risk was moderate, the intervention was not effective (Lazar *et al.* 1989).

Neither drugs nor cerclage can be proposed as routine preventive methods. Use of drugs must be restricted to cases in which the advantages outweigh the disadvantages and dangers. Cerclage is appropriate only in very rare cases.

Results of policies for prevention

It was possible to reduce the incidence of preterm births among all women of the French population for whom a prevention policy was proposed in 1971. The reduction in incidence was more marked for very early preterm births and a major reduction in the number of very low birth weight babies was noted.

The proportion of deliveries before 37 weeks fell from 8.2 per cent in 1972 to 6.8 per cent in 1976, 5.6 per cent in 1982, and 4.9 per cent in 1988 (Breart *et al.* 1991).

These results explain the marked reduction in infant mortality in France during the last 20 years (Table 19.4, 19.8, 19.9, 19.10) as assessed by the Haguenau study.

Table 19.8 Preterm births in the longitudinal study of Haguenau 1971–1982 (16 300 women with single pregnancy included)

	1971–1974	1975–1978	1979–1982	*p*-value
Women followed	5619	4820	5861	
Preterm births				
N	328	210	236	
%	5.8	4.4	4.0	0.001
Stillbirths among preterm births				
N	29	18	26	
%	0.5	0.4	0.4	NS
Live births				
N	299	192	210	
%	5.3	4.0	3.6	0.001

Table 19.9 Preterm births after direct standardization for maternal age, parity and years of schooling by study period: Longitudinal study of Haguenau.

	1971–1974	1975–1978	1979–1982	*p*-value
Crude rate (%)	5.8	4.4	4.0	0.001
Standardized rate				
Maternal age	5.8	4.5	4.2	0.001
Parity	5.8	4.4	4.0	0.001
Education level	5.8	4.3	4.0	0.001

The most important results were in deliveries at less than 34 weeks: these decreased on national representative samples (Breart 1991) from 2.4 per cent of deliveries in 1972 to 1.7 per cent in 1976, to 1.2 per cent in 1981, and 0.9 per cent in 1988. The incidence of very low birth weight babies decreased from 0.8 per cent in 1972 to 0.7 per cent in 1976 and 0.4 per cent in 1981; it remained stable or increased to 0.5 per cent in 1988.

The neonatal death rate (deaths in the first month of life), a major component of the infant death rate, fell from 11.2 per 1000 in 1972 live births to 5.6 per 1000 in 1988. This result is related in large part to the reduction in very early preterm births (Breart *et al.* 1991).

In a teaching department in Clamart, France where I was the head from 1973 to 1990, the introduction of the prevention program was rapidly followed by a reduced rate of preterm births. In a private hospital in France, the number of preterm births was 150 (1.7 per cent) among 8869 women from 1979 to 1981. This could not be explained by the demographics of the women in the sample, which

Table 19.10 Low birth weight and very low birth weight births by study period and by gestation length: longitudinal study of Haguenau

	1971–1974	1975–1978	1979–1982	*p*-value
N	5835	4991	5963	
Less than 2500 g	302	207	248	0.01
%	5.2	4.4	4.2	
Less than 1500 g	53	38	26	
%	0.91	0.76	0.42	0.01
Less than 2500 g and 37 + weeks	110/5616	80/4819	112/5850	
%	2.0	1.7	1.9	NS
Less than 2500 g and less than 37 weeks	173/5616	124/4819	129/8850	
%	3.1	2.6	2.2	0.001

were no different from the demographics of all women of reproductive age in the country. But the obstetricians at this hospital emphasized prenatal care, with particular attention to risk analysis and education for prevention (Dalloul 1983).

During 1981–1993, the stable rate of very low birth-weight births has hidden a new and important phenomenon. As new techniques have become available, the obstetrical team is more frequently able to recognize growth retardation of the fetus. It then becomes possible to prevent accidents related to growth retardation, particularly fetal death. This leads to a new type of medical intervention: deliberate inducement of preterm delivery in order to prevent fetal death. It has thus become necessary to distinguish the spontaneous preterm birth from the preterm birth by medical decision.

In the USA, several programs were successful in reducing preterm births. The *sine qua non* is to address the program to all women in a given population (Herron *et al.* 1982, Reis *et al.* 1987; Morrisson *et al.* 1987; Yawn and Yawn 1989). In Yawn and Yawn's study, the intervention was conducted on 784 pregnant women in a rural practice. The rate of preterm birth (before 36 weeks) was 2.6 per cent, significantly less than the rate in a comparable control period with 1257 births, at 3.6 per cent. Prevention of preterm birth was attempted in Dundee, UK among women carrying twins; the rules were similar to those applied to single pregnancies. A remarkable improvement in the perinatal death rate was achieved, but not because the overall proportion of preterm deliveries decreased (it did not). Rather, the preventive programs achieved a reduction in the number of births at very short gestation: there were fewer births before or at 28 weeks and of less than 1500 g birth weight, which explained the improvement in the perinatal death rate for twins (Osbourne and Patel 1985).

The advantages for the baby of being less at risk of preterm birth include not only a lower risk of death in the first month of life, but also a lower risk of impairment and handicap. In a community in Norway, a study of 34 756 births from 1970 to 1984 showed that a reduction in the numbers of very low birth weight babies was followed by a reduced risk of handicap (Meberg 1990).

Many obstetrical teams in the USA do not believe that preterm births are preventable (Tucker *et al.* 1991), because controlled trials of prevention failed among high-risk women. In inner-city Philadelphia, 943 indigent Black women were studied and no benefit could be measured (Main *et al.* 1989). A similar negative result was observed in a parallel controlled trial on 1000 high-risk women, mostly Black, in Birmingham, Alabama (Goldenberg *et al.* 1990).

We would have reached the same conclusions in our settings had our program been addressed only to high-risk women. We were unable to reduce the risk of preterm delivery in women with a major risk factor, such as previous preterm birth or bleeding in the second or third trimester or teenagers not included in a shelter program or women over 35 years of age (Huel *et al.* 1989). Clearly, prevention does not work on high-risk women. This is not surprising, as primary prevention only works before the disease occurs.

A different approach is needed to address those women at high risk. This has been well established in the management of other health problems, such as coronary heart disease (Lewis *et al.* 1986). Confusion develops because the same word—prevention—is used to refer to secondary prevention, which is the reduction of disease in people with high-risk factors (obsesity, high blood pressure, high levels of cholesterol in blood), and primary prevention, which is the reduction of risk in people without high-risk factors. Secondary prevention is addressed to individuals; primary prevention is addressed to all people in a given population. No physician would recommend jogging as exercise for a 50 year old obese man with high blood pressure, for whom the risk factors are obvious. But physicians would recommend more exercise to all young and healthy members of a population in order to prevent the appearance of risk factors.

Our prevention program for preterm births did exactly what it was supposed to do. It achieved a risk reduction. Obvious risk factors were reduced, resulting in fewer preterm births and fewer women with episodes of bleeding in the second or third trimester (Huel *et al.* 1989 Bouyer and Papiernik 1989).

References

Ahlborg, G. J. R., Bahn, L., and Hogsted, T. C. (1990). Heavy lifting during pregnancy: a hazard to the fetus? A prospective study. *International Journal of Epidemiology*, **19**, 90–7.

Alexander, G. R., Tompkins, M. E., Altekruse, J. M., and Hornung, C. A. (1985). Racial differences in the relation of birth weight and gestational age to neonatal mortality. *Public Health Report*, **100**, 539–47.

Bakketeig, L. S. and Oakley, A. (1986).

Methodological issues in evaluation of perinatal care. In *Perinatal health services in Europe: searching for a better childbirth* (ed. J. M. L. Phaff), pp. 160–71. Croom Helm, London.

Berardi, J. C., Benslama, F., and Alexandre, B. (1988). La prévention communautaire de la prématurité: Etude sur une communauté de migrantes maghrébines. *Journal of Gynecology Obstetrics and Biology of Reproduction*, **17**, 851–9.

Bishop, E. H. (1964). Pelvic scoring for elective induction. *Obstetrics and Gynecology*, **24**, 266–8.

Blondel, B., Le Coutour, X., Kaminski, M., Breart, G., and Sureau, C. (1991). Comparison of vaginal examinations findings in two antenatal clinics. *European Journal of Obstetrics and Gynecology*, **39(1)**, 51–4.

Bouyer, J. and Papiernik, E. (1989). Risk factors identified during prenatal consultations. In *Effective prevention of preterm births: the French experience measured at Haguenau* (March of Dimes Original Article Series, Vol. 25, Number 1) (ed. E. Papiernik, L. Keith, J. Bouyer, J. Dreyfus, and P. Lazar), pp. 37–72. March of Dimes Birth Defects Foundation, White Plains NY.

Bouyer, J., Papiernik, E., Dreyfus, J., Collin, D., Winisdoerffer, G., and Guegen, S. (1986). Maturation signs of the cervix and prediction of preterm birth. *Obstetrics and Gynecology*, **68**, 209–14.

Bouyer, J., Papiernik, E., Guegen, S., Lecomte, M., and Bonithon-Kopp, C. (1989). The decline in preterm deliveries in Haguenau. In *Effective prevention of preterm birth: the French experience measured at Haguenau* (March of Dimes Original Article Series, Vol. 25, Number 1) (ed. E. Papiernik, L. Keith, J. Bouyer, J. Dreyfus, and P. Lazar), pp. 107–14. March of Dimes Birth Defects Foundation, White Plains NY.

Breart, G., Beaufils, M., and Uzan, S. (1991). Low-dose aspirin and nulliparae. *Lancet*, **338(8771)**, 892.

Brustman, L. E., Raptoules, M., Langer, O., Anyaegtunam, A., and Merkatz, I. R. (1989). Changes in the pattern of uterine contractility in relation to coitus during pregnancies at low and high risk for preterm labor. *Obstetrics and Gynecology*, **13**, 166–8.

Butler, N. R. and Alberman, E. P. (ed.) (1969). Maternal factors affecting duration of pregnancy. In *perinatal problems* (Second report of the 1958 British Perinatal Mortality Survey). Livingstone, Edinburgh.

Cabrol, D. (1991). Cervical distensibility changes in pregnancy term and preterm labor. *Seminars in Perinatology*, **15**, 133–9.

Chamberlain, R., Chamberlain, G., Howlett, B., and Clareaux, A. (ed.) (1975). The first week of life. In *British Births 1970* Vol. 1, p. 51. William Heinemann, London.

Chambers, S., Pons, J. C., Richard, A., Chisa, M., and Papiernik, E. (1990). Vaginal infections, cervical ripening and preterm delivery. *European Journal of Obstetrics, Gynecology and Reproductive Biology*, **38**, 103–8.

Chapalain, M. T. (1978). Perinatality: French cost benefit studies and decisions on handicap and prevention in major mental handicap: methods and costs of prevention. In *Ciba Foundation Symposium 59*, pp. 193–206. Elsevier, Amsterdam.

Clewell, W. H. (1979). Prematurity. *Journal of Reproductive Medicine*, **23**, 237–44.

Dalloul, C. (1983). Prévention de la prématurité. Evolution du taux de prématurité dans une maternite de la région Centre. *Revues Medicale de Tours*, **17**, 811–5.

Debre, R., Jouannon, P. and Crémieu-Alcan, M. T. (1934). Enquête internationale sur la mortalité foeto-infantile (organisée sous les auspices du Comité d'Hygiène de la Société des Nations). *Revue d'Hygiéne*, **1**, 6–32.

Dehan, M., Vodovar, M., Goujard, J., Crost, M., Rougeot, M., Gautier, J. P., *et al.* (1990). Devenir des prématurés de moins de 33 semaines d'âge gestationel: résultats d'une enquête menée en 1985 dans la région parisienne. *Journal of Gynecology, Obstetrics and Biology of Reproduction*, **19**, 25–35.

Dollfus, C., Patetta, M., Segel, E., and Cross, A. W. (1990). Infant mortality: a practical approach to the leading causes of death and risk factors. *Pediatrics*, **86**, 176–83.

Donnely, J. F., Flowers, C. E., and Creadick, R. N., (1964). Maternal, fetal and environmental factors in prematurity. *American Journal of Obstetrics and Gynecology*, **88**, 918–31.

Douglas, J. W., (1950). Some factors associated with prematurity: the results of a national survey. *Journal of Obstetrics and Gynaecology of the British Empire*, **57**, 143.

Fedrick, J. and Anderson, A. B. (1976). Factors associated with spontaneous preterm birth. *British Journal of Obstetrics and Gynaecology*, **83**, 342–50.

Garn, S. M., Shaw, H. A., and McCabe, K. D. (1977). Effects of socio-economic status and race on weight-defined and gestational prematurity in the United States. In *The epidemiology of prematurity* (ed. D. M. Reid and F. J. Stanley), pp. 127–44. Urban and Schwarzenberg, Baltimore.

Gibson, D. L., Sheps, S. B., Schechter, M. T., Wiggins, S., and McCormick, A. G. (1989). Retinopathy of prematurity: a new epidemic. *Pediatrics*, **83**, 486–92.

Goldenberg, R. L., Davis, R. O., Copper, R. L., Corliss, D. K., Andrew, J. B., and Carpenter, A. H. (1990). The Alabama preterm birth prevention project. *Obstetrics and Gynecology*, **75**, 933–9.

Grant, A. (1989). Cervical cerclage to prolong pregnancy. In *Effective care in pregnancy and childbirth* (ed. I. Chalmers, M. Enkin, and M. J. N. C. Keirse), pp. 633–46. Oxford University Press.

Hack, M. and Fanaroff, A. A. (1988). How small is too small? Considerations in evaluating the outcome of the tiny infant. *Clinics in Perinatology*, **15**, 773–88.

Hagberg, B., Hagberg, G., Olow, I. and Van Wendt, X. X. (1989). The changing panorama of cerebral palsy in Sweden: in the birth years period 1979–82. *Acta Paediatrica Scandinavica*, **17**, 283–90.

Hartikainen-Sorri, A. L. and Sorri M. (1989). Occupational and socio-medical factors in preterm birth. *Obstetrics and Gynecology*, **74 (1)**, 13–16.

Herbst, A. L., Hubby, M. M., Biough, R. R., and Azizi, F. (1980). A comparison of pregnancy experience in DES exposed and DES unexposed daughters. *Journal of Reproductive Medicine*, **24**, 62–9.

Hernandez, J. A., Ofutt, J., and Buitterfield, L. S. (1986). The cost of care of the less than 1000 g infant. *Clinical Perinatology*, **13**, 461–76.

Herron, M. A., Katz, M., and Creasy, R. K. (1982). Evaluation of a preterm birth prevention program: preliminary report. *Obstetrics and Gynecology*, **59**, 452–6.

Homer, C. J., Sherman, A. J., and Siegel, T. (1990). Work related to psychosocial stress and risk of preterm low birthweight delivery. *American Journal of Public Health*, **80**, 173–7.

Huel, G., Keller, E., Guegen, S., Robert, C., Bouyer, J., and Papiernik, E. (1989). Effective perception of preterm birth : the French experience measured at Haguenau *Birth Defects*, **25(1)**, 1–234.

Ierodiaconon, E. (1986). Maternity protection in European countries. In *Perinatal health services in Europe* (ed. J. M. L. Phaff, the Regional Office for Europe of the WHO), pp. 134–9. Croom Helm, London.

Jones, J. M., Sweetnam, P., and Hibbard, B. M. (1979). The outcome of pregnancy after cone biopsy of the cervix: a case control study. *British Journal of Obstetrics and Gynaecology*, **86**, 913.

Keirse, M. J. N. C. Grant, A., and King, J. T. (1989). Preterm labour. In *Effective care in pregnancy and childbirth* (ed. I. Chalmers, M. Erkin, and M. J. N. C. Keirse), pp. 694–745. Oxford University Press.

Klebanof, M. A., Shiono, P. H., and Rhoads, G. G. (1990). Outcomes of pregnancy in a national sample of resident physicians. *New England Journal of Medicine*, **323**, 1040–5.

Klug, P. W., Rayer, H. C. G., and Standach, A. (1988). Die Sociographische und palpatorische Beurteilung des zervikalen Verscluss appareters. *Geburtsch und Frauenheik*, **48**, 143–9.

La Guardia, K. D., Druzin, M. L. and Eades, C. (1989).

Maternity shelter care for adolescents: its effect on incidence of low birth weight. *American Journal of Obstetrics and Gynecology*, **161**, 303–6.

Laumier, L. J., Vilar, J., Kestler, T., and Deomis, M. (1990). The effect of maternal work on fetal growth and duration of pregnancy: a prospective study. *British Journal of Obstetrics and Gynaecology*, **97**, 62–70.

Lazar, J., Guegen, S., Dreyfus, J., Renaud, R., Pontonnier, G., and Papiernik, E. (1989). Multicentered controlled trial of cervical cerclage in women at moderate risk of preterm delivery. *British Journal of Obstetrics and Gynecology*, **91**, 731–5.

Lewis, S., Rann, J. I., and Rancinni, M. (1986). Reducing the risks of coronary heart disease in individuals and in the population. *Lancet*, **i**, 956–9.

Main, D. M., Richardson, D. K., Hadley, C. B., and Gabbe, S. G. (1989). Controlled trial of preterm labor detection program, efficacy and costs. *Obstetrics and Gynecology*, **74**, 873–7.

Mamelle, N., Munoz, F., Collin, D. *et al.* (1981). Quantification de la charge de travail féminin pendant la grossesse. *Arch Mal Prof*, **42**, 211–6.

Mamelle, N., Munoz, F., Collin, D. *et al.* (1981). Fatigue professionnelle et prématurité. *Arch Mal Prof*, **42**, 205–10.

Mamelle, N., Laumon, B., and Lazar, P. (1984). Prematurity and occupational level during pregnancy. *American Journal of Epidemiology*, **119**, 309–22.

Mamelle, N., Laumon, B., Munoz, F., and Collin, D. (1989). Life style. In *Effective prevention of preterm birth: The French experience measured at Haguenau* (March of Dimes Original Article Series, Vol. 25, Number 1) (ed. E. Papiernik, L. keith, J. Bouyer, J. Dreytus, and P. Lazar), pp. 73–86. March of Dimes Birth Defects Foundation, White Plains NY.

McCormick, M., Brooks-Gunn, J., Wosterman-Danisch, K., Turner, J. A., and Pekman, G. J. (1982). The health and developmental status of very low birth weight children at school age. *Journal of the American Medical Association*, **267**, 2204–8.

McCormick, M., Shapiro, S., and Starfield, B. (1985). The regionalization of perinatal services. *Journal of The American Medical Association*, **253**, 799–804.

McCormick, M. C., Brooks-Gunn, J., Workmon-Daniels, K., Turner, J., and Peckham, G. J. (1992). The health and developmental status of very low-birth-weight children of school age. *Journal of American Medical Association*, **267(16)**, 224–8.

McDonald, A. D., McDonald, J. C., Armstrong, B., Cherry, N. M., Nolin, A. D., and Robert, D. (1988). Prematurity and work in pregnancy. *British Journal of Industrial Medicine*, **45**, 56–62.

Meberg, A. (1990). Declining incidence of low birth weight—impact on perinatal mortality and incidence of cerebral palsy. *Journal of Perinatal Medicine*, **18**, 195–200.

Morrisson, J. C., Martin, J. M., Martin, R. W., Gookin, K. S., and Wiser, W. L. (1987). Prevention of preterm birth by ambulatory assessment of uterine activity: a randomized study. *American Journal of Obstetrics and Gynecology*, **156**, 536–43.

MRC–RCOG Working Party on Cervical Cerclage (1988). Interim report of the Medical Research Council. *British Journal of Obstetrics and Gynaecology*, **95**, 437–45.

Neilson, J. P., Vercuyl, D. A. A., Crowther, C. A., and Bannerman, C. (1988). Preterm labor in twin pregnancies; prediction by cervical assessment. *Obstetrics and Gynecology*, **72**, 719–23.

Niswander, K. R. and Gordon, M. (1972). *The women and their pregnancies; the collaborative perinatal study of the national Institute of neurologic disease and stroke, NIH*. W. B. Saunders, Philadelphia.

Osbourne, C. K. and Patel, N. B. (1985). An assessment of perinatal mortality in twin pregnancies in Dundee. *Acta Genenica Medicina Gemellolog*, **34**, 193–9.

Papiernik, E. (1969). Le coefficient de risque d'accouchement prématuré. *La Presse Médicale*, **77**, 793–4.

Papiernik, E. and Kaminski, M. (1974). Multifactorial study on the risk of prematurity at 32 weeks of gestation. I: A study on the frequency of 30 predictive characteristics. *Journal of Perinatal Medicine*, **2**, 30–5.

Papiernik, E. and Tresmontant, R. (1984). Prévention primaire de la naissance prématurée: demonstration par la quasi-disparition du gradient socio-économique. *Archives Française Pediatrie*, **41**, 237–40.

Papiernik, E., Cohen, H., Richard, A., Monted de Oca, M., and Feingold, J. (1986a). Ethnic difference in duration of pregnancy. *Annals of Human Biology*, **13**, 259–65.

Papiernik, E., Bouyer, J., Yaffe, K., Winisdoerffer, G., Collin, D., and Dreyfus, J. (1986*b*). Women's acceptance of a preterm prevention program. *American Journal of Obstetrics and Gynecology*, **155**, 939–46.

Papiernik, E., Bouyer, S., Guegen, S., Collin, D., Winisdoerffer, G., and Dreyfus, J. (1986*c*). Precocious cervical ripening and preterm labor. *Obstetrics and Gynecology*, **67**, 238–42.

Pinard, A. (1895). Note pour sevir à I'histoire de la puericulture. *Bulletin de la Société de Médecine et d'Hygiène Professionnelle*, **18**, 326–32.

Reis, P. J., Ernest, J. M., Moove, M. L., Michiclutte, R., Sharp, P. O., and Buescher, P. A. (1987). Regional program for prevention of premature birth in northwestern North Carolina. *American Journal of Obstetrics and Gynecology*, **157**, 550–6.

Robertson, P. A., Sniderman, S. H., Laros, R. K., Cowan, R., Heilbron, D., Goldenberg, R. L., *et al.* (1992). Neonatal morbidity according to gestational age and birth weight from five tertiary centers in the United States 1983 through 1986. *American Journal of Obstetrics and Gynecology*, **166**, 1629–45.

Rumeau-Rouquette, C., Breart, G., Du Mazaubrun, C. *et al.* (1978). Evolution de la pathologie périnatale et de la prévention en France: enquêtes nationales INSERM, 1972–1976. *J Gynécol Obstét Biol Reprod*, **7**, 1905–16.

Rumeau-Rouquette, C., Breart, G., Du Mazaubrun, C., and Crost, M. (1979). *Naitre en France: enquetes nationales sur la grossesse et l'accouchement, 1972–1976.* INSERM, Paris.

Rumeau-Rouquette, C., Goujard, J., Ancelin, C., Gracco de loy, M., and Maillard, F. (1985). Registres and recherches. *Progress in Clinical Biological Research*, **163B**, 23–6.

Saurel-Cubizolles, W., Subtil, D., and Kaminski, M. (1991). Is preterm delivery still related to physical working conditions in pregnancy? *Journal of Epidemiology and Community Health*, **45**, 29–34.

Stahlman, M. T. (1989). Medical complications in premature infants: is treatment enough? *New England Journal of Medicine*, **32**, 1551–3.

Stewart, A. L. (1955). A note on the obstetrics effects of work. *British Journal of Preventive and Social Medicine*, **9**, 159–61.

Stillman, R. J. (1982). *In utero* exposure to diethyistilboestrol: adverse effects on reproductive performance in male and female offspring. *American Journal of Obstetrics and Gynecology*, **142**, 905–10.

Tucker, J. M., Goldenberg, R. L., Davis, R. O., Copper, R. L., Winckler, C. L., and Hauth, J. C. (1991). Etiology of preterm births in a indigent population: is prevention a logical expectation? *Obstetrics and Gynecology*, **77**, 343–7.

Turnbull, A. C. (1989). The early diagnosis of impending premature labour. *European Journal of Obstetrics, Gynecology and Reproductive Biology*, **33**, 11–24.

US Congress Office of Technology Assessment (1987). *Neonatal care for low birth weight infants: costs and effectiveness*, Health Technol Case Study 38. US Congress, Washington DC.

Veen, S., Evsdokkum, M. H., Schender, A. M., Veeloove-Vanhorick, S. P., Braud, R., and Ruys, J. H. (1991). Impairements, disabilities and handicaps of very preterm and very low birth weight infants at five years of age. *Lancet* **338**, 33–6.

Verloove-Vanhorick, S. P., Verwey, R. A., Braud, R., Bennehoe, K., Gravenhorst, J., Keirse, M. J. N. C., and Ruys, J. H. (1986). Neonatal mortality risk in relation to gestational age and birthweight: results of a national survey of preterm and very low birth weight infants in the Netherlands. *Lancet*, **i**, 55–7.

Vignier, B., Chapelain, M. T., and Papiernik, E. (1971). La périnatalité: étude de rationalisation des choix budgétaires. In Pour une politique de la Santé. Ministere de la Santé Publique et de la Sécurité Sociale, La Documentation Francaise, Paris.

Wood, C., Bannerman, R. H., and Booth, R. T. (1965). Prediction of premature labour by observation of the cervix and external tocography. *American Journal of Obstetrics and Gyneology*, **91**, 396–402.

World Health Organization (1980). *International classification of impairements disabilities and handicaps*. WHO, Geneva.

Yawn, B. P. and Yawn, R. A. (1989). Preterm birth prevention in a rural practice. *Journal of the American Medical Association*, **262**, 230–3.

Zuspan, V., Leyronnas, D., and Dehan, M. (1991). Dysplasie broncho-pulmonaire. *Revue des Maladise Respiratoires*, **8**, 351–65.

20 Infections in pregnancy that may affect the development of the baby

Catherine S. Peckham

Introduction

About one in 20 women is likely to experience an infectious illness in pregnancy. Most of these infections are harmless, but a small minority may cause damage to the fetus or newborn infant. The fetus may become infected *in utero* (congenital infection), or the newborn may acquire infection at the time of birth through contact with infected blood or vaginal secretions (intrapartum infection). Maternal infections that are associated with congenital or intrapartum infection and which may result in damage are listed in Table 20.1 and include rubella (German measles), cytomegalovirus, toxoplasmosis, hepatitis B, and herpes simplex infection.

Complications of maternal infection include spontaneous abortion, stillbirth, premature labor, and abnormalities that may either be obvious at birth or that may not become manifest or even develop for months or years (Table 20.2). The timing of the maternal infection and the route by which it is acquired by the infant have important implications for management. Some infections such as rubella only affect the fetus when acquired early in the pregnancy, whereas others, such as cytomegalovirus, may exert their effect throughout the pregnancy. Maternal

Table 20.1 Infections in pregnancy that affect the fetus and newborn

Rubella	Syphilis
Cytomegalovirus	Listeria monocytogenes
Hepatitis B virus	Neisseria/gonorrhoeae
Herpes simplex virus	Group B streptococcus
Varicella-zoster	Toxoplasma gondii
Human immunodeficiency virus	Chlamydia trachomatis
Human T-cell leukaemia virus type 1	
Parovirus B19	

Table 20.2 Infections in pregnancy

Outcome
Abortion and stillbirth
Congenital abnormalities
Acute illness or death in the neonatal period
Damage
Obvious at birth
Late development or manifestation
Asymptomatic infection
Normal child

infections such as hepatitis B or herpes simplex, may present a problem when acquired by the infant around the time of delivery.

In 1941, an Australian ophthalmologist first noted the association between rubella in pregnancy and congenital abnormalities (Gregg 1941). These abnormalities included congenital cataracts, heart defects, brain damage, and deafness. Gregg's observation, which was soon confirmed by others, was of particular importance since knowledge that an infection as mild as rubella could cause congenital defects meant that there was scope for prevention. A rubella vaccine was subsequently developed and congenital rubella is now a preventable condition. It was anticipated that many other virus infections might also cause congenital malformations but this has not proved to be the case. Indeed, infections in pregnancy probably account for fewer than 3 per cent of all congenital anomalies.

Infections in pregnancy are a cause of great anxiety to both women and their doctors and knowledge about the possible effects that they may have on the fetus and infant are of great practical importance. A pregnant women exposed to a specific infection needs to understand the implications this has for her pregnancy and to be offered the most appropriate management. Policy makers also require sound clinical and epidemiological data to assist them in developing appropriate strategies for prevention, for example in assessing the need for a vaccine or considering the introduction of a new prenatal screening programme. For each infection, information needs to include the local prevalence of the infection in pregnancy, the risk of maternal–fetal transmission, and the consequences of congenital or perinatal infection in relation to pregnancy outcome and subsequent disability. Before any screening programme is introduced, both risks and benefits of treatment or preventive measures, as well as the financial implications, require full assessment. In addition, the safety and validity of screening and diagnostic tests must be established, as well as the efficacy of the intervention.

Public concern and expectations must also be taken into account. However, even here there can be conflicting demands. The need for a screening programme to identify a particular infection in pregnancy may seem obvious when the individual experience of affected families is considered. But, this may run contrary to other public expectations about reducing medicalization of pregnancy and birth. As new diagnostic tests become available and more invasive techniques such as amniocentesis and fetal blood sampling are being recommended for perinatal diagnosis of infections such as cytomegalovirus and toxoplasmosis, decisions which have important implications for the population must not be made without adequate assessment of all the available information. Decreasing potential disability must be weighed against increasing intervention in the antenatal period. It is important for doctors and decision makers not to forget that screening is about the prevention of disability and disease, not simply the detection of infection.

The diagnosis of infections in pregnancy can pose particular problems as many infections that may cause fetal damage are not associated with symptoms and signs in the mother or in her congenitally infected newborn infant. In view of this most congenitally infected children are not identified and when problems arise later in childhood it is often not possible to distinguish congenital infection from infections acquired later in childhood which may be unrelated to the problem. In other situations where symptoms and signs are present and congenital infection is suspected, as may be the case with HIV infection or toxoplasmosis, it may not be possible to determine conclusively whether or not the infant is infected at birth because of the presence of maternal antibodies (passively acquired by transfer across the placenta from mother to fetus), or a lack of sensitive and specific laboratory investigations. In this situation, the infant will need to be followed clinically and serologically for many months before a definitive diagnosis of congenital infection can be made.

Cytomegalovirus infection

Cytomegalovirus (CMV) is a member of the herpes family of viruses. An important property of these viruses is that once infection has been acquired the virus remains latent in the cells and may reactivate intermittently throughout life. In healthy individuals CMV infection is usually mild and without specific signs and symptoms, but when the infection is acquired in pregnancy it may cause fetal damage. CMV is the most common congenital infection and an established cause of congenital handicap.

In non-industrialized countries most women of child-bearing age are seropositive, having acquired CMV infection early in life. In contrast, in industrial countries about 50 per cent of women of child-bearing age are seronegative, susceptible to infection, and at risk of acquiring an infection for the first time (a primary infection) in pregnancy. The birth prevalence of congenital CMV infection varies in different parts of the world from 0.2 to 2.2 per cent of live births (Stagno *et al.* 1983). Most maternal infections are not diagnosed because there are no presenting symptoms and because fewer than 10 per cent of congenitally infected infants show signs of infection at birth, the vast majority pass unrecognized.

The clinical manifestations in affected newborns may include a rash, prolonged jaundice, hepatomegaly, splenomegaly, intrauterine growth retardation, microcephaly, pneumonitis, thrombocytopenia, and intracranial calcifications. Most of the infants with clinical evidence of infection at birth suffer long-term complications which are often multiple and may include brain damage with signs of cerebral palsy, mental handicap, or sensorineural hearing loss (Pass *et al.* 1980). Of the 90–95 per cent of infected children who are asymptomatic at birth, only a small proportion, 5–10 per cent, will have long-term neurological sequelae, sensorineural hearing loss being the most frequent problem (Peckham 1991).

In a large prospective study of CMV in pregnancy in London, the congenital infection rate, based on over 30 000 consecutive births, was three per 1000 (Peckham 1991). Only four of the 103 infants with congenital infection identified had any symptoms or signs of infection in the neonatal period and all four suffered serious permanent sequelae, including sensorineural hearing loss, cerebral palsy, mental handicap, and microcephaly. Of the 99 children who were well in the neonatal period, 96 were followed to at least 3 years of age and six children were found to have a bilateral or unilateral sensorineural hearing loss, which was associated with a movement disability in two. The IQ scores of the 90 per cent of infected children with no discernible disabilities at 2 years were similar to those of matched controls who did not have congenital infection, at both 2 and 5 years. This is encouraging and suggests that children with no obvious neurological handicap develop normally (Pearl *et al.* 1986).

Congenital CMV infection does not only occur after a primary infection in pregnancy: intrauterine transmission of CMV infection also commonly follows recurrent maternal infection, even in the presence of substantial maternal immunity (presence of antibodies). Congenital infection resulting from a recurrence of CMV in pregnancy is less likely to result in fetal damage than primary infections (Stagno *et al.* 1982), although defects compatible with congenital CMV infection have been reported (Rutter *et al.* 1985).

Prospective studies suggest that about 1 per cent of women who are susceptible to CMV infection will acquire the infection at some stage during their pregnancy. About 40 per cent of those who acquire the infection will pass the virus on to their fetus (Fig. 20.1). Based on this risk of mother–fetus transmission and on a 10 per cent risk of CMV-associated damage in a congenitally infected infant, a woman who acquires a primary CMV infection in pregnancy has a risk of approximately one in 25 of having a child with CMV-associated handicap. Studies in Sweden (Ahlfors *et al.* 1979) and Canada (Saigal *et al.* 1982) show similar results to those from the UK, although studies from the USA (Fowler *et al.* 1992) show a higher rate of damage in congenitally infected children. It is important to put this into perspective, as 3 per cent of normal pregnancies may be complicated by a congenital abnormality.

There is some evidence, mainly from the USA, that nursery staff may be at occupational risk of acquiring CMV (Adler 1989; Pass *et al.* 1980; Murph *et al.* 1991). Studies have suggested that routine infection control procedures are protective in health care settings like hospitals and laboratories, but nursery staff and others involved in the daily care of groups of very young children work in a more domestic setting. Whether an occupational risk exists may depend on many different factors, including size of nursery, the age of children catered for, strains of virus circulating, and general hygiene, and there is no evidence that occupational exposure to CMV is a particular problem in the UK. However, about 20 per cent of children acquire the infection, usually from their mothers, in the first year of life; most of these children are unrecognized and have no CMV-related problem, but will intermittently shed virus in urine and saliva.

While there is no justification for routinely screening children, nursery staff should assume that any child might be infectious and pregnant staff should minimize the kind of contact that might involve the transfer of saliva, and wash their hands thoroughly after changing nappies or other similar tasks. There must therefore be proper facilities for reasonable hygiene, realistic health education about common infections in the community like CMV, and sensitive management of pregnant staff with particular anxieties.

If a primary infection is identified early in pregnancy, termination of the pregnancy could be considered an option, but prediction of outcome is not straightforward. Unlike rubella, there is no stage in pregnancy beyond which infection can be said to pose little risk and fetal damage may follow maternal infection in any of the trimesters of pregnancy. In the absence of symptoms, maternal infection is unlikely to be diagnosed. However, as laboratory analysis of blood samples may reveal an acquired infection, antenatal screening with repeat testing of blood samples from susceptible women has been proposed. At

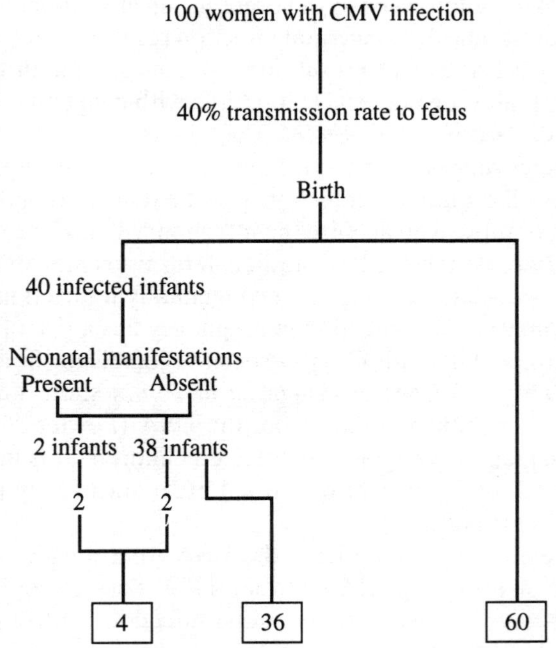

Fig. 20.1 Consequences of a primary CMV infection in pregnancy.

present, there is no treatment for a women with CMV infection in pregnancy and prenatal screening to identify women who acquire a primary CMV infection with a view to offering them a pregnancy termination is not recommended in the UK. Such a programme would not be able to identify infections occurring in late pregnancy, nor recurrent infections, and would fail to identify most pregnancies where fetal damage had occurred.

Toxoplasmosis

Toxoplasmosis is caused by infection with the protozoan parasite *Toxoplasma gondii*. Infection is acquired by the ingestion of toxoplasma tissue cysts in undercooked meat or from exposure to toxoplasma oocysts in feline faeces, either directly or through contaminated soil or unwashed vegetables. When toxoplasmosis is acquired in pregnancy, it can cause fetal infection, with potentially serious consequences for the newborn infant.

The prevalence of infection varies markedly from country to country and between groups within a country (Remington and Desmonts 1990). The best estimate of the incidence of toxoplasmosis in the UK is around two per 1000 pregnancies (Ades 1992) but higher rates of infection have been reported from France, the USA and other countries. There is some evidence from Europe that there may be a downward trend in the incidence of toxoplasmosis in the population generally (Walker *et al.* 1992).

In most healthy women, newly acquired infection is not recognized as it may not be associated with illness or may present with non-specific signs or symptoms. As with CMV, infections in pregnancy can only be detected by repeat blood tests. It is generally held that fetal infection is only associated with acute toxoplasmosis in the mother and not with chronic infection. Based on this precept, serological screening programmes have been adopted in some countries, notably in France and Austria.

Estimates of the rate of transmission of infection from mother to fetus vary, but are about 40 per cent. The risk of fetal infection depends, however, on the stage of pregnancy at the onset of maternal infection: the rate is low (10 per cent) when infection occurs in the first 2 weeks after conception but rises to over 90 per cent following infection in the last 2 weeks of pregnancy. In contrast, the likelihood of an infected fetus being damaged is much higher when infection occurs in early pregnancy (Desmonts and Couvreur 1974).

If toxoplasmosis is diagnosed in pregnancy, the management includes either termination of the pregnancy or treatment with the antibiotic spiramycin to reduce the risk of fetal infection. However, the efficacy of spiramycin remains uncertain; evidence of benefit is based on historical comparisons of transmission rates and a randomized trial has never been performed. Health education remains the best approach to prevention (Hall 1992).

There is little information on the incidence of congenital toxoplasmosis in different countries and evidence suggests that it is extremely low in the UK

(Hall 1992). About 10 per cent of babies with congenital toxoplasmosis have clinical manifestations of infection at birth. These include a spectrum of clinical effects ranging from the classic triad of hydrocephaly, chorioretinitis, and intracranial calcification, to non-specific manifestations including intrauterine growth retardation, hepatosplenomegaly, jaundice, thrombocytopenia, and convulsions (Desmonts and Couvreur 1974). However, there is little information on long-term outcome in the 90 per cent of congenitally infected neonates who are well at birth and in the neonatal period. It is often argued that the incidence of retinochoroiditis is high, but there is little evidence to support this assumption and the risk has not been assessed. There have only been a few prospective studies of neonates with asymptomatic infection and these have included very small numbers of children with no controls. It is virtually impossible, therefore, to generalize about the risk to the neonate on the basis of these studies (Peckham and Logan 1993).

There is no one simple test that will identify acute toxoplasmosis infection after conception and even when the classic signs of congenital toxoplasmosis are present the diagnosis may be problematic. This depends on the identification of IgM antibody specific for toxoplasmosis in cord or neonatal blood samples or the demonstration of persistent IgG antibody. Toxoplasma IgM assays are relatively insensitive and a negative result does not exclude infection. Sequential measurements are therefore necessary for at least the first year of life in order to demonstrate changes in IgG antibody titer that differentiate between antibody acquired passively from the mother and true fetal infection.

Hepatitis B virus

Hepatitis B virus (HBV) infection is an important cause of morbidity and mortality world-wide (Krugman 1985). This results from the direct effect of acute hepatitis or the long-term sequelae of chronic infection, cirrhosis of the liver, and hepatocellular cancer. In Southeast Asia and sub Sahara Africa the prevalence of HBV infection is high and most infection is acquired in childhood. While the high prevalence in the Far East is maintained by vertical transmission from mother to baby during the perinatal period (Stevens *et al.* 1975), in Africa infection is usually acquired horizontally from other routes (Davis *et al.* 1989). In populations where the prevalence is high, a substantial number of women (10–20 per cent) are chronic symptomless carriers of HBV and at risk of passing the infection on to their baby around the time of delivery.

In Europe and North America, where the prevalence is low, fewer than 10 per cent of adults have experienced HBV infection and the number of pregnant women who are chronic carriers of the virus is also low, about 0.5 per cent. In low prevalence areas, most infections are acquired through sexual contact or drug use and perinatal infection is uncommon. However, immigrants in low prevalence countries have similar HBV carrier rates to those in their country of origin. Women who are silent chronic carriers of HBV can infect their newborn babies and prenatal testing for hepatitis B surface antigen may be performed to identify carriers of the virus.

Newborns usually acquire HBV infection at the time of birth from contact with infected vaginal secretions or maternal blood and intrauterine infections are uncommon. The virus does not cross the placenta and the few intrauterine infections which occur are probably due to leakage of maternal blood into the fetal circulation. The risk of the infant becoming infected varies from country to country and seems to be related to ethnic groups. Infectivity is related to the presence of a high titer of hepatitis B surface antigen (HBsAg) in the mother's circulation and of the presence of hepatitis Be antigen (HBeAg). The prevalence of HbeAg varies in different populations and is particularly high in Southeast Asia. More than 90 per cent of infants born to mothers who are HBeAg positive become infected, 80–90 per cent of them becoming chronic carriers themselves. The risk of infection in infants born to carrier mothers who are HBeAg negative is much lower, about 10 per cent (Stevens *et al.* 1979). The earlier an infant acquires HBV infection the greater the risk of developing chronic infection (Fig. 20.2).

Fortunately, with the development of an HBV vaccine it is now possible to prevent transmission of infection from a mother to her newborn baby. The cost-effectiveness of antenatal screening and intervention depends on the prevalence of HBV infection in the population. In areas of high prevalence and this often includes inner cities in countries with a low prevalence, the most effective approach to prevention is the universal testing of pregnant women for HBV carrier status. Infants identified as at risk of infection can then be protected with a single dose of specific immunoglobulin given at birth and HBV vaccine in a three injection schedule (at birth, 3 months, and 5 months). In areas of low endemicity a more effective approach might be selected testing of pregnant

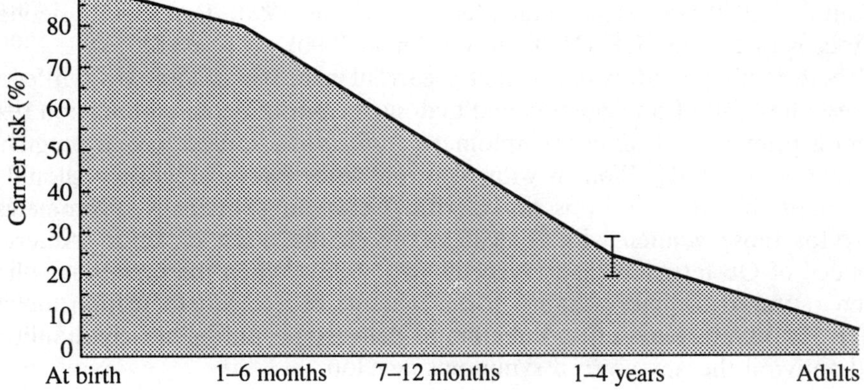

Fig. 20.2 The risk of becoming a carrier is related to the age at the time of onset of infection. The most at risk are the very young. (Source: Hepatitis B vaccine attacking a pandemic. WHO November, 1988).

women considered to be at risk, such as women from countries where HBV infection is endemic or injecting drug users.

Herpes simplex infection

Herpes simplex virus (HSV) can be separated into two types, HSV-1 and HSV-2. HSV-1 infection is usually acquired early in life, whereas HSV-2 generally follows puberty and is associated with the onset of sexual activity. HSV-1 is most commonly isolated from the mouth, nose, and throat, and HSV-2 from the genital mucosa. However, both types can affect either or both sites and as with the other members of the herpes virus group, such as CMV, both HSV-1 and HSV-2 can remain latent in the cells and reactivate throughout life.

There have been isolated case reports of maternal infection in the first 20 weeks of pregnancy associated with congenital abnormality, but evidence that transplacental transmission of HSV causes abnormalities is inconclusive. HSV in early pregnancy is not an indication for termination of a pregnancy.

Maternal infection acquired around the time of delivery presents a much more serious problem since the newborn may acquire HSV infection during passage through an infected birth canal or by ascending infection after rupture of the membranes. Neonatal HSV infection is a potentially serious condition, associated with high mortality and morbidity (Whitley *et al.* 1980). It may present with isolated skin lesions, localized neurological disease, or disseminated disease involving multiple organs. Disseminated infection is associated with a high mortality and infection confined to the brain has a poor prognosis. Many of the surviving infants have severe damage. Neonatal infection may result from both HSV-1 and HSV-2, but there is no apparent difference in the severity of the disease. The exact incidence of neonatal HSV infection is unknown, but it has been estimated that in the USA, with about 3.5 million deliveries a year, there are about 700–1000 cases of neonatal infection (Whitley 1990). Fortunately, neonatal herpes is rare in the UK (Hall and Glickman 1990).

There is now good evidence that recurrent maternal genital HSV infection poses a low risk of transmission and that most cases of neonatal infection result from a primary and often asymptomatic, infection acquired in late pregnancy (Brown *et al.* 1991). Women with recurrent infection in pregnancy should be reassured that their baby is not at risk. Cesarean delivery is recommended only for those women with clinical lesions at the onset of labor (American College of Obstetricians and Gynecologists 1988). When the membranes have been ruptured for more than 4 h the benefits of a cesarean section are less clear. All infants exposed to infection at delivery should be closely monitored and antiviral therapy given if symptoms develop.

Summary

A considerable body of information is now available on the risk of damage to the fetus or newborn following specific infections in pregnancy. It is important that this knowledge is widely disseminated so that women, as well as the medical profession and health service managers are aware of the implications of infections in pregnancy and of the preventive measures that are available. Where possible the avoidance of infection in pregnancy is a priority, but when a pregnant woman is exposed to or acquires an infection, appropriate management decisions must be reached without delay.

The prevention of congenital rubella has been a major success story and in countries where national rubella vaccination programmes have been implemented there has been a marked reduction in its incidence. With a low background rate of rubella in the community it is still important for women planning a pregnancy to be aware of the need to be protected.

As most infections that can adversely affect the fetus are not clinically recognizable, serological screening in pregnancy is sometimes advocated to identify pregnancies at risk. This is justified on the basis that treatment can be initiated or that a woman can be given the opportunity to have the pregnancy terminated if the fetus is at risk. Most pregnant women already experience some anxiety as to whether the baby will be normal and this can often be exacerbated when blood tests are taken as part of the routine antenatal procedure to identify infections. It is important to ensure that women are adequately informed about the purpose of the antenatal tests they undergo and that they understand the implications of a positive test. There is often a failure to explain adequately why tests are being done and this may result in a well woman being informed unexpectedly that her pregnancy is complicated by a silent infection that could damage her baby.

At present, routine antenatal tests are done for syphilis and rubella. These two tests, however, have quite different aims. Screening for syphilis identifies those women who are infected so that effective treatment can be offered and the serious consequences of congenital syphilis prevented. On the other hand, rubella screening has no effect on the management of the current pregnancy, but it identifies those women who have no rubella antibodies and are susceptible to infection so that rubella vaccine can be offered to them in the postpartum period. A positive rubella screening test is sometimes mistakenly assumed to infer that infection did not occur in pregnancy but this is not necessarily the case and all women with a history of rubella or rubella contact need to be fully investigated, even if they give a history of rubella immunization.

Universal screening of pregnant women to identify those who are HBV carriers is recommended in the USA and Canada and more recently in the UK where there was evidence that selective screening of pregnant women at risk of infection failed to identify many carrier women. Treatment at birth of the infants born to carrier women with hepatitis B immunoglobulin and vaccine dramatically reduces the incidence of acute and chronic infections in newborns.

For full protection a further two doses of vaccine must be given at stipulated intervals. Such a policy has been shown to be cost-effective in the USA and aims to interrupt the transmission of HBV and prevent the serious consequences of infection.

With the rapid development of new laboratory tests to identify infections and improvements in prenatal diagnosis following amniocentesis and fetal blood sampling, consideration is being given increasingly to extending antenatal screening to include toxoplasmosis and CMV infection. Screening for other infections such as chlamydia, herpes simplex, and group B streptococcal infection (an important cause of perinatal bacterial infections), is also under discussion. Decisions to introduce prenatal diagnosis must be based on the prevalence of the infection, its consequences, and the availability and effectiveness of any treatment. This must be carefully balanced against the possible harm that might ensue, including problems associated with false-positive results and unnecessary medical interventions.

Indeed, what is appropriate policy for one country may not be for another. For example, a Multidisciplinary Working Group (1992) in the UK recently concluded after detailed review of the evidence available that it would not be appropriate at the present time to introduce nation-wide prenatal screening for toxoplasmosis. The group considered that screening for acute infection in pregnancy was not of proven benefit and there was a possibility that such a program might cause more harm than benefit. Active surveillance of symptomatic congenital toxoplasmosis in the UK had suggested that this was a rare condition and it was concluded that further studies were required on the current incidence of toxoplasmosis infection in pregnancy, the incidence of congenital infection, the relative frequency of symptomatic and asymptomatic infected neonates, and the prevalence of long-term sequelae, disability, and handicap. Improved screening and diagnostic tests for detection and timing of recent infection in pregnancy were also required to minimize false-positive results and thereby avoid unnecessary further investigations in a large number of women if a screening programme was initiated. At the present time the most appropriate approach to the prevention of congenital toxoplasmosis is health education to avoid infection.

Similarly there is no national prenatal screening for CMV in the UK and evidence available would not support such a policy. No vaccine is available and there is no consensus as to the prevention of congenital CMV except to advise women that sexual and other intimate contact, including possibly close family-type contact with children, could be implicated as a source of infection. There is still a lack of knowledge among many health professionals and the public about CMV infection.

In pregnancy, screening must not be confused with the diagnosis and treatment of symptomatic or suspected infections in individual women. Indeed, if a pregnant woman develops an infection she should be given the most up-to-date information available so that she can make an informed decision as to whether to continue the pregnancy based on the risk of adverse sequelae and the available treatment options.

References

Ades, A. E. (1992). Methods for estimating the incidence of primary infection in pregnancy: a reappraisal of toxoplasmosis and cytomegalovirus data. *Epidemiology of Infectiou*, **108**, 367–75.

Adler, S. P. (1989). Transfusion acquired CMV injection in premature infants. *Transfusion*, **29(3)**, 278–90.

Ahlfors, K., Ivarsson, S., Johnsson, T., and Svanberg, L. (1979). A prospective study on congenital and acquired cytomegalovirus infections in infants. *Scandinavian Journal of Infectious Disease*, **11**, 177–8.

American College of Obstetricians and Gynecologists (1988). Pernatal herpes simplex injection. ACOG Technical Bulletin, Washington, DC.

Brown, Z. A., Benedetti, J., Ashley, R., *et al* (1991). Neonatal herpes simplex virus infection in relation to asymptomatic maternal infection at the time of labor. *New England Journal of Medicine*, **324**, 1247–52.

Davis, L. G., Weber, D. J., and Lemon, S. M. (1989). Horizontal transmission of hepatitis B virus. *Lancet* **i** 889–93.

Desmonts, G. and Couvreur, J. (1974). Congenital toxoplasmosis: a prospective study of 378 pregnancies. *New England Journal of Medicine* **290**, 1110–6.

Fowler, K. B., Stagno, P. H. S., Pass, R. F., Britt, W. J., Boll, T. J., and Alford, C. A. (1992). The outcome of congenital cytomegalovirus infection in relation to maternal antibody status. *New England Journal of Medicine*, **326**, 663–7.

Gregg, N. M. (1941). Congenital cataract following German measles in the mother. *Transactions of the Ophthamological Society of Australia* **3**, 35–46.

Hall, S. M. (1992). Congenital toxoplasmosis. *British Medical Journal*, **305**, 291–7.

Hall, S. M. and Glickman, M. (1990). Report from the British Paediatric Surveillance Unit. *Archives of Diseases of Childhood*, **65**, 807–9.

Krugman, S. (1985). Viral hepatitis update: 1985. *Pediatrics Reviews*, **7**, 3–11.

Multidisciplinary Working Group (1992). *Prenatal screening for toxoplasmosis in the UK*. Royal College of Obstetricians and Gynaecologists, London.

Murph, J. R., Baron, J. C., Brown, C. K., Ebelhack, C. L., and Bale, J. F., Jr (1991). The occupational risk of cytomegalovirus injection among day-care provders. *Journal of the American Medical Association*, **265(5)**, 603–8.

Pass, R. F. (1991). Day-care Centers and the spread of Cytomegalovirus and parovirus B19 *Pediatric Annals*, **20(8)**, 419–26.

Pass, R. F., Stagno, S., Myers, G. J., and Alford, C. A. (1980). Outcome of symptomatic congenital cytomegalovirus infection: results of long-term longitudinal follow-up. *Journal of Pediatrics*, **66**, 758–62.

Pearl, K., Preece, P., Ades, A., and Peckham, C. (1986). Neurodevelopmental assessment after congenital cytomegalovirus infection. *Archives of Diseases of Childhood*, **61**, 323–6.

Peckham, C. S. (1991). Cytomegalovirus infection: congenital and neonatal disease. *Scandinavian Journal of Infection*, **Suppl. 78**, 82–87.

Peckham, C. S., and Logan, S. (1993). Screening for toxoplasmosis during pregnancy. *Archives of Diseases of Childhood*, **68**, 3–5.

Remington, J. S. and Desmonts, G. (1990). Toxoplasmosis. In *Infectious Diseases of the Fetus and Newborn Infant*, (3rd edn), (ed. J. S. Remington and J. O. Klein J O), PP. 89–195. W B Saunders, Philadelphia.

Rutter, D., Griffiths, P., and Trompeter, R. (1985). Cytomegalic inclusion disease after recurrent maternal infection. *Lancet*, **ii**, 1182.

Saigal, S., Lunyk, O., Larke, R. P. B., and Chernesky, M. A. (1982). The outcome in children with congenital cytomegalovirus infection. *American Journal of Diseases of Children*, **136**, 896–905.

Stagno, S., Pass, R. F., and Dworsky, M. E. (1982). Congenital cytomegalovirus infection: the relative importance of primary and recurrent maternal infection. *New England Journal of Medicine*, **306**, 945–9.

Stagno, S., Pass, R. F., Dworsky, M. E., and Alford, C. A. (1983). Congenital and perinatal cytomegalovirus infections. *Seminars in Perinatology*, **7**, 31–42.

Stevens, C. E., Beasley, R. P., Tsui, J., and Lee, W. L. (1975). Vertical tranmission of hepatitis B antigen in Taiwan. *New England Journal of Medicine*, **292**, 771–4.

Stevens, C. E., Neurath, R. E., Beasley, R. P., and Szmuness, W. (1979). HBe Ag and anti-HBe detection by radioimmunoassy: correlation with vertical transmission of hepatitis B virus in Taiwan. *Journal of Medical Virology*, **3**, 237–41.

Walker, J., Nokes, D. J., and Jennings, R. (1992). Longitudinal study of toxoplasma seroprevalence in South Yorkshire. *Epidemiology of Infection*, **108**, 99–106.

Whitley, R. J. (1990). Herpes simplex virus infections. In *Infectious diseases of the fetus and newborn infant*, (3rd edn), (ed. J. S. Remington and J. O. Klein), PP. 282–305. W B Saunders, Philadelphia.

Whitley, R. J., Nahmias, A. J., Soong, S. J., Galasso, G. G., Fleming, C. L., and Alford, C. A. (1980). Vidarabin therapy of neonatal herpes simplex virus infection. *Pediatrics*, **66**, 495–501.

21 Screening for the abnormal baby

Philip R. Reilly

Techniques for prenatal screening

During the last two decades, striking advances in our ability to search for warning signs about a developing fetus have helped many pregnant women. In this chapter I shall describe several major screening programs that have or may become standard practice. I shall also consider some legal and public policy issues that have arisen concerning prenatal screening. But at the outset it is important to understand the crucial distinction between diagnosis and screening. Diagnosis pertains to the effort to understand an illness in a particular patient; screening pertains to the search of a healthy population whose members may be at some special risk of having an undiagnosed condition that could lead to illness in themselves or, in prenatal screening, their offspring.

Advanced maternal age and amniocentesis

The oldest, best known, and most widely practiced form of prenatal screening is also the simplest: asking the pregnant woman her age. For many decades, doctors have known that older women are more likely to have a child with Down's syndrome. The presence of an extra chromosome 21 in each cell causes a baby with this condition to be mentally handicapped, and to have some of a wide range of physical abnormalities. Since about 1970 the development of amniocentesis, in which a needle is used to remove some fluid from the pregnant woman's womb, and karyotyping (the ability to grow the fetal cells in that fluid and study their chromosomes under a microscope) have led to the point where it is now routine to offer prenatal testing to all women who will be 35 or older at their date of delivery. This age cut-off is arbitrary, but not without logic. It reflects the fact that a 35 year old woman's risk of carrying a child with Down's syndrome (about one in 270) is about the same as her risk of pregnancy loss or fetal injury through amniocentesis. In younger women, the risk of fetal loss after amniocentesis is greater than the likelihood that the test will identify a fetus with abnormal chromosomes and serious birth defects.

In the USA each year about 250 000 women undergo amniocentesis, the vast majority simply because of their age. About 2 weeks after they undergo the procedure, about 98 per cent of these women will learn that their fetuses have a normal looking set of chromosomes. Of those who learn of an unexpected fetal abnormality, most will face the intensely emotional dilemma of whether to terminate a wanted pregnancy. Although the subject has not been studied in great detail, it appears that among women who seek amniocentesis for advanced maternal age, 80–90 per cent of those who discover that the fetus has been diagnosed with Down's syndrome—the most commonly discovered serious chromosomal abnormality—do undergo an abortion.

Chorionic villus sampling and early amniocentesis

In recent years a new technology, chorionic villus sampling (CVS) has emerged as an important alternative to amniocentesis. Chorionic villi are a type of tissue from the uterus of the pregnant woman that contains fetal cells. The physician removes a sample by passing a flexible plastic catheter through the vagina or a needle through the abdomen using ultrasound for guidance. The choice may depend on the location of the placenta. The main advantages of CVS over standard amniocentesis are (1) that it is performed during weeks 9–12 of gestation, considerably earlier than amniocentesis and (2) that more tissue can be obtained. Thus if a woman is at risk of bearing children with a severe genetic disorder for which a test is available, she can obtain a diagnosis earlier—which is important if she is considering termination of the affected fetus.

Especially during the early 1980s there was concern that women who underwent CVS were more likely to miscarry than women who underwent amniocentesis. A 1989 study comparing 2278 women who underwent CVS with 671 who underwent amniocentesis at 16 weeks found that the fetal loss rate for CVS was less than 1 per cent higher than for amniocentesis, not a significant difference (Jackson 1992).

Perhaps most troubling has been the concern that there is an increased risk of abnormalities of the limbs and facial bones among fetuses born after CVS. One study found five such cases among 289 pregnancies and the investigators speculated that CVS could cause reduced blood flow to the fetus (Firth 1991). However, other studies did not find an increased incidence of such abnormalities and no causal relationship has been established. A large study completed in 1994 found no evidence of an increased risk of limb defects in fetuses exposed to CVS. Chromosomal analysis of chorionic tissue is more difficult than analysis of cells derived from amniotic fluid, but in experienced hands not significantly so. These slightly increased risks must be weighed against the benefits of earlier diagnosis.

The American College of Obstetricians and Gynecologists has concluded that: 'Transcervical CVS, when performed by expert operators is a relatively safe procedure and may be considered an acceptable alternative to mid-trimester genetic amniocentesis' (Committee on Obstetrics: Maternal and Fetal Medicine 1989).

Clearly, the earlier that women can safely undergo amniocentesis for diagnostic purposes the better. A growing number of physicians now perform amniocentesis before the fifteenth week of pregnancy with about the same success rate in obtaining tissue for analysis as with CVS. There have been no controlled trials of the safety of early amniocentesis and given that an early procedure withdraws a larger percentage of the amniotic fluid, it may be hazardous. A sharply reduced volume of amniotic fluid may, for example, compromise development of the fetal lungs (D'Alton and DeCherney 1993).

Screening for neural tube defects

Unquestionably the largest prenatal screening effort in the world is that intended to identify women at increased risk for carrying a fetus with a neural tube defect. This condition, usually called spina bifida, is caused by the failure of the embryonic tissue to fold properly into what is destined to be the spinal column. Babies with the most severe cases (those involving the top of the spine and the brain) die shortly after birth. People born with defects in the lower spine may be relatively mildly affected (requiring braces to walk and having bladder problems) or be quite severely affected and this fact greatly complicates how a woman analyzes the diagnosis of this condition in her fetus.

Spina bifida is a common birth defect, occurring in as many as one in 500 births in parts of the UK and in about one in 1000 births in the USA. During the 1970s, it was discovered and confirmed that fetuses with open spina bifida leak high levels of a protein known as α-fetoprotein or AFP into the amniotic fluid, which then crosses the placenta to enter the mother's bloodstream. This discovery provided the basis for a screening test known as the maternal serum α-fetoprotein test. The screening protocol is fairly complicated but, in essence, it is based on the fact that comparing the level of AFP in a mother's blood at about week 16 with typical values based on experience from thousands of other pregnancies can show whether she (regardless of her age) is at increased risk for giving birth to a child with spina bifida (American Society of Human Genetics 1987).

The test is only a screening tool; it does not diagnose the condition and it may miss women carrying a fetus with a small spinal defect. But properly done, it does identify the majority of such pregnancies. A key problem, however, is that to detect the real cases (true positives), the level of AFP used to signal that a woman is at risk is set so low (usually 2.5 multiples of the median value), that most women singled out by the screen turn out *not* to be carrying an affected fetus. These women have test results that are falsely positive. Unfortunately, they must undergo repeat blood testing, ultrasonic study of the fetus and, sometimes, amniocentesis to clarify the suspicion raised by screening. If the amniotic fluid AFP is high, the laboratory tests for a chemical called acetylcholinesterase. If this is also high, there is a strong possibility that the fetus has an open spinal lesion (American College of Obstetricians and Gynecologists 1991).

Despite the fact that many women who undergo the AFP screen are made unnecessarily anxious by a false-positive result, the screening program (and further refinements of it) are rapidly becoming a standard of practice. For example, several years ago California enacted a law requiring physicians to inform pregnant women about the availability of this screening test. About 70 per cent of the more than 500 000 women who give birth each year in California undergo AFP screening. A reasonable guess is that in the USA far more than 1 000 000 pregnant women had this screening test in 1992.

Recently, the test has been altered in some important ways. In the 1980s it was discovered quite by chance that the AFP values of blood drawn from women carrying fetuses with Down's syndrome were often quite low (the opposite of the results expected from a fetus with spina bifida) (Dimaio 1987). Subsequently, researchers identified two other compounds that could be used in conjunction with AFP to make a more powerful statement about the risk that a given fetus had Down's syndrome. These were human chorionic gonadotropin and unconjugated estriol.

Together, the three markers provide a way to screen women regardless of their age to ascertain if they are at increased risk for bearing a child with Down's syndrome. For example, a 25 year old woman with no relevant family history has a one in 890 chance of bearing a child with Down's syndrome. If her AFP level at 16 weeks gestation is 0.36 multiples of the median, her risk increases to about one in 180. If her human chorionic gonadotropin and unconjugated estriol levels are also abnormal, her risk may be further increased. As is the case with spina bifida screening, the test will miss some women who are carrying an affected fetus and most women flagged as being at high risk will in fact not have a baby with Down's syndrome. Nevertheless, since 85 per cent of babies with this disorder are born to women under 35, the emergence of an age-independent screen means that it is now possible to identify a higher percentage (up to 60–65 per cent) of the pregnancies at risk. It was during 1990 that the power of this multi marker test became apparent and during 1992 a large number of obstetricians began to use it instead of the AFP test. The company that does the largest volume of such prenatal tests in the USA has reported that it has largely replaced the single-marker test.

Carrier screening for common genetic disorders

Among the thousands of different disorders caused by defects in a single gene, several are of particular interest to prenatal screening. This is because the abnormal genes are quite common among specific ethnic groups. For example, Tay–Sachs disease, a rare, fatal childhood disorder, is far more common among Ashkenazi Jews than Europeans in general. Sickle cell anemia is far more common among Africans and their descendants in America than Caucasians, and cystic fibrosis is found significantly more frequently among people of northern European than people in the rest of Europe, the near East, and Africa.

Each of these disorders is an autosomal recessive condition, which means that an individual who carries a single copy of the mutation does not have the condition. But if he or she chooses a partner with the same mutant gene, there is a one in four risk of each of their children having the disease. Thus, it is hardly surprising that screening programs have tested members of relevant ethnic groups to determine if they carry a mutant gene which may put them at risk of bearing a child with one of these serious disorders. During the 1970s screening programs to identify Tay–Sachs carriers and carriers of the sickle trait were widely set up.

The screening strategies and their outcomes differed dramatically (Mackta 1985). This history provides important lessons about how best to develop screening initiatives—a topic I will take up in concluding this chapter.

Programs designed to identify sickle cell carriers often used mandatory laws (such as making testing a condition of school entry or obtaining a marriage license) to accomplish their goal. Such laws were enacted between 1970 and 1972 in 13 American states, but frequently did not provide adequate resources for educating and counseling. Some were so poorly drafted that they stigmatized screening. For example, one sickle cell screening law was written as an amendment to the law requiring prenatal testing for syphilis! In 1972, a federal law was enacted that made money available to state-based programs that embraced voluntarism, respected privacy, and provided counseling. Although this law largely overrode the state laws, the sickle cell screening experience of the early 1970s left a legacy of mistrust and may explain in part why screening is not more highly used in the African American community today (Reilly 1977).

In contrast, Tay–Sachs testing was never based on legislative initiative. From the start, it was community-based, largely self-supported, and completely voluntary. Perhaps because Ashkenazi Jews make up only about 5 per cent of the population and tend to be economically secure and because of the grave nature of their disorder (Tay–Sachs disease is uniformly fatal in early childhood), the program has been quite successful. Most Ashkenazi Jewish couples undergo screening and the number of children born with the disease in this group has dropped by 90 per cent in a generation. Pregnancy termination is almost always chosen when tests indicate that the at-risk fetus is affected.

β-Thalassemia, a severe blood disease caused by the genetic errors in the ability to make hemoglobin, is quite common among peoples of Mediterranean origin. Although widespread screening has not taken hold in the USA, the experience in places such as Cyprus and Sardinia, where the abnormal gene is unusually common, has been remarkable. Church, state, and the medical community have altered cultural traditions to help reduce the number of marriages at risk of bearing children with this fatal disorder.

Currently, medical geneticists are studying the question of whether to make screening to identify carriers of the gene for cystic fibrosis (CF) a routine part of health care. CF is a serious disorder of the lungs and pancreas, and one in 25 White Americans of northern European extraction carries a CF mutation. One of every 2500 newborns has the disorder. CF screening represents a new era, because it is the first screening test that is DNA based. That is, new techniques from molecular biology are being used to examine the genetic material itself (not protein coded for by the gene) for the presence or absence of the more common mutations. Unfortunately, there are more than 300 different mutations that can cause CF and it is only (at the moment) practical to screen for 10–30 of them. Currently available tests can identify about 90 per cent of all carriers. Thus, a negative result does not absolutely rule out being a carrier, but rather reduces the risk from one in 25 to about one in 250 (Special Report 1990).

It is neither the technical limits of the test (which are certain to improve) nor its price (which is sure to decrease) that lies at the heart of the debate over CF screening. Many medical geneticists worry that we lack the resources to provide enough counselors to support large-scale CF screening programs. They fear that a test result will often be misinterpreted, leading a couple to worry unnecessarily or even to make wrong choices. During 1992–94, the National Institutes of Health funded six pilot projects to study the best way to screen and counsel large numbers of people about whether they carry the CF gene and to determine how test results affect their reproductive plans. A number of university groups and genetic testing companies are conducting similar studies. As I discuss below, the decision as to whether or not to routinely offer CF screening to young adults has significant medico-legal implications, so the current deliberations are justified.

Ultrasonography

During the last decade transabdominal ultrasonography has almost become a screening tool because it has become so widely used as part of the care of healthy women at no special increased risk for bearing babies with birth defects.

An ultrasonographic study of a fetus early in the second trimester (week 16) can discern a great deal. Ultrasonographers study fetal anatomy, movement, and the size of the different parts, as well as the amniotic fluid volume, the uterus, and the placenta. They are particularly looking for the absence of expected structures, the presence of unexpected masses, dilatation beyond an obstruction, for example in the bowel or kidneys, herniation (an opening of a normally closed space with extrusion of an organ), and abnormal organ size. Experienced ultrasonographers can sometimes make specific diagnoses (such as Down's syndrome or trisomy 18) based on a constellation of findings or identify an isolated problem such as cleft palate. Although it is not quite proper to characterize fetal ultrasonography as a screening test, continued technological advances, the availability of a large number of well trained physicians and technicians, and declining cost could some day make it so. On the other hand there is some evidence that the procedure is not a valuable screening tool (D'Alton and DeCherney 1993).

Public policy on prenatal screening

Any discussion of prenatal and carrier screening raises challenging issues in constitutional law, malpractice law, public policy, and medical ethics. It is beyond the scope of this chapter to analyze each in detail, but it may be helpful to consider some of the more important topics.

Constitutional law: the right to privacy and abortion

Prenatal screening is intended to alert women to the possibility that they may be carrying a fetus with a serious genetic disorder or birth defect, which is often incurable or essentially untreatable. Most women who seek prenatal diagnosis do so with the understanding that they may be confronted with a finding that will lead them to choose abortion. The United States Supreme Court has narrowed

Roe v. Wade—the 1973 decision that defined the constitutional right to privacy to include a woman's right within certain bounds to terminate her pregnancy—now allowing each state the power to greatly limit access to abortion. Recent legislative efforts in Guam, Louisiana, and in Utah make it clear that, in a sizeable minority of jurisdictions (perhaps as many as ten states), the right to terminate a pregnancy may be so restricted that even women who know they are carrying a fetus with severe, untreatable birth defects may be denied freedom of choice.

Recognizing that such restrictive laws greatly diminish the value of prenatal testing to their patients, in 1990 the American Society of Human Genetics adopted language for model legislation intended to preserve that right. Of those members voting, 97 per cent supported the wording. The relevant words are:

> Regardless of any other provisions of this statute or other laws of this jurisdiction, any pregnant female whose pregnancy has not reached the point of viability and who has been informed by a licensed or certified health care professional that her fetus (or fetuses) is likely to have a serious genetic or congenital disorder shall have the right, among other options, to choose to terminate her pregnancy. This right shall extend to situations where the female is at significantly increased risk for bearing a child with a serious disorder for which precise prenatal diagnosis is not available (American Society of Human Genetics 1991).

Even the most restrictive state abortion statutes have included exceptions in the cases of rape and incest. Is not the emotional and economic price attached to the obligation of lifetime care for a child with profound birth defects as high as for those special categories? It should be noted that less than 1 per cent of the abortions performed each year are the result of prenatal screening. I expect that if the regulation of abortions is returned to the states, most will honor a woman's freedom to choose when she is carrying a fetus with a serious defect.

Sex Selection

One of the most troubling ethical issues in prenatal diagnosis is to determine under what circumstances, if any, it is appropriate to use this technology solely to permit a woman to ascertain the sex of the fetus, which she may claim is critical to her decision about whether or not to continue her pregnancy. For a time in certain regions in India this practice was rather widespread and resulted overwhelmingly in the abortion of female fetuses. Geneticists in Western nations are occasionally confronted with requests by couples who have an exceedingly strong preference for a child of a particular gender. For couples at risk for bearing boys with severe X-linked disorders, a female fetus is a virtual guarantee that they will have a child who is not burdened with that disorder. Prenatal diagnosis for sex selection has been made available to such couples because for them gender is coupled with high (50 per cent) risk of disease in a male child.

Gender is not a disease and the vast majority of physicians are unwilling to provide prenatal diagnosis solely to plan the gender or gender order of offspring. Of course, within legal limits, women may terminate a pregnancy for whatever reason they wish. This, however, does not mean that society should allocate resources to women who wish to use prenatal diagnosis for this purpose. Further, it may be unethical to perform an invasive medical procedure on a woman for purposes other than those related to concern for disease.

A particular worrisome issue arises in rare instances when a woman states she will terminate her pregnancy unless she is informed that the fetus is of the desired sex. In this case the provision of prenatal diagnosis creates the possibility that the fetus will be taken to term whereas refusal to provide sex selection is likely to lead to abortion. It is unethical to hold physicians hostage in this way. A US presidential commission that considered this issue concluded that: 'although physicians are free to follow the dictates of conscience, public policy should discourage the use of amniocentesis for sex selection' (President's Commission for the Study of Ethical Problems in Medicine and Biochemical and Behavioral Research 1983).

Malpractice law: new standard of care

The advent of prenatal screening in the 1970s spawned a small but widely studied new branch of malpractice law: wrongful birth litigation. Such lawsuits are initiated by women who give birth to children with disorders for which the risk was relatively high and for which a test was available, but who were not informed about the test by their physicians. A classic case might involve a 38 year old woman who has given birth to a child with Down's syndrome. The first such cases appeared in the mid-1970s and are routinely filed today. Virtually every state appellate court that has considered the matter has recognized a cause of action for wrongful birth (Shaw 1984).

The difficult judicial problem is to decide the dimensions of the physician's duty to recognize women at some special risk for which helpful tests do exist and to inform them. The duty to inform women aged 35 and older of the risk that the fetus will have Down's syndrome and to warn Ashkenazi Jews of the risk of Tay—Sachs disease is clearly established. The same duty probably holds for warning Black couples about the risks of sickle cell anemia. It may soon be established in regard to informing women of the value of maternal serum AFP screening for identifying fetuses at high risk of having neural tube defects. Few such cases go beyond the trial court level, so there are not enough appellate decisions from which to infer the emergence of new medico-legal duties on a disease by disease basis.

Although courts are the ultimate arbiters of physicians' duties to their patients, professional groups can expert great influence by publishing their views of what constitutes appropriate practice. Medical geneticists and obstetricians have been quite active in this regard. The American Society of Human Genetics and the American College of Obstetricians and Gynecologists (ACOG), as well as several regional groups, have issued statements attempting to define standards of care for maternal serum AFP screening. Although there was some ambiguity in earlier publications, the ACOG (1991) *Technical bulletin* on α-fetoprotein is clear: 'Since most NTD [neural tube defects] occur in the absence of (family) history, all gravida should be offered screening for elevated MSAFP'. The bulletin also makes clear that a low maternal serum AFP value must trigger consideration that the fetus may have Down's syndrome. Elsewhere in the document ACOG asserts that as of April 1991 it regarded the use of multiple markers to enhance screening as 'investigational'. More recently (February 1992) the New England Regional Genetics Group concluded that while the markers were no longer under investigation, they 'should not be considered standard of care at this time'.

The debate over standard of practice issues has spilled into other areas as well. The American Society of Human Genetics has twice stated that physicians should not be required to alert patients with no family history of the disorder to the existence of CF testing. The New England Regional Genetics Group has asserted that a rapid chromosomal screening technology known as fluorescent *in situ* hybridization (FISH) should not yet be viewed as a laboratory standard test upon which a final diagnosis may rely.

There will probably be more statements purporting to define standards of practice. Such documents have two impacts. On the one hand they permit physicians to be conservative in deciding when a test has become a standard of practice; on the other hand, once articulated, they become a powerful legal weapon against those who fail to follow their tenets.

Public policy: reimbursement for screening tests

As was pointed out initially, screening programs do not usually lead to diagnosis, rather, they point the way. In fact, the yield (true positives) in virtually any prenatal screening program is quite low. Given the other pressures on health insurers, it should not be too surprising to hear that many are reluctant to pay for screening tests, even for those of well-established value such as Tay–Sachs carrier testing. Finances figure prominently too in the CF carrier screening debate; it would cost about \$100 000 to identify a couple who face a one in four risk of bearing an affected child. Although many geneticists think genetic testing will greatly enhance preventive medicine, the cost of screening by means of these tests still needs to be substantially reduced.

Prenatal screening: the 1990s

The discovery and implementation of new prenatal diagnostic tests will accelerate throughout the 1990s (See Chapter 26). Most of these tests will be designed to identify genetic disorders that are so rare that it would not be cost-beneficial to use them as part of routine prenatal screening. Of course, that determination depends in part on the burden of the particular disorder and the cost of the test. One genetic test that may become a routine part of prenatal care is a DNA-based screen for fragile X syndrome.

This common heritable cause of mental handicap occurs in about one in 1000 males and about one in 2000 females, making it as common as Down's syndrome. The inheritance pattern is not the same as classical X-linked disorders such as hemophilia (in which healthy carrier females have a 50 per cent chance of bearing affected sons). Rather, in at-risk families, healthy men may carry a 'premutation', an elongated stretch of DNA that is still not long enough to cause problems. They pass this mutation to their daughters who are also healthy. However, during development of the daughters' eggs the premutation can expand to a full mutation that somehow disrupts the function of a key gene, resulting in the birth of mentally handicapped sons or daughters (for complicated reasons, sons with the full mutation are almost certain to be affected, but only about half of the daughters with the same mutation will be affected) (Shapiro 1991).

A highly informative test to identify fetuses affected with this condition became available in 1992. Because the test will be relatively cheap and the disorder is relatively severe, I expect that soon obstetricians who are offering amniocentesis to women because of their age will also inform them that a test for fragile X syndrome can be done at the same time. Insurers may at first be reluctant to reimburse for the test, largely because of the relatively low risk of the disorder. However, the price of the test will be sufficiently low to counter that concern and the cost of finding an affected fetus will be quite reasonable. It is likely that cost-conscious health maintenance organizations may be the first routinely to use this test.

As has been the case in the CF screening debate, there is already much concern about how properly to educate patients about the implication of a positive fragile X test. The level of mental retardation in affected persons ranges widely, from mild to severe. Furthermore, we know less about the condition than we do about Down's syndrome. Clearly, it will take time and some effort to make couples aware in advance of the diagnostic uncertainties and to provide competent counseling to those who learn they carry an affected fetus.

The elements of an ideal prenatal screening program

Prenatal screening efforts are in essence programs to warn women about a developmental defect in the fetus. In a society that respects personal autonomy, they have the greatest chance of success when

(1) the program is voluntary;

(2) the test offered is reliable;

(3) the quality of the testing laboratories is reasonably high;

(4) the woman has an opportunity to be fully informed about the limits on the accuracy of the test and about the clinical expression of the disorder(s) being screened;

(5) test results are communicated in a timely manner that allows a woman whose test is positive adequate time to choose her course of action;

(6) competent post-test counseling is readily available;

(7) test results are treated as confidential;

(8) the option of safe, legal pregnancy termination is available.

Past experience has shown that the omission of any of these elements greatly impairs the screening efforts (Reilly 1992).

References

American College of Obstetricians and Gynecologists (1991). Alpha-fetoprotein. *Technical Bulletin*, **154**.

American Society of Human Genetics (1987). Policy statement for maternal serum alpha-protein screening programs and quality control of laboratories performing maternal serum and amniotic fluid alpha-fetoprotoin assays. *American Journal of Human Genetics*, **40**, 75–82.

American Society of Human Genetics (1991). Statement on clinical genetics and freedom of choice. *American Journal of Human Genetics*, **48**, 10.1.

Committee on Obstetrics: Maternal and Fetal Medicine (1989). Chorionic villus sampling. ACOG Committee Opinion Number 69.

D'Alton, M. E. and DeCherney, A, (1993). 'Prenatal diagnosis'. *New England Journal of Medicine*, **328**, 114–20.

Dimaio, M. S. (1987). Screening for Down's syndrome in pregnancy by measuring maternal serum alpha-fetoprotein levels. *New England Journal of Medicine*, **317**, 342–6.

Firth, H. V., Bogd, P. A., Chambeslain, P., Mackenzie, I. Z., Linderbaum, R. H., and Husan, S. M. (1991). Servere limb abnormalities after chorion villus sampling at 56–66 days gestation. *Lancet*, **337(8744)**, 762–3.

Mackta, J. (ed.) (1985). *What every family should know. Tay-Sachs and the allied diseases*, (ed. The National Tay-Sachs and Allied Diseases Association, Inc), pp. 1–19. Cedarhurst, New York.

President's Commission for the Study of Ethical Problems in Medicine and Biomedical and Behavioral Research (1983). *Screening and counseling for genetic conditions*, US Government Printing Office Washington, DC. p. 58.

Jackson, L. G., Zacharay, J. M., Fowler, S. E., Desnick, R. J., Gelbus, M. S., and Ledbetter, D. H. (1992). A randomized comparison of transcervical and transabdominal chorionic virus sampling. The US National Institute of Child Health and Human Development Chorionic Villus Sampling and Amniocentesis study Group. *New England Journal of Medicine*, **329(9)**, 594–8.

Reilly, P. R. (1977). *Genetics, law and social policy. Harvard University Press*, Cambridge.

Reilly, P. (1992) American Society of Human Genetics statement on genetics and privacy: testimony to United States Congress. *American Journal of Human Genetics*, **50**, 640–2.

Shapiro, L. R. (1991). The fragile X syndrome. *New England Journal of Medicine*, **325**, 1736–7.

Shaw, M. W. (1984). To be or not to be? That is the question. *American Journal of Human Genetics*, **35**, 1–9.

Special Report (1990). Statement from the National Institutes of Health workshop on population screening for the cystic fibrosis gene. *New England of Medicine*, **323**, 70–1.

[illegible]

[illegible] *Academy* [illegible]

[illegible]

[illegible]

V Impact of Adverse Infant Outcomes

22 Infant mortality: confronting disciplinary fragmentation in research and policy

Paul H. Wise

It is a curious paradox that infant mortality is as much a public concern today as it was in the mid-nineteenth century, despite the fact that the rate has fallen by more than 95 per cent since then. In a sense, concern persists because interpretation of infant mortality demands context and in each era a society derives its own context from its perceptions of the causes of infant mortality and what it considers to be its capacity to respond.

The basic premise of the discussion in this chapter is that our current search for context and the most appropriate ways to respond are seriously hindered by a growing fragmentation in the methods and purpose each discipline employs to address infant mortality. Although the complexity and unique public stature of infant mortality has always generated a rather pluralistic set of scientific and programmatic approaches, the intensity of the emerging divisions now appears in many ways to be greater and their impact more disturbing than before. The unprecedented specialization of clinical and investigative expertise, coupled with severe fiscal pressures to prioritize interventions, make it very likely that this disciplinary parochialism will ultimately find expression in destructive antagonisms in concept and praxis.

The nature of the problem

The infant mortality rate can be defined as the number of deaths to liveborn children before they reach 1 year of age, divided by the total number of live births in the same population and time span. In most areas, data for the calculation is derived from vital statistics registries; the numerator is drawn from death certificate files, while the denominator is acquired from birth certificate files.

Interpretation of infant mortality rates requires not only consideration of the absolute magnitude but also a comparison with the rates of other populations or periods. These distinctions are important since mixed interpretations are possible for any given rate. For example, infant mortality in the USA in 1988 was ten per 1000 live births, which was the lowest ever recorded there. However, this rate ranked the USA behind 22 other countries in an international comparison. Moreover, the overall rate obscured the profound disparity in infant mortality between racial groups in the USA. For the same year, the rate among Black Americans was 18.5, while that for their White counterparts was 8.4.

The task in analyzing infant mortality is therefore to ensure that the basis of comparison is legitimate. Birth and death definitions and recording practices must be sufficiently standard to allow meaningful comparisons, while explanations for observed differences must fully respect the large number of factors that determine infant mortality. In many ways, the latter is the more troublesome task, for it requires a level of disciplinary flexibility that rarely accompanies empirical investigation, particularly when so much social meaning is attached.

One strategy for understanding the observed differences in infant mortality rates is to recognize that they are really a composite of a series of component rates. Neonatal mortality refers to death before 28 days of age. Because so much of infant mortality is due to severe conditions that are evident at birth, particularly prematurity and lethal congenital anomalies, neonatal mortality accounts for the majority of infant deaths in most industrialized countries. Postneonatal mortality encompasses deaths occurring between 28 days and 1 year of age. Although it represents a minority of infant deaths, postneonatal mortality is a major contributor to differences in infant mortality between some communities. These component rates can be further stratified by a variety of attributes, including birth weight, gestational age, and cause of death.

Given the fact that infant mortality is multifactorial, it is not surprising that many disciplines and ideologies have provided important insights. Therefore, analysis of the problem ultimately depends on integrating these diverse insights, and recognizing fully that while social determinants have a pervasive impact, clinical medicine has a profound capacity to respond.

The historical roots of antagonism between disciplines

Biblical references provide early insights into the social meaning of infant death. Pharaoh proclaimed that 'Every son that is born ye shall cast into the river (Exodus 1:22) and Herod's order to slay the young children of Bethlehem in a vain attempt to kill 'the babe' destined to be 'King of the Jews' (Matthew 2:16) is commemorated as the Feast of the Holy Innocents. Indeed, reconciling the promise of childbirth and the tragedy of young child death has long been a subject for both traditional religious thought and mysticism.

However, current medical and social concern for infant mortality largely emerged from the social reform movements of the early and mid-nineteenth century. During the 1830s, Victorian reformist efforts began to rely on increasingly sophisticated analyses of social differences in illness and mortality in

Europe's burgeoning industrial cities (Eyler 1979). By 1839, a national vital registration system had been established in England. Under the direction of William Farr, the registry began to publish annual reports that documented a disturbing picture of grossly elevated mortality in poor urban populations. These reports and other health-related social analyses culminated in the publication of the seminal *Report on the sanitary condition of the labouring population of Great Britain*, written principally by Edwin Chadwick and published in 1842. Perhaps more than any single document, it altered the political debate on the urban poor by linking deplorable sanitary conditions to their physical and moral well-being and by documenting unequivocally that poverty meant more than hardship; it also meant death. Ground-breaking analyses by Villerme (1828) in France and Virchow (1872) in Germany provided additional strong evidence linking mortality to social status.

A special focus on young child mortality soon emerged from the developing capacity to address social issues with health-related statistics, because the rates of mortality among the young were seen to be alarmingly high and because the causes of young child death were deemed to be inherently sensitive to sanitary conditions (Flinn 1965) and other social factors. On a political level, the innocence and frailty of young children endowed young child mortality with an emotional content that made it easier to advocate for social reform. In a speech, Chadwick (1860) contended that the mortality rate of young children was 'the best single test of the sanitary condition of a place or population, as that test is least affected by occupation, immigration, or migration, and as children are most affected by aerial impurity. Farr (1866) pointed out that approximately 80 per cent of the total excess mortality in poor districts was due to death in children under 5 years. Like Chadwick, Farr also contended that the comparison of young child mortality rates provided an unmatched measure of local health conditions. Villerme (1834) argued a similar point in his classic study of the French marshlands (Coleman 1982), while Virchow (1874) pointed to the special sensitivity of infants to improved sanitary conditions.

The adoption of infant mortality as a special social indicator was not based on technical considerations alone. Although the horror of the conditions documented in the statistical reports met with general concern, specific proposals for sanitary and social reform were not universally embraced. It was soon clear that highlighting the plight of children could help overcome the widespread public ambivalence about the causes of poverty and the role of government in fashioning an appropriate response. When technical insights were coupled to political utility, infant mortality was embued with a special character in public discourse (Meckel 1990). In one simple statistic, the legitimacy of empirical science and the urgency of a profound human tragedy were combined.

The growing significance of infant mortality as a health statistic fueled tensions over how it should be interpreted and addressed. An important group of sanitary reformers, which included Chadwick and Florence Nightingale, held that the concentration of disease in urban neighborhoods was due to direct environmental contamination. Consequently, concern for the desperate conditions of poor urban areas could be raised with little regard for the qualities or social claims of the affected inhabitants (Himmelfarb 1983). The comparison of data from different regions, cities, and neighborhoods, was less social epidemiology than social geography of morbidity and mortality, emphasizing the dangers of urbanization rather than industrialization. Indeed, Chadwick and his colleagues elevated hygiene above privation, sanitation above injustice, and—while serving the cause of reform—constrained its purview to the effects of unsanitary local conditions, not the economic forces that created them.

Not surprisingly, the remedies that emerged from this position were primarily technical. A strong emphasis was placed on public works, including sewage systems, street paving and cleaning, and improved water supplies. Solutions were derived from civil—not social—engineering, although the importance of generating public support for requisite government action was recognized. The focus on technical interventions allowed the improvement of urban conditions to be functionally separated from more fundamental questions regarding the poor and generated a number of mainstream sanitary activities which in England culminated in the passage of the Public Health Act of 1848 (Eyler 1979; Himmelfarb 1983).

Although this direct focus on reducing illness and mortality lay at the heart of the sanitary reforms of the mid-nineteenth century, an important dissident group used the emerging mortality data as evidence of broader societal problems, including inequitable economic relations and social injustice. Frederick Engels (1845) in *The condition of the working class in England* used published mortality data to argue for more fundamental change. With special attention to young child mortality, Engels and others used differences in mortality to look beyond technical or programmatic interventions to more basic changes in the fabric of industrial Europe.

The growing sophistication of statistical analyses and the rapidly expanding power of the medical establishment intensified the differences in interpretation and use of infant mortality data. By the early part of the twentieth century, new state institutions had become leaders in the struggle to address infant mortality (Muncy 1991). In the 1920's in the USA, the Children's Bureau chose infant mortality as the subject of its first major study. Significantly, this effort expressly linked analysis to action and recommended technical programs while at the same time strongly typing infant mortality to social deprivation. By the early 1930s, however, the inclusive vision and administrative power of the Children's Bureau had largely been replaced by increasingly forceful representatives of the mainstream medical community and its tight focus on technical solutions (Muncy 1991).

The dominance of the medical community in defining responses to infant mortality increased with the phenomenal growth of the Medicaid program in the late 1960s and 1970s. This massive shift from the traditional maternal and child health system to the mainstream medical system for the health care of poor children coincided with unprecedented advances in medical knowledge and clinical capacity. Together, these trends only intensified the isolation of the pediatric, obstetric, and public health disciplines and set in motion the analytic and political antagonisms that have continued to characterize our societal approach to the reduction of infant mortality.

Conceptual expressions of disciplinary fragmentation

Social versus medical explanations

The disciplinary antagonism in addressing infant mortality is exemplified by the pervasive tension between social and medical explanations for observed differences in outcome. At many levels, this has often been framed as a choice between 'social' and 'medical' models of infant mortality causation. Social models stress the power of social variables and the importance of structural change in determining infant survival. Medical models stress pathophysiology and potential ways of interrupting pathological processes through clinical interventions. In this framework, social factors such as poverty are cast as alternative explanations to clinical factors such as chorioamnionitis or respiratory distress syndrome. This conceptual tension between social and medical explanations is expressed in empirical research, clinical care, and the development of public policy.

The disciplinary isolation between the social and biologic sciences is disturbing. A vast sociologic, anthropologic, and demographic literature exists on the causes of infant mortality. However, it is rarely tapped in the exploration of clinical pathways to reducing infant mortality. Similarly, the social sciences continue to make poor use of the clinical literature in refining the search for relevant social and behavioral influences.

Programs and policies directed at reducing infant mortality have also been plagued by deep divisions between advocates of social strategies such as community development and proponents of expanded clinical services such as enhanced prenatal monitoring for high-risk women. Too often, the effort to elevate the role of social determinants is framed by the indictment of clinical technologies as failed strategies. The danger of depreciating the value of clinical interventions is that it diverts attention from the essential goal of providing them equitably to all those in need. Antagonism between social and medical explanations, therefore, is not merely a conceptual concern. It emboldens disciplinary provincialism and impedes the development of effective policy.

Preventive versus therapeutic approaches

Tensions have also emerged between preventive and therapeutic arenas of intervention. Although preventive strategies are intuitively more desirable but that does not mean that therapeutic strategies have not been effective in improving infant mortality (Meckel 1990). There seems to be an underlying public impression that poor children somehow benefit less from therapeutic—particularly high technology—interventions than do their wealthier counterparts. There is little question that preventive efforts have been seriously ignored and must be broadly enhanced. Yet therapeutic services—particularly, neonatal intensive care—have been extremely important in improving survival of poor and wealthy infants alike (Paneth *et al.* 1982; Wise *et al.* 1985).

The notion that therapeutic efforts have been ineffective is false. In fact, 60–80 per cent of the total decline in neonatal mortality in the USA over the past two decades has been ascribed to improved management of high-risk deliveries and intensive care for ill newborns (Paneth *et al.* 1982; Williams and Chen 1982). Rather, profound social inequities have often made therapeutic efforts inaccessible. Provision of intensive care in many developing countries is inadequate and in some areas in the USA regionalized neonatal intensive care systems break down when patients are unable to pay. This effect deserves attention, since even small social disparities in access to high technology care can lead to differences in outcome for infants.

The schism between the clinical and public health disciplines

The tensions between social and medical explanations of disparate infant outcome have given rise to a schism between clinical and public health communities. Public health efforts to address infant health have generally focused on enhancing use of health care by means of financial mechanisms and community-based initiatives, including outreach, home visitation, and social service programs (National Governors Association 1992). Often, however, these programs have been developed and implemented without linkages to clinical services or facilities. Indeed, clinical providers may not even be aware that large portions of their patient populations may be enrolled in such programs. Under such circumstances, the potential for fragmentation of services is significant. In addition, enhanced outreach efforts may only aggravate already strained clinical facilities (Rosenbaum *et al.* 1988). This lack of collaboration represents a lost opportunity for the clinical and public health communities to advocate jointly for an expanded commitment to improving infant health.

Confronting racial disparities in infant mortality

Disciplinary fragmentation has taken its greatest toll in the search for the causes of racial disparities in infant mortality. This has largely been due to the unavoidable linkage of a complex scientific field to deeply held beliefs regarding the dynamics of societal inequality and **the concept of equal justice**. In the USA, the issue of social disparities in infant mortality has often been framed by the issue of race, because race continues to be associated with powerful differences in economic well-being and social position. In addition, because vital statistics data in the USA contains information on race but not on social status, race has become a proxy variable for the analysis of social differentiation (Liberatos *et al.* 1988; Navarro 1990). For the year 1989, infant mortality for Blacks was 18.6 deaths per 1000 live births, while the rate for whites was 8.1—a risk ratio of 2.3 (National Center for Health Statistics 1992*a*). In general, the trend over the past three decades has been for the absolute difference between rates for Black and White infants to fall while the relative disparity has continued to grow.

For many, the racial disparity in infant mortality is a direct reflection of disparate social conditions. Recently, however, a diverse literature has emerged that has been interpreted as questioning this social explanation. Not surprisingly, given the troubled history of defining race (Gould 1981), and the intensely political nature of disparate infant mortality, public discussion of the empirical work behind this literature has been highly fractious and deeply affected by conceptual antagonisms and fragmented disciplinary approaches (Eberstadt 1991). Although the elements of this process are manifold and at times quite subtle, two general issues seem central to the debate.

Examining the social meaning of race

In one series of studies, multivariate techniques were used to assess the influence of race on infant outcome while controlling for a series of social variables such as income or education (Wise *et al.* 1985; Shiono *et al.* 1986; Gould and LeRoy 1988). In general, these studies have reported persistently higher rates of poor birth outcomes among African Americans even when selected social and economic variables are taken into account. In addition, the relatively low rates of low birth weight and infant mortality among Mexican American populations despite significant social deprivation (Kleinman *et al.* 1991) has also been interpreted as suggesting non-social causes for higher rates among African Americans. In a sense, these studies are perceived as statistically stripping race of its social character, leaving a residual biologic component behind.

The concern with this interpretation is that the social variables used in these analyses have been quite crude and are not likely to have captured fully the social meaning of race in American society. Health researchers have not adequately sought out the insights of the social sciences in analyzing racial influences and have often not fully recognized the subtle social character of race, which has been so well documented in the sociologic, psychologic, and anthropologic literature (Cooper and David 1986). Even with similar family incomes, Black families possess far fewer assets than their White counterparts, are less likely to own their homes, and receive less intensive care services in hospital. College-educated Whites have significantly higher incomes than Blacks with the same levels of education (Byrd and Leuchter 1989). In addition, whether complex psychosocial effects associated with racial discrimination can influence birth outcomes remains poorly explored (Institute of Medicine 1985). Indeed, the persistence of racial disparities in health outcomes despite the simultaneous analysis of social variables is more the rule than then exception and has characterized patterns of mortality due to pedestrian injury and homicide, among many others (Wise *et al.* 1985). The empirical experience of a variety of disciplines suggests that the social character of race is exceedingly complex and that the interpretation of persistent racial effects should be approached with informed caution.

The reification of birth weight

Approximately two-thirds of the difference between Black and White infant mortality in the USA is due to differences in neonatal mortality. Slightly more than two-thirds of this neonatal differential is in turn accounted for by the greater numbers of Black neonates with birth weights of less than 1500 (National Center for Health Statistics 1992). This association has led to strong interest in factors that can influence birth weight.

The central reason to measure birth weight is because it is a powerful predictor of infant morbidity and mortality. As its importance as an analytic tool has grown, however, there has been a tendency to ignore the elasticity of the relationship of birth weight to infant outcome, particularly prematurity (Kramer 1990) and treat it as a concrete outcome itself. Examination of racial disparities in infant mortality has increasingly been plagued by this transformation of birth weight from predictor to outcome. Certain findings on birth weight have been highlighted as essential that in fact have little relevance to the fundamental issue of disparate mortality. There is great concern with the suggestion that race-specific standards be used to compare the birth weight distributions of Blacks and Whites (Wilcox and Russell 1990). The primary fear is that such adjustments would reduce the racial disparities in low birth weight rates, which in turn would be construed as being tantamount to adjusting away the observed differences in mortality. In reality, such an adjustment would merely make birthweight a less useful predictor of mortality. Altering birth weight standards to account for race cannot change the magnitude of the overall difference in infant death.

It is also important to distinguish between factors that may influence mean birth weight and those that can affect the risk of pathologic conditions associated with very low birth weight. This seems particularly important in assessing the relevance of any possible inherited racial effects on birth weight, as well as potential effects of a mother's birth weight on her offspring's birth weight (Emanuel *et al.* 1989). The search for possible influences on birthweight may include measurement of differences in mean birth weight, but such differences do not necessarily hold any importance to morbidity or mortality. Significantly, recent insight into the clinical epidemiology of very low birth weight suggested that the excess among Blacks was due to an elevation in the risk of almost all conditions associated with preterm birth (Kempe *et al.* 1992). Thus, if genetic or intergenerational effects are operative, they have a profoundly heterogeneous expression.

Technical expressions of fragmentation

International comparisons

Infant mortality in different nations is frequently compared. In the USA, this exercise is usually associated with calling attention to its relatively poor standing in relation to other industrialized countries. In 1988, US infant mortality was ranked twenty-third in the world at ten per 1000 live births (National Center for Health Statistics 1992*a*). Japan reported an infant mortality rate of 4.8 per 1000, the lowest in the world. Perhaps more disturbing is the fact that the rate of infant mortality is decreasing in the USA significantly more slowly than in most of the industrialized world, hovering around 2 per cent per annum (Kleinman 1990).

Although these comparisons undoubtedly provide a broad comparative framework for assessing national infant mortality, their legitimacy is increasingly being questioned. Concern focuses upon differences in reporting practices, particularly in regard to fetal deaths and extremely premature newborns (National Center for Health Statistics 1992*b*).

In 1986 in the USA, 26 per cent of infant deaths were attributed to extremely low birth weight (less than 1000 g); 20 per cent weighed more than 1000 g and died as the result of congenital abnormalities. In France, the UK, and Japan, infants who are born weighing less than 1000 g and die soon afterwards are more likely than in the USA to be classified as stillbirths and therefore are excluded from the infant mortality statistics. Furthermore, these countries permit third trimester termination of pregnancy when congenital abnormalities are detected. When the US infant mortality rate is adjusted for extremely low birth weight infants and cases of congenital abnormalities, it compares favorably with rates in Western European countries. The fact that the US infant mortality rate includes these cases should not be viewed as a failure of our healthcare system, but rather as a reflection of the strength of our perinatal services and our commitment to attempting to aid every infant's survival. International comparisons of reproductive health should include weight-specific fetal and infant mortality rates and delineate causes of death (Sachs *et al.* in press).

Analyzing causes of infant death

The fragmented approach to infant mortality has also taken its toll in the analysis of the causes of infant death. In general, causes of death have been categorized according to their underlying pathology or their perceived amenability to prevention. Classification schemes that emphasize pathology tend to be more useful in exploring the underlying pathophysiology of perinatal death. Systems that categorize causes by their amenability to intervention are generally most useful in guiding discussions of public health policy. However, both types of designs have been characterized by somewhat insulated perspectives, which in turn have limited their utility to the confines of their disciplines of origin.

Classification schemes that define infant death in clinical and pathological terms alone often have little capacity to address social determinants. Their use must therefore be accompanied by a greater emphasis on building linkages with social and behavioral influences.

Classification schemes based on pathological or clinical causes are also relatively unable to link obstetrical and neonatal conditions coherently. For example, a widely used perinatal mortality classification scheme developed in Aberdeen, UK in the early 1950s focuses on obstetrical diagnoses with little attention to neonatal conditions other than congenital anomalies (Baird *et al.* 1954; Cole *et al.* 1986; Whitfield *et al.* 1986). Although ground breaking in its approach to obstetric conditions, the only distinctions between deaths due to prematurity and those occurring in term newborns were in the unexplained categories. In the studies that have used this system, this category accounts for the largest portion of all perinatal deaths.

An associated system based on autopsy findings highlights asphyxial conditions and does not directly address obstetrical conditions resulting in premature birth

(Hey *et al.* 1986). A more detailed system that makes use of information derived from placental examination has been proposed (Naeye 1977). Although a major improvement in analyzing obstetrical conditions resulting in perinatal death, this scheme is not designed to distinguish between neonatal diagnoses. In addition, because it attempts to link placental and clinical findings, this system in some ways falls victim to its interdisciplinary requirements. This system's use—but not necessarily its utility—has been limited by a lack of consensus regarding the integration of placental and clinical findings in determining relevant diagnoses, as well as by the practical requirements for local interdisciplinary collaboration.

A system derived from annual reports of infant death from the US National Center of Health Statistics (1992) emphasizes neonatal conditions and gives little insight into causative obstetrical conditions. Based on death certificates, this classification system responds largely to clinical diagnoses, and many important diagnostic categories, such as perinatal conditions, short gestation and low birth weight, and respiratory distress syndrome, appear somewhat arbitrarily defined. Viewed together, the pathology-based systems provide useful analytic frameworks when their use is framed by tightly conceived objectives. However, this caveat implies that a comprehensive assessment must integrate both obstetrical and neonatal causes.

Schemes designed to use cause-of-death information to assess the nature and scope of ameliorative interventions have similarly suffered from disciplinary constraints. A system proposed by Wigglesworth (1980) relies on the linkage of clinical and birth weight information and is clearly designed to provide insight into clinical needs. Although useful in organizing diverse conditions into clinically relevant categories, this system does not provide much insight into obstetrical causes. Other more expansive classification systems that attempt to use clinical diagnoses as proxies for 'preventability' are also hindered by disciplinary parochialism. For example, clinicians who care for newborns are likely to advocate schemes that declare deaths of infants weighing less than 750 or 500 g to be non-preventable (Rosenblatt *et al.* 1991). However, this excludes potentially preventable maternal conditions that increase the risk of delivering such an infant. On the other hand, schemes that list all infant deaths due to prematurity as preventable (Elbom *et al.* 1991) ignore the heterogeneity of the causes of prematurity and are unlikely to be used in refined public health and policy analyses.

Deaths due to congenital abnormalities have commonly been considered non-preventable (Elbom *et al.* 1991; Rosenblatt *et al.* 1991). Exposures to teratogens may be highly preventable, however. In addition, prenatal diagnostic advances may permit the prevention of infant deaths from these causes in some populations. Moreover, classification of congenital anomaly mortality as non-preventable disregards the ability of services and clinical strategies to improve the health and well-being of severely affected young children.

The sudden infant death syndrome (SIDS) should also not be universally viewed as non-preventable. A significant portion of SIDS deaths occur in infants born prematurely, often because of preventable maternal conditions. In addition, if sleep positioning becomes an accepted preventive measure, the interpretation of subsequent SIDS deaths must clearly be amended.

Overall, the primary problem with current cause-of-death classification schemes is not so much their technical validity but that each scheme is valid for a rather constrained arena of causation (Golding 1991). Current methodology not only creates significant confusion in the interpretation of social and biologic interactions but also impairs our our ability to develop comprehensive approaches to improve perinatal and infant outcome.

Creating a cross-disciplinary approach

Reconciling social and medical concepts of causation

Reconciling social and medical models of causation must begin with recognition that they are not conceptually distinct. Poverty is a social phenomenon. Infant death is a biologic event. This implies a process of transformation whereby primary social phenomena are translated into inherently biologic outcomes.

At a basic level, social conditions influence the likelihood of a poor health outcome through two general mechanisms: the elevation of risk and the reduction of access to interventions that could modulate the impact of elevated risk on outcome. These two mechanisms or 'dual currencies' of social influence affect both preventive and therapeutic arenas of intervention (Wise 1990).

Interestingly, however, the relative strength of risk or differences in access in determining differentials in outcome is ultimately determined by the efficacy of the intervention in question. Thus, interventions wholly without efficacy are not likely to create disparities in outcome even if differences in access exist. For interventions with minimal efficacy, social differences in risk status will dominate differences in outcome. For interventions of high efficacy, differences in access to these interventions will dominate differences in outcome.

This analytic framework is useful because it makes no distinction between social and biologic influences on outcome. Biologic etiologies can be altered profoundly by social influences; social etiologies, through their clinical expression, may provide opportunities for clinical intervention. Rather than sharply distinguishing between biologic and social influences, it is more useful to recognize their inherent linkage, which is largely mediated by the efficacy of any potential intervention. For example, phenylketonuria is a potentially lethal disorder of genetic origin. However, given that an effective intervention exists (dietary alterations) any observed disparities in mortality are likely to be social in origin.

Case reports

Case 1

A 17 year old woman presents to a teritary care hospital's emergency room in active labor at 28 weeks' gestation. She has no steady income, lives with an abusive boyfriend, and has had minimal prenatal care. Despite efforts to stop the labor, an 850 g infant is delivered, which dies after 9 h of life, despite maximal intervention in the neonatal intensive care unit. The woman experiences no medical sequelae and is discharged as per protocol at 24 h postpartum. She is told to get a check-up in about 6 weeks.

If this case characterized a population, the described social circumstances would probably result in an elevated risk for preterm birth. The inadequate use of prenatal care in the face of elevated risk would further increase the tendency for preterm birth. The rate of very low birth weight infants in this population would therefore be elevated. However, the immediate impact of intensive clinical care would generally be to reduce birth weight-specific mortality rates and so lessen the impact of increased social risks for preterm birth. However, the inadequate plan for follow-up care in this case reflects a poorly integrated reproductive health system, which fails to coordinate clinical and social interventions for women who remain at high risk.

Case 2

A 33 year old woman in previous good health presents to a rural community hospital in active labor at 39 weeks. Although her employer does not provide health insurance, she has received good prenatal care. After 12 h of labor, she delivers a 3450 g infant which begins to exhibit significant respiratory distress and cyanosis soon after birth. Based on clinical and laboratory examination, a complex cardiac anomaly is suspected. Transfer to the closest referral center is attempted, but its quota of beds dedicated to uninsured patients is currently filled. After 6 h of searching, placement at another referral center is arranged. However, before the transport team arrives, the child experiences a cardiorespiratory arrest and, despite resuscitative efforts, dies at 7 h of age.

In this case, social influences are expressed not through effects on birth weight itself, but rather through birth weight-specific increases in mortality, since access to neonatal intensive care is closely tied to mortality within birth weight strata (Paneth *et al.* 1982). Although in this case the elevation in mortality would be reflected in the normal birth weight category, the social influence on access to tertiary care could as easily affect high-risk infants in other birth weight categories.

Linking social and medical strategies

In a setting of disadvantage, the purpose of medical care is largely to uncouple poverty from its implications for health. To the extent that clinical interventions can reduce the effect of social forces on infant outcomes, analytic and policy-based efforts to improve infant survival must recognize the congruence of social and medical influences. Social etiologies of infant death must ultimately act via clinical pathways. The tension between social and medical explanations appears to stem not from fundamental concerns but rather from differences in disciplinary purviews and professional self-interests. Strategies to reduce illness and mortality through clinical intervention need not conflict with efforts to resolve underlying social determinants. Efforts to expand preventive initiatives should not devalue therapeutic interventions. Indeed, it seems far more useful to develop integrated strategies that strive for equity in the provision of whatever preventive and therapeutic interventions may exist.

Reassessing classification and reporting methods

As international and social comparisons take on new importance, it seems appropriate to ensure that definitions and recording procedures are not significantly contributing to observed differences. This is particularly important given the growing contribution of extremely premature infants to mortality rates, since this group is most likely to be subject to differences in classification.

Beyond the issue of differences in classification, it also seems appropriate to link traditional measures of infant mortality to other indicators of reproductive loss, such as late fetal deaths and spontaneous abortions. Wider use of measures that recognize the continuum of reproductive loss could provide a basis for exploring the cascade of risk over the course of a woman's reproductive lifetime and help integrate the fragmented arenas of women's health care services.

Improving women's health

Historically, an essential impulse of child advocacy has been to elevate the needs of the child above those of the parent (Wise 1990). Not surprisingly, the child's special status has deeply affected the manner in which infant mortality has been framed politically and addressed programatically. It has also strengthened disciplinary boundaries in how the basic scientific questions regarding infant outcome have been approached. The struggle to understand and address the causes of poor birth outcome has been primarily confined to prenatal issues.

Given this emphasis on the prenatal period, concern for the health of women has largely been addressed only to the extent that it affects that of the newborn. The numerous programs designed to improve birth outcomes have invariably been publicly touted as programs focused on infant well-being despite the fact that they all operate by providing services to women. In research as well, a tight focus on direct intrauterine effects has resulted in a striking paucity of information on the impact of conditions that exist before a woman becomes pregnant. Even the concept of preconceptual care refers to the infant.

It seems long overdue that we more actuely recognize that, in some measure, problems with infant health may be a legacy of poor women's health generally. Cross-disciplinary investigations that examine interactions between the general health of women and childbearing seem particularly important. This effort is likely to require first the development of measures with the disciplinary scope to adequately assess this cascade of risk, use of care, and health status. Issues of reproductive health—including contraception, sexually transmitted diseases, and abortion services—should no longer be as dramatically separated from the mainstream of infant mortality investigations and programs as they are today. The adverse effects of unhealthy behaviors, such as smoking and substance abuse, on birth outcome should be more closely linked to concerns for their effects on the health of the woman. An expanded focus on women's health would also probably enhance the effectiveness of current prenatal care initiatives. Perhaps the best guarantee for the early initiation of prenatal care is for the pregnant women to have had a strong relationship with a high-quality health care system long before conception occurred.

In essence, an expanded commitment to women's health would help transform prenatal care from what it essentially is today—the first component of child health care—to merely one component, albeit an important one, of women's health care over a lifetime. Such an effort would require significant collaborations across disciplines and a far more intensively integrated system of women's health care than exists today.

Summary

The power of infant mortality to command attention is derived from its intense emotional content as a profound human tragedy and its capacity to capture in one simple health statistic the multitude of social and biologic interactions that reflect a society's capacity to provide for its members. Yet these same attributes have made infant mortality vulnerable to profound disciplinary fragmentation and false antagonisms in policy. Ignoring the social roots of infant mortality can trivialize the meaning of both individual and populations of infant deaths. Depreciating the value of clinical care can only serve to undermine pleas for enhanced access to it, a result that virtually all those concerned for infant health would see as profoundly counterproductive. The challenge is to seek the inclusive political and disciplinary embrace that will best ensure that societal strategies to confront persistent elevations in infant mortality ultimately prove both effective and just.

Acknowledgment

This chapter is in part modified from a paper presented to the Workshop on Preterm Delivery Among African–American Women: Psychosocial Factors and Physiologic Responses, Atlanta, 1992 and published in *American Journal of Preventive Medicine*, 1993, Suppl. 6, 7–16, with permission.

References

Baird, D., Walker, J., Thomson, A. M. (1954). The causes and prevention of stillbirths and first week deaths. *Journal of Obstetrics and Gynaecology of the British Empire*, **61**, 433–7.

Byrd. V., and Leuchter, M. A. (1989). Race and Money. *Money*, December, pp. 154–72.

Chadwick, E. (1860). Address on public health. *Transactions of the National Association for the Promotion of Social Science*, 580.

Cole, S. K., Hey, E. N., Thomson, A. M. (1986). Classifying perinatal death: an obstetric approach. *British Journal of Obstetrics and Gynaecology*, **93**, 1204–8.

Coleman, W. (1982). *Death is a social disease*. University of Wisconsin Press, Madison.

Cooper, R., and David, R. (1986). The biological concept of race and its application to public health and epidemiology. *Journal of Health Politics Policy, and Law*, **11**, 97–116.

Eberstadt, N. (1991). America's infant-mortality puzzle. *Public Interest*, **3**, 30–47.

Elbom, P. N., Stark, H. G., and Kilmer, G. G. (1991). A classification system for preventable infant mortality. *Pediatrics*, **4**, 744–8.

Emanuel, I., Hale, C. B., and Berg, C. J. (1989). Poor birth outcomes of American black women: an alternative explanation. *Journal of Public Health Policy*, **10**, 299–308.

Engels, F. (1845). *The Condition of the Working-Class in England*. Progress, Moscow (republished 1973).

Eyler, J. M. (1979). *Victorian social medicine*. Johns Hopkins University Press, Baltimore.

Farr, W. (1866). Mortality of children in the principal states of Europe. *Journal of the Statistical Society of London*, **29**, 15–8.

Flinn, M. W. (ed.) (1965). *Report on the sanitary condition of laboring population of Great Britain*. Edinburgh. University Press, Edinburgh.

Golding, J. (1991). The epidemiology of perinatal death. In *Reproductive and Perinatal Epidemiology* (ed. M. Kiely) pp. 401–37. CRC Press, Boca Raton.

Gould, J. B. and LeRoy, S. (1988). Socioeconomic status and low birth weight: a racial comparison. *Pediatrics*, **82**, 896–904.

Gould, S. J. (1981). *The mismeasure of man*. Norton, New York.

Hey, E. N., Lloyd, D. J., and Wigglesworth, J. S. (1986). Classifying perinatal death: fetal and neonatal factors. *British Journal of Obstetrics and Gynaecology*, **93**, 1213–5.

Himmelfarb, G. (1983). *The idea of poverty*. Knopt, New York.

Institute of Medicine. (1985). *Preventing low birthweight*. National Academy Press, Washington DC.

Kempe, A., Wise, P. H., Barkan, S. E., Sarrenfield, W. M., Sachs, B. P., and Gortmaker, S. L. (1992). Clinical determinants of the racial disparity in very low birth weight. *New England Journal of Medicine*, **327**, 969–73.

Kleinman, J. (1990). The slowdown in the infant mortality decline. *Paediatric and Perinatal Epidemiology*, **4**, 373–81.

Kleinman, J. C., Fingerhut, I. A., and Prager, K. (1991). Differences in infant mortality by race, nativity status, and other maternal characteristics. *American Journal of Diseases in Childhood*, **145**, 194–9.

Kramer, M. S. (1990). Birthweight and infant mortality: perceptions and pitfalls. *Paediatric and Perinatal Epidemiology*, **4**, 381–90.

Liberatos, P., Link, B. G., and Kelsy, J. L. (1988). The measurement of social class in epidemiology. *Epidemiological Review*, **10**, 87–121.

Meckel, R. A. (1990). *Save the babies*. Johns Hopkins University Press, Baltimore.

Muncy, R. (1991). *Creating a female dominion in American Reform*: 1890–1935. Oxford University Press, New York.

Naeye, R. L. (1977). Causes of perinatal mortality in the US Collaborative Perinatal Project. *Journal of the American Medical Association*, **238**, 228–32.

National Center for Health Statistics. (1992*a*). *Health, United States, 1991*. Public Health Service, Hyattsville.

National Center for Health Statistics. (1992*b*). *International Collaborative Effort*. Public Health Service, Hyattsville.

National Governors Association (1992). *Gaining ground: state initiatives for pregnant women and children*. National Governors Association, Washington DC.

Navarro, V. (1990). Race or class versus race and class: mortality differentials in the United States. *Lancet*, **336**, 1238–40.

Paneth, N., Kiely, J. L., Wallenstein, S., Marcus, M., Pakter, J., and Susser, M. (1982). Newborn intensive care and neonatal mortality in low birth weight infants: a population study. *New England Journal of Medicine*, **307**, 149–55.

Rosenbaum, S., Hughes, D. C., and Johnson, K. (1988). Maternal and child health services for medically indigent children and pregnant women. *Medical Care*, **26**, 315–32.

Rosenblatt, R. A., Mayfield, J. A., and Hart, L. G. (1991). Neonatal mortality clusters: a new tool for classifying neonatal outcomes. *Journal of the American Board of Family Practitioners*, **4**, 299–306.

Sachs, B. P., Fretts, R. C., Ritter, R., Hellerstein, S., Wampler, N., and Wise, P. A Reappraisal of infant mortality as an healthcare indicator: the importance of women's health. (In Press).

Shiono, P. H., Klebanoff, M. A., Graubard, B. I., Berendes, H. W., and Rhoads, G. G. (1986). Birth weight among women of different ethnic groups. *Journal of the American Medical Association*, **255**, 48–52.

Villerme, L. R. (1828). Memoire sur la mortalité en France dans la classe aisee et dans la classe indigente. *Memories de l'Academie Royale de Medicine*, 97.

Villerme, L. R. (1834). De l' influence des marais sur la vie. *Annales d'Hygiene Publique et de Medecine Legale*, **11**, 342–62.

Virchow, R. (1872). On mortality in Berlin. *Berliner Klinische Wochenschrift*, 51.

Virchow, R. (1874). *General report on the findings of the Municipal Mixed Committee for the Investigation of Problems Relating to Canalization and Removal of Wastes*. Berlin.

Whitfield, C. R., Smith, N. C., Cockburn, F., and Gibson, A. A. M. (1986). Perinatally related wastage—a proposed classification of primary obstetric factors. *British Journal of Obstetrics and Gynaecology*, **93**, 694–7.

Wigglesworth, J. S. (1980). Monitoring perinatal mortality: a pathophysiological approach. *Lancet*, **ii**, 684–6.

Wilcox, A. and Russell, I. (1990). Why small black infants have a lower mortality rate than small white infants: the case for population-specific standards for birth weight. *Journal of Pediatrics*, **116**, 7–10.

Williams, R. L. and Chen, D. M. (1982). Identifying the sources of the recent decline in perinatal mortality rates in california. *New England Journal of Medicine*, **306**, 207–14.

Wise, P. H. (1990). Poverty, technology and recent trends in the United States infant mortality rate. *Paediatric and Perinatal Epidemiology*, **4**, 390–401.

Wise, P. H. (1992). The social context of maternal and child health care reform. In *The case for universal maternity care in the US* (ed. J. B. Kotch, C. H. Blakely, S. S. Brown, F. Y. Wong) pp. 9–25. American Public Health Association, Washington DC.

Wise, P. H., Kotelchuch, M., Wilson, M. L., and Mills, M. (1985). Racial and socioeconomic disparities in childhood mortality in Boston. *New England Journal of Medicine*, **313**, 360–6.

23 Small for gestational age infants

Robert L. Goldenberg

Introduction

While it has long been recognized that the weight of a baby at birth is highly correlated to both survival and freedom from handicap, only in the last two decades have researchers clearly distinguished the concept of born too early from the concept of born at the right time, but too small. The latter infants are frequently labeled as being small for gestational age (SGA) or having intrauterine growth retardation. While some writers attempt to distinguish between SGA and intrauterine growth retardation, with SGA meaning a birth weight less than an arbitrary standard for gestational age and intrauterine growth retardation referring to an infant whose size at birth is 'less than its potential', for the purpose of this chapter both terms will be used to described infants whose weight at birth is below some arbitrary cut-off point for their gestational age.

It should be emphasized that SGA is not a disease itself or even necessarily a poor outcome. The condition is a cause for concern only because it is associated with various morbidities or mortality. A pregnancy resulting in an infant born small but healthy, who grows up with no handicap, should not be considered a poor outcome.

The attention paid to pregnancies associated with an SGA infant has soared in recent years, probably for several reasons. Most important has been the repeated observation that SGA fetuses are more frequently born dead, die in the neonatal period, and suffer from an excess of both short-term morbidity and long-term neurologic handicap. The availability of newer technologies has also contributed to this increased attention to SGA pregnancies. Ultrasound, for example, has the potential to measure fetal size; doppler flow measurement and various types of fetal heart rate monitoring also make it possible to monitor fetuses with this condition and potentially identify those at risk for fetal death and morbidity due to asphyxia.

Central to any discussion of SGA is its definition. Over the years, various authors have used many definitions, including two standard deviations below the mean, and the 3rd, 5th, 10th, and 15th percentile birth weight for gestational age, as well as definitions based measurements of the neonate which exclude gestational age, such as weight for length and an arm: head circumference ratio. In addition to this plethora of definitions, the population standards from which the percentile birth weights are drawn differ markedly, and differences of hundreds of grams in the cut-off points are found depending on the standard used. Furthermore, while gestational age is a crucial component of most definitions of SGA, there is little consistency from one study to the next in this very important parameter because of different methods for determining gestational age, including reliance only on the last menstrual period, variations in the use of ultrasound, and differences in rounding of weeks. The result of these discrepancies is that essentially no two studies of SGA—whether focusing on risk factors, mortality, long-term handicap, or the influence of various interventions—have examined equivalent groups of fetuses or infants.

In recent years, a consensus has developed that the 10th percentile birthweight for gestational age should define SGA. Despite the wide variability in the ranges of poor outcomes associated with SGA for the reasons discussed above, most authors would agree that fetal death is approximately five times more common, neonatal death two to three times more common, short-term neonatal problems five to ten times more common, and long-term neurologic handicap approximately five times more common in SGA infants than in infants with a birth weight above the 10th percentile.

Because of the confounding elements of birth weight and gestational age, it is not easy to show an improvement in outcome for SGA infants over time. However, a comparison of papers published in the 1960s with those published in the 1970s and 1980s does seem to show an improvement in specific low birth weight for gestational age mortality over time. Stillbirth rates have also decreased since the mid-1960s. Whether these rates decreased among SGA fetuses is difficult to determine, but we suspect that these improvements do include decreasing mortality for SGA infants as well. There is no evidence, either positive or negative, that long-term morbidity for SGA infants has changed over time.

One of the major difficulties in understanding the variations in obstetric outcome associated with an SGA infant is that the etiology of the decreased growth is almost certainly more important to the eventual outcome of the pregnancy than the decreased growth itself. For example, an infant who is SGA in association with a chromosomal abnormality or a congenital infection or secondary to maternal alcoholism or drug use is likely to have a very different outcome than an SGA infant of equivalent weight and gestational age born to a mother whose only risk factors for growth retardation is short stature. In order to better understand outcomes associated with SGA, far more attention must be paid to the maternal risk factor as they interact with size at birth.

The risk factors associated with SGA can be divided into several categories, although rarely is it possible to say that a specific factor caused a specific case of SGA. In developed countries, pre-eclampsia and related conditions associated with decreased blood flow to the uterus and placenta are responsible for about one-third of SGA infants. Maternal nutritional deprivation is probably less important, but certainly maternal thinness and failure to gain weight, as well as specific deficiencies of vitamins and minerals such as folic acid and zinc, have been related to decreased fetal growth. Poor life-styles as manifested by smoking, alcohol, or drug use influence infant size at birth. Cigarette smoking, in fact, is thought to account for as much as one-third of all SGA births. About 25 per cent of all pregnant women in the USA are smokers, as are a disproportionate number of women of low socio-economic status.

The picture in underdeveloped areas is significantly different. First, a much larger proportion of all births tend to be SGA. Second, SGA births more frequently appear to be related to a combination of poor maternal nutritional status and chronic infection. Furthermore, growth patterns in SGA newborns in underdeveloped areas tend to be different than in those from developed areas. In underdeveloped areas, approximately 80 per cent of the SGA newborns are symmetrically growth retarded (that is, short, but not particularly thin), while in developed areas, the reverse is true, with nearly 80 per cent of SGA infants being asymmetric (that is, thin but of normal length). Furthermore, these symmetric SGA newborn are more likely to be associated with congenital infections, anomalies, or toxic intake.

Maternal nutrition and SGA

Numerous authors have emphasized that glucose, which the fetus receives by diffusion across the placenta, is the primary substrate for fetal growth. Fetal growth, therefore, depends on an adequate substrate supply of glucose, vascular competence to receive it, and an appropriate fetal hormonal milieu, so that the fetus may appropriately use its glucose supply. There are several studies which show that maternal hypoglycemia may be related to SGA in the fetus.

The role of nutritional deprivation in determining the size of the infant at birth and, consequently, the rate of SGA in the population is difficult to determine. There is no doubt, for example, that tall women have longer and therefore heavier babies and that heavy women (whether heaviness is determined by weight alone or a weight for height ratio) have heavier babies. Therefore, using the 10th percentile definition of SGA, short and thin women have more SGA babies. However, in societies where there is a reasonable food supply without significant starvation, even if the diet is not ideal by contemporary nutritional standards, there is little evidence that thin women can be fed out of having an SGA baby. In developed countries, for example, studies have shown that most nutritional supplementation programs, even in lower socio-economic populations, result in a mean newborn weight gain of only 25–50 g. In addition, there is reasonably good evidence that supplementation programs that include high levels of protein are associated with smaller babies and worse outcomes.

In underdeveloped countries, however, especially where there is substantial food deprivation and where maternal energy expenditures are very great, nutritional supplementation substantialy increases the size of the newborn at birth, therefore reducing the rate of SGA in the population. These more recent experimental data confirm epidemiologic data obtained during famines in the Netherlands and in Leningrad during the Second World War. These older studies showed that poor maternal nutrition, especially during the third trimester, can greatly reduce birth weight. These studies also showed that maternal deprivation in the first half of pregnancy has little impact on birth weight. Babies will achieve normal birth weight and normal long-term neurologic development when the mother has sufficient calories toward the end of the pregnancy even if she suffered massive deprivation during the first and early second trimesters.

These types of studies suggest that SGA associated with maternal nutritional deprivation alone is a very different condition than that associated with maternal vascular conditions such as pre-eclampsia. In the former, the only deficit confronting the fetus appears to be calories. In the latter, because of a decreased utero-placental blood flow, the fetus is deprived not only of calories but also of oxygen. The reason why the Dutch and Leningrad deprived infants, although growth retarded, consistently scored as normal on neurological tests as they matured is almost certainly that they received a normal supply of oxygen. In contrast, the high rate of long-term neurological abnormalities associated with SGA births in pre-eclamptic women is probably related to chronic and/or acute oxygen deprivation. This suggests very strongly that in studies of long-term outcome, it is no longer appropriate to categorize SGA by measurements of the neonate alone. Instead, whenever possible, maternal risk factors associated with the development of the SGA should be documented.

Screening for SGA

Many factors may contribute to the etiology of an SGA fetus; those which are in some way statistically related to SGA and can be deduced prior to birth are considered risk factors. These would include a birth of a previous SGA infant or a fetal death, substance abuse, a very high or low hematocrit or hemoglobin level, medical conditions such as hypertension, renal disease, or sickle cell disease, and present pregnancy complications such as bleeding or twins. Physical factors which tend to put women at high risk for giving birth to an SGA infant may include short stature, low prepregnancy weight and failure to gain weight, and lower than average uterine fundal height measurements. Various risk-scoring systems based on combinations of these factors have been developed to screen for SGA. There have also been a whole series of biochemical and biophysical measures which are reported to be reasonable predictors of SGA, including Doppler flow studies, a positive roll-over test, measurement of various estrogens, serum cystine aminopeptidase, human placental lactogen, factor VIII-related antigen, and the exogenous dehydroepondrosterone sulfate half-life. None of these measurements appear to be superior to routine clinical and ultrasound measurements and none have been adopted into general clinical use.

In recent years, the major test for diagnosing SGA prior to birth has been the ultrasound examination in which one or more fetal measurements are compared with some standard. In fact, ultrasound imaging has become so sophisticated that nearly any fetal structure can be visualized, measured, and, to a degree, found to be smaller in babies who turn out to be growth retarded. Routine measurements now include the biparietal diameter, head circumference, abdominal circumference, femur length, various ratios of the above measurements, a qualitative or quantitative measurement of amniotic fluid, and a qualitative determination of placental maturation. At one time or another, measurement of nearly all of these parameters and many others as well have been proposed as the best test of fetal growth retardation.

The papers reviewed suggest that there should be two levels of screening for SGA. The first should be clinical and include both the appraisal of medical and life-style risk factors and measurement of fundal height. Known risk factors for SGA should raise the clinician's suspicion. With these risk factors, especially if they occur in conjunction with a fundal height measurement that is less than the 10th percentile for gestational age, a second-level screening test for SGA (an ultrasound examination) is probably indicated. In such high-risk populations, the true positive rate for SGA for the ultrasound examination should be about 70 per cent. In addition, about 60 per cent of all cases of SGA will be found in this group. In low-risk populations, if the second stage of the screening procedure is performed, the detection rate is still very low, but the false-positive rate is greater than 90 per cent. For these reasons ultrasound screening for SGA should not be routinely performed in low-risk populations.

There is little information in the literature from which to determine the gestational age best suited for screening for SGA. One study, however, shows the specificity for fundal height measurements predicting SGA to be greatest at about 32 weeks. Even less information is available about the most appropriate timing of ultrasound measurements. It appears that the closer it is done to delivery, the greater the likelihood of predicting SGA, but there is then the possibility that it will be too late to prevent death or damage to the fetus. The best timing is unknown; any recommendation between viability and maturity can probably be defended. For the reasons discussed above, however, one author recommends ultrasound screening for SGA in high-risk cases at about 34 weeks.

Prevention and treatment

A number of clinical goals can be related to the prevention and treatment of SGA pregnancies. Most important, but somewhat outside the scope of this review, is to make sure that every pregnancy at substantial risk for SGA is intended and wanted. In addition, since many women at risk of having SGA babies can be identified before they conceive, an adequate contraceptive program should be instituted so that high-risk women who are currently unenthusiastic about having a baby will be able to avoid or delay conception. Furthermore, since prepregnancy nutritional status (especially low weight for height) appears to be such an important predictor of an SGA birth, the aim would be to delay pregnancies in these women until they achieve a better nutritional status.

The major problem in defining a prenatal care protocol to prevent or treat the SGA problem is that few, if any, specific treatments or management plans have been shown to be effective in randomized controlled studies. Potentially useful methods of prenatal therapy for SGA include bed-rest, reduction of maternal risk factors, nutritional supplementation, and the use of drugs to improve utero-placental blood flow. Bed-rest has been recommended to improve uterine blood How. However, despite reasonable evidence that bed-rest in the left lateral position may improve blood flow and possibly protect against asphyxia in labor, there is no evidence that it ameliorates SGA or prevents its occurrence. Its use, although widely recommended, is controversial even in hypertensive pregnancies.

Decreasing work or physical activity has also been suggested as a means of protecting against poor fetal growth, but again, no controlled studies are available which support this treatment in pregnancies at risk for SGA. Furthermore, although the use of tobacco, alcohol, and illicit drugs are all statistically associated with SGA births, there are few reports showing that, once SGA is suspected, growth can be improved by eliminating these risk factors. However, there is reasonable evidence that before growth is delayed, behavioral changes such as stopping or reducing alcohol consumption and drug and tobacco use or increasing weight gain, can enhance fetal growth. More important, it appears that the earlier the behavioral patterns are changed (and in the case of toxic substances, the less is consumed), the greater the likelihood of achieving a more normal growth pattern. However, since most pregnant women who abuse tobacco, alcohol, or drugs do not achieve permanent behavioral changes even when enrolled in programs designed to decrease use, the chances of achieving a major impact on the rate of SGA in these populations is small. Nevertheless, more than half the cases of SGA do not have their origins in maternal medical disease, but rather, in various maternal behavioral characteristics. Life-style changes, which include eliminating the use of toxic substances and achieving an appropriate dietary intake, are of very low risk to the mother, are likely to benefit her health as well as her baby's and should therefore be recommended, even though their effect on reducing the incidence of SGA is limited.

For most diseases associated with SGA, there is little evidence that treatment of the disease will reduce the incidence of SGA. For example, there is an extensive literature on treatment of various types of hypertension in pregnancy, but little evidence to show that the risk of SGA associated with hypertension can be reduced by treatment. On the other hand, it appears that in women with sickle cell disease, appropriate transfusion may lower the risk of SGA and improve outcome. Appropriate management of maternal heart disease may achieve similar results.

Other than case reports, there is also little evidence that any pharmacologic treatment will improve fetal growth in SGA fetuses. As an example, there are several uncontrolled studies claiming benefit of anticoagulant therapy in women with a history of an SGA infant in a previous pregnancy. Similarly, in an uncontrolled study, it has been suggested that correcting maternal hypotension will reduce the incidence of SGA. Until randomized studies are carried out, the benefit of these and other approaches will remain unknown.

One exception to the absence of randomized studies and of great recent interest is the prophylactic administration of low-dose aspirin to reduce the incidence of SGA. Studies by Wallenburg and others suggest that in women at risk, low-dose aspirin enhances fetal growth and may reduce the rate of SGA.

Furthermore, there are encouraging case reports of mothers with a previous SGA infant or a fetal death in association with lupus anticoagulant, in whom a combination of low-dose aspirin and steroids have resulted in an improved pregnancy outcome.

Because of the general lack of success in preventing SGA or in improving fetal growth once it is discovered, the goal in managing SGA pregnancies tends to center on screening for risk of asphyxia or intrauterine death, with the endpoint being delivery of a non-asphyxiated, living fetus. Some authors recommend early delivery, not only to achieve this goal, but also because the intrauterine environment is believed to be hostile and the fetus is 'better out than in'. However, no studies have demonstrated that early delivery with a goal other than reducing the likelihood of intrauterine death is beneficial. The risk of stillbirth in a population of prenatally detected SGA fetuses is almost certainly higher than that in the general population and it can almost certainly be reduced by early delivery. However, the risk of stillbirth in SGA fetuses not delivered before term is relatively low, probably in the range of 1–5 per cent. If early delivery becomes the method for prevention of stillbirth, then for every fetal death averted by early delivery, 95–99 fetuses not destined to die will be delivered early. The risks or benefits to the mothers and to the fetuses of such intervention is unknown. Therefore, selecting a subset of SGA fetuses at higher risk of fetal death for early delivery appears to be a reasonable plan, although there is still little evidence that this substantially improves outcome. Another important consideration is that virtually all tests for detecting SGA *in utero* have a substantial false-positive rate; early delivery must therefore be implemented only with extreme caution, because of the potential to intervene in a normal pregnancy in a potentially harmful manner.

A number of tests and measurements have been proposed to determine which fetuses at risk for SGA are also at risk for fetal death and asphyxic damage before or during birth. These include measurements of biochemical substances such as estrogens, subjective measurements of fetal movement, Doppler flow measurements, and various fetal monitoring measurements, such as the non-stress test (which counts accelerations in the heart rate with fetal movement), and the contraction stress test (which monitors declerations in the fetal heart rate). More recently, a biophysical profile has been proposed as a mechanism to predict which fetuses are at risk for death and asphyxia. Components of the profile include ultrasound measurement of fetal activity, fetal breathing, fetal tone, and the volume of amniotic fluid, plus a non-stress test. It is not yet clear which component of the biophysical profile is most effective in predicting fetal death, but nearly all scoring systems have a false-negative rate of less than 1 per cent, and a negative test should allow the pregnancy to proceed without intervention.

The meaning of a positive test is less clear, although the risk of fetal death within 1 week is certainly increased. Therefore, if fetuses with abnormal monitoring tests, such as oligohydramnios, are selected for early delivery, it is almost certain that some fetal deaths will be prevented. Whether these infants are destined to die in the neonatal period or to have long-term neurologic difficulty not preventable

Table 23.1 Some recommendations for SGA births

Standardize the definition of SGA among governmental and professional organizations
Encourage research studies which evaluate potential therapies and short-and long-term outcome in relationship to risk factors for SGA as well as size at birth
Place major emphasis on reducing the damage done to fetuses by life-style risk factors for SGA
Consider SGA to be a symptom sometimes associated with a problem, and not a problem in itself

by early delivery is unknown. Furthermore, it is unlikely that a group of fetuses with a risk of fetal death of more than 25 per cent can be found, regardless of the criteria used to define risk. In those fetuses with abnormal monitoring tests, therefore, at least 75 per cent will have an induction or cesarean section that will not change their outcome (in terms of fetal death) and may place the fetus at other risks, especially those associated with prematurity.

Summary

In summary, the recent literature dealing with SGA births, although voluminous, is not very instructive. Disappointingly, there is only suggestive evidence that the incidence of SGA can be reduced or that the outcome of SGA pregnancies can be improved. There are few convincing randomized studies demonstrating improved outcome in SGA pregnancies managed in certain ways. Nevertheless, substantial data suggests that early delivery of certain fetuses discovered to be at high risk for stillbirth will improve survival. SGA pregnancies with decreased fetal movement, non-reactive, non-stress tests, positive contraction stress tests, or a positive biophysical profile, and those with oligohydramnios appear to fall into this group. There is no way to determine the negative aspects of intervention in these cases, however. Reported complications of induced early delivery include maternal morbidity and mortality, as well as neonatal morbidity and mortality associated with prematurity, and neonatal asphyxia secondary to the iatrogenic delivery. There is also no way at present to even estimate the damage done to those non-SGA false-positive fetuses who are judged at risk for fetal death or asphyxia.

References

Bakketeig, L. S., Hoffman, H. J., and Harley, E. E. (1979). The tendency to repeat gestational age and birth weight in successive births. *American Journal of Obstetrics and Gynecology*, **135**, 1086.

Fitzhardinge, P. M. and Steven, E. M. (1982). The small-for-date infant. II. Neurological and intellectual sequelae. *Pediatrics*, **50**, 50.

Goldenberg, R. L. Cutter, G. R. Hoffman, H. J. Foster, J. M., Nelson, K. G., and Hauth, J. C. (1989*a*). Intrauterine growth retardation: standards for diagnosis. *American Journal of Obstetrics and Gynecology*, **161**, 271.

Goldenberg, R. L., Cutter, G. R., Hoffman, H. J., Brumfield, C. G., and Foster, J. M. (1989*b*). Prematurity, post dates, and growth retardation. The influence of ultrasound utilization on the reported gestational age. *American Journal of Obstetrics and Gynecology*, **160**, 462.

Hales, C. N., Barker, D. J. P., Clark, P. M. S., Cox, L. J., Fall, C., Osmond C., Winter, P. D. (1991). Fetal and infant growth and impaired glucose tolerance at age 64. *British Medical Journal*, **303**, 1019–22.

Kramer, M. S. (1987). Determinants of low birth weight Methodological assessment and meta-analysis. *Bulletin of the World Health Organization*, **65**, 663.

Low, J. A., Galbraith, R. S., Muir, D., Killen, H. L., Pater, E. A., and Karchmar, E. J. (1983). Intrauterine growth retardation: a study of long-term morbidity. *American Journal of Obstetrics and Gynecology*, **142**, 670.

McCormack, M. (1985). The contribution of low birthweight to infant mortality and childhood morbidity. *New England Journal of Medicine*, **312**, 81.

Miller, H. C., and Merritt, T. A. (1979). *Fetal growth in humans*. Year Book Medical Publishers, Inc., Chicago.

Miller, H. C. and Merritt, T. A. (1979). *Fetal growth in humans*. Year Book Medical Publishers, Inc., Chicago.

Starfield, B., Shapiro, S., McCormick, M., and Bross, D. (1982). Mortality and morbidity in infants with intrauterine growth retardation. *Journal of Pediatrics*, **101**, 978.

Stein, Z., Susser, M., and Rush, D. (1978). Prenatal nutrition and birth weight experiments and quasi-experiments in the past decade. *Journal of Reproductive Medicine*, **21**, 287.

Villar, J., and Belizan, J. M. (1986). The evaluation of the methods used in the diagnosis of intrauterine growth retardation. *Obstetrical and Gynecological Survey*, **41**, 187.

Wallenburg, H. C. S. and Rotmans, N. (1987). Prevention of recurrent idiopathic growth retardation by low dose aspirin and dipyridarnole. *American Journal of Obstetrics and Gynecology*, **157**, 1230.

Wen, S. W., Goldenberg, R. L. Cutter, G. R., Hoffman, H. J., and Cliver, S. P. (1990). Intrauterine growth retardation and preterm delivery: risk factors in an indigent population. *American Journal of Obstetrics and Gynecology*, **162**, 213.

24 Cerebral palsy

Karin B. Nelson

Since its earliest description as an entity, in a report by John Little (1861) to the Obstetrical Society of London, cerebral palsy has been attributed to difficult or premature birth and often to deprivation of oxygen during birth. Although there were early arguments against such a point of view—most notably from Sigmund Freud (1897)—the impression has developed that birth asphyxia is the dominant cause of cerebral palsy and that good obstetric care should usually be able to prevent asphyxia and thus prevent the condition.

More recently a different point of view has emerged (Lancet 1989): 'There is no evidence for the widespread belief that intrapartum care commonly influences the risk of cerebral palsy.' The reasons for the change in perception have been discussed elsewhere (Nelson 1989; Stanley and Blair 1991), and I mention here only a few factors. Obstetrics has advanced greatly since John Little's day and is indeed one of the great success stories of modern medicine. Our knowledge of birth asphyxia and outcomes that can credibly be ascribed to it has advanced. The sciences of epidemiology and statistics have also advanced, so that standards of medical and scientific evidence and quality of studies have improved. New studies have increased our knowledge and some have asked a wider range of questions and employed techniques of analysis that have provided more sophisticated answers.

Thus, thinking about the possibility of reducing the incidence of cerebral palsy by altering obstetric management has been clouded by ill-founded assumptions inherited from the past. It has also been impeded by the difficulty of collecting good evidence about causes (see below) and particularly in the USA, complicated by pressures stemming from lawsuits against obstetricians (Rostow *et al.* 1989; Acheson 1991). Litigation charging obstetrical care givers with failing to prevent neurologic impairment in the child and fear of litigation have adversely affected access to health services for women and have contributed to a higher rate of diagnostic and therapeutic interventions, including those without demonstrated clinical benefit (Rostow *et al.* 1989).

Definition and distribution of cerebral palsy

The term cerebral palsy refers to a group of chronic neurologic disorders manifested by abnormal control of movement, beginning early in life and not due to underlying progressive disease. In addition to their motor disability, people with cerebral palsy often have other neurologic problems such as mental retardation, epilepsy, and disorders of vision and hearing. About 12 per cent of affected people acquire their disability after the first month of life; they will not be considered further in this chapter.

Between 1.2 and 2.5 per 1000 children of early school age have cerebral palsy. A recent population-based study suggested that at least 5000 people with moderate or severe handicap due to congenital cerebral palsy are added to the population of the USA each year (Cummins *et al.* 1993).

Studies in countries which monitor the numbers of people with cerebral palsy indicate that, despite improvements in obstetrics and neonatal care, attested to by marked improvements in survival, the condition is not less frequent today than in the past. In fact, as mortality has declined among infants of very low birth weight, the rate of cerebral palsy among those who survive has increased (Mutch *et al.* 1992).

Life expectancy in people with cerebral palsy is related to the severity of their movement disorder and the presence and severity of mental disability (Evans *et al.* 1990; Eyman *et al.* 1991). With good medical care, the majority of even the most severely affected people now survive into adult life.

Cerebral palsy is expensive. In 1988, costs to the state of California for diagnostic services and care—excluding physical and occupational therapy which are themselves expensive—was nearly $200 million (California Birth Defects Monitoring Program 1992). In addition, there were economic and non-economic costs to affected people and their families.

Causes of cerebral palsy

The etiology of cerebral palsy is difficult to study. It cannot be diagnosed until years after birth, so prolonged and expensive follow-up studies are required to relate pregnancy and birth factors to outcome. Medical histories of birth events, elicited after the condition is recognized, are subject to serious biases that make retrospective studies unreliable. Since cerebral palsy is fortunately relatively uncommon, studies that follow children from birth to the stage where it can be determined whether or not they have it must be very large and therefore very cumbersome and costly. The likelihood that it has more than a single cause, that causative factors might interact, and that some factors once thought to be causes are really early effects, means that studies must employ sophisticated techniques for analysis if confident conclusions are to be reached. Examining the relationship of cerebral palsy to asphyxia is complicated by problems with identifying asphyxia before or during birth, as discussed below.

For these reasons and others, relatively few methodologically appropriate studies of the etiology have been performed to date. In existing studies, the range of questions asked about causes of cerebral palsy is narrow, most having been concerned almost exclusively with complications of pregnancy and birth. Not surprisingly, then, few other causative factors have been identified. Yet when other associations have been sought, promising leads have been found (Nelson and Ellenberg 1985*a*; Torfs *et al.* 1990).

Physical trauma

In earlier periods and in some countries now, physical trauma at delivery probably contributed significantly to cerebral palsy. Trauma is no longer a major factor in developed countries. Babies born weighing 4000–4500 g, whose relatively large size made them especially susceptible to obstetric trauma in the past, now have the lowest rate of cerebral palsy of any birth weight group (Cummins *et al.* 1993).

Prematurity

Early birth and low birth weight are among the most important risk factors known for cerebral palsy. Cases arising in low birth weight infants constitute a large and an increasing sector of the total number. The lowest birth weights are associated with greatest risk. An infant born weighing less than 1000 g has a hundred times the risk of a baby whose birth weight is 3000–3499 g, the most common weight group (Cummins *et al.*, 1993). Weight between 2000 and 2499 g, which is much more common than more severe degrees of low birth weight, is associated with a much lower risk of cerebral palsy than extremely low weight at birth.

In a recent American cohort (Cummins *et al.*, 1993), babies born weighing less than 1000 g constituted 0.17 per cent of singleton survivors but contributed 8.7 per cent of the cerebral palsy in singletons and babies between 1000 and 1500 g contributed another 16 per cent.

The best predictor of low birth weight is low weight of a previous child born to the same mother. Three other factors that contribute to the likelihood of low birth weight and are also strongly associated with risk of cerebral palsy whatever the birth weight, are congenital malformations, inflammation of the placenta, and twinning.

Malformations within and outside the central nervous system are more common in children with cerebral palsy than in the general population (Nelson and Ellenberg 1985*a*), and are considerably more common among infants of low and very low weight at birth. Among low birth weight infants, those with congenital malformations are at special risk of cerebral palsy (Nelson and Ellenberg 1985*b*).

Inflammation of the placenta is an important risk factor for cerebral palsy in babies of all birth weights. The frequency of such inflammation is strongly and inversely associated with premature birth and evidence of inflammation is present in 50–80 per cent of very premature births (Steer 1991). Among low birth weight infants, those with placental inflammation are at especially high risk of cerebral palsy (Nelson and Ellenberg 1985*b*). Thus, both congenital maldevelopment and placental inflammation contribute to cerebral palsy over and above their contribution to low birth weight, and are also associated with the condition in term babies (Nelson and Ellenberg 1985*b*).

Another factor associated with low birth weight that predisposes to cerebral palsy is twinning. In addition to their tendency to be low in birth weight, twins—and especially monozygotic twins—have other problems including excesses of congenital malformations and connections between the blood vessels of co-twins within the placenta. If one twin dies, there is a substantial risk of neurologic complications in the surviving twin, often along with other organ defects, including atresia of the intestine or kidney and limb reduction defects (Szymonowicz *et al.* 1986; Paludetto 1991). In a recent American study, twins, who constituted 1.9 per cent of the population, contributed 10 per cent of the cerebral palsy (Grether *et al.* 1992).

The disappearance during pregnancy of one member of a twin pair whose earlier existence was documented by early ultrasound examination or placental examination at the time of delivery is not infrequent and has been linked in some cases with brain and systemic defects in survivors (Landy *et al.* 1986). Product liability suits have been brought against pharmaceutical companies for limb reduction defects, but it is theoretically possible that some were related to the unrecognized early disappearance of a twin in those pregnancies and that some otherwise unexplained cerebral palsy might arise by this mechanism; only a large and carefully designed prospective study will provide information about these possibilities.

With the use of fertility-enhancing medical treatments, the frequency of twins and triplets has increased strikingly, leading to what Papiernik has described as an epidemic of multiple births (quoted in *New York Times*, 26 May 1992). In a population-based Australian study (Petterson *et al.* 1990), the risk of cerebral palsy in triplets was high (32 per 1000 live births; the risk per pregnancy was presumably still higher). Most of the affected triplets were born after hormonal stimulation of ovulation or *in vitro* fertilization. An increase in the rate of cerebral palsy, as well as of costs (Keith *et al.* 1991), is likely to be the dark shadow of medical science's success in bringing help to previously childless couples. Further studies quantifying and further analyzing these risks will be important for management decisions in the future.

Birth asphyxia

Birth asphyxia can only be measured directly in the brain of the fetus or newborn in a very few facilities in the world. Everywhere else, the presence of asphyxia is inferred from the history and a variety of clinical measures; these correlate poorly with the obstetrical history and with one another, are dubiously related to deprivation of oxygen, and are poor predictors of outcome. In the past, asphyxia was often thought to have occurred whenever an infant was noted to be neurologically depressed. However, neurologic depression, as evinced by low Apgar scores, need for resuscitation, poor muscular tone, and depressed responsivity and reflexes, is not specific to asphyxia, but occurs with a variety of other problems; non-specific clinical indicators like low Apgar scores and hypotonia permit the recognition of illness in the newborn infant but are not informative as to the cause of that illness.

With the development of magnetic resonance spectroscopy, it is likely that we will have for the first time a gold standard by which to recognize birth asphyxia and its consequences in the brains of neonates. Very complicated and expensive, this technique will never be widely available, but it will serve as the basis for validation of other measures. Other approaches, such as near infrared spectroscopy, may be developed for wider application. In the near future, then, some of the uncertainty surrounding identification of abnormal gas exchange and its effect on fetal and neonatal brain will probably become resolvable. However, questions may remain concerning whether hypoxemia is part of the primary pathology or a late secondary complication.

Experimental evidence and clinical studies using the measures available to date indicate that the mammalian fetus withstands a degree of asphyxia during birth that would destroy the brain of an older creature; if that were not so, cerebral palsy would be far more common than it is. Asphyxia in the fetus or neonate can damage the brain irreversibly, but does so only if it is severe and prolonged. Additional pathogenic factors, especially marked drops in blood flow, may be required before brain damage is likely. Such reduced blood flow is not specific to disorders that begin with deprivation of oxygen but can be the result of a variety of pathogenic mechanisms, including infectious or immune processes, because these processes involve the release of endogenous substances that dilate blood vessels.

Population-based studies in developed countries indicate that about 80 per cent of people with cerebral palsy did not have even these non-specific indicators of serious asphyxia during or immediately after birth (Nelson and Ellenberg 1986; Blair and Stanley 1988; Emond *et al.* 1989; Torfs *et al.* 1990). Studies that take into account the presence before labor of potentially brain-damaging factors such as intrauterine infection and malformation suggest that perhaps as little as 3 per cent of cerebral palsy is due to birth asphyxia (Nelson and Ellenberg 1986). The form of the condition most convincingly linked with birth asphyxia—although not specific to it—is spastic quadriparesis with movement disorder. Hemiparesis may often be due to strokes occurring before birth or in the perinatal period.

Term infants whose brains have been irreversibly injured by deprivation of oxygen during delivery are ill in the newborn period. Babies at special risk of cerebral palsy are those with immediate postbirth neurologic depression who develop other neurologic signs, including neonatal seizures within the first 2 or 3 days after birth; such infants account for an important but small proportion of cases of cerebral palsy, 16 per cent in one series (Ellenberg and Nelson 1988). Term babies who are depressed but do not have seizures and those with seizures but no marked depression are much less at risk. Children who survive severe neurologic depression without cerebral palsy do not tend to have low IQs (Seidman *et al.* 1988) or an increased rate of mental handicap or epilepsy (Nelson and Ellenberg 1981).

Newborns whose neurologic illness arises through birth asphyxia also show evidence of asphyxial injury in other organ systems, including the kidneys, intestines, heart, and lungs. This clinical picture is not specific to asphyxial states (Nelson and Leviton 1991). In an infant who was not seriously neurologically and systemically ill in the newborn period, birth asphyxia is unlikely to have been the cause of any later discovered defect; the consistency of the evidence and the magnitudes of the differences in risk based upon these considerations make it reasonable to apply this criterion to judging causation in individual cases.

Electronic fetal monitoring in labor was introduced in part in the hope of increasing information on oxygenation state of the fetus and thereby permitting earlier intervention to prevent cerebral palsy. However, as discussed below and in Chapter 17, the information provided by fetal monitoring has not been shown to be a valid predictor of cerebral palsy.

Other factors

As a group, children with cerebral palsy have an excess of congenital malformations both within and outside of the brain. Magnetic resonance imaging in one recent series suggested that nearly one-third of people with cerebral palsy who were born at term had cortical dysgenesis secondary to abnormal neuronal migration (Truwit *et al.* 1992).

Athetoid cerebral palsy was once relatively common, as a result of marked hyperbilirubinemia caused by Rhesus incompatibility. Techniques to prevent sensitization, phototherapy, or exchange transfusion to prevent high levels of bilirubin, have now made this form of the condition uncommon. Rubella virus can cause brain injury resulting in cerebral palsy, and toxoplasmosis and cytomegalovirus infection can produce motor sequelae. Intrauterine exposure to methyl mercury and to exogenous thyroid hormone and estrogen (Nelson and Ellenberg 1985*a*), and neonatal exposure to benzyl alcohol (Benda *et al.* 1986) have been associated with the condition. Maternal conditions, including mental handicap (Emond *et al.* 1989), unusual menstrual cycles (Nelson and Ellenberg 1985*a*) and thyroid disorders (Nelson and Ellenberg 1985*a*) have also been associated with increased risk. More investigation of these and other factors is needed.

In developing countries, infection, malnutrition, maternal hemorrhage, iodine deficiency, neonatal hypothermia, physical trauma at delivery, and other factors are likely to play significant roles. Documentation concerning most of these is sparse because few epidemiologic studies from these countries exist.

Prevention of cerebral palsy

Prematurity and low birthweight

Previous work (chapters 19 and 23 of this book) and Alexander *et al.* (1991) assesses efforts to prevent prematurity and low birth weight, which are important risk factors for cerebral palsy. There was no decrease in the rate of low or very low weight births in the USA between 1950 and 1989. Few randomized trials have shown an effect on birth weight sufficient to make much difference to cerebral palsy risk. Since the risk is highest at extremely low birth weights, small improvements nearer to the normal level—for example, increasing birth weight from 2400 to 2550 g—would not be expected to lead to much change in risk for cerebral palsy. An important goal is significant improvements at the lowest birth weights, but it is not clear that we know how to achieve this (Alexander *et al.* 1991).

We still lack information about the degree to which short gestation or poor fetal growth or both contribute to later neurologic morbidity in babies born at low weights. It will be necessary to know this, and to identify major antecedents of the specific patterns that represent greatest risk, if we are to design and test new management strategies.

Gibbs *et al.* (1992) have recently reviewed evidence that placental infection, clinical or subclinical, is often the trigger to premature birth. Infection can also lead to release of endogenous substances that may be harmful to the brain of the infant (Selma and Raine 1988; Brenneman *et al.* 1992; Romero *et al.* 1992). Thus, the cause of preterm birth may also be a cause of brain injury in the prematurely born infant.

Some factors that can cause low birth weight, such as cigarette smoking, do not affect risk of cerebral palsy. It is often assumed that earlier prenatal care can prevent low birth weight and thereby prevent cerebral palsy. In a recent American study, time in pregnancy when women first sought prenatal care was not different in women who did and in those who did not give birth to children with congenital cerebral palsy (Cummins *et al.* 1993). The causes of marked prematurity and of cerebral palsy are probably not sufficiently understood or susceptible to intervention by modern prenatal care for earlier care to make as much difference as has been hoped.

Birth asphyxia

It is not known to what extent birth asphyxia of a degree sufficient to cause cerebral palsy is obstetrically preventable. The large majority of infants who survive recognizable obstetric complications, including 'anoxigenic' complications, are later normal; in attempting to judge the need for intervention in pregnancy and labor, medical care givers need means to recognize significant degrees of asphyxia. But the tools at the obstetrician's disposal for assessing fetal well-being during labor are inadequate (Pattinson 1992).

Indicators of fetal distress correlate so poorly that doubt has been raised as to whether these constitute a syndrome (Steer *et al.* 1989). Severe slowing of the fetal heart rate to less than 60 beats per minute, as observed by auscultation, is associated with some increase in risk of cerebral palsy (Nelson and Ellenberg 1985*a*). It had been hoped that refining observations of fetal heart rate in labor by means of electronic fetal monitoring would permit earlier recognition of significant asphyxia and thereby permit interventions that would decrease the rate of cerebral palsy. However, in the three randomized trials that followed infants long enough to identify eventual abnormal neurologic status, such abnormal status was not less frequent with the use of electronic fetal monitoring than with intermittent auscultation (Langendoerfer *et al.* 1980; Grant *et al.* 1989; Steer *et al.* 1989). In fact, in one trial it was significantly higher (Shy *et al.* 1990). Children with cerebral palsy are not known to have abnormal monitoring characteristics more often than normal children. Two studies suggest that internal fetal monitoring may contribute to chorioamnionitis (Newton *et al.* 1989; Soper *et al.* 1989), itself a risk factor for cerebral palsy (Torfs *et al.* 1990). Monitoring contributes to increasing the rate of interventions, which poses additional risks to mother and child.

Measurements that can be done in newborns are not good predictors of long-term outcome, either. Most are not specific to a single etiology. Bacterial infection of placental membranes can mimic many of the features often thought to mark birth asphyxia, such as low umbilical arterial pH and a low Apgar score; this can be so even in the absence of clinical evidence of chorio-amnionitis or of prolonged rupture of the fetal membranes (Meyer *et al.* 1992). Apgar scores must be severely depressed for a relatively long while to be associated with substantial risk of cerebral palsy (Nelson and Ellenberg 1981). Acid–base measurements must also be severely abnormal to show much relationship to neurologic status, even within the neonatal period (Goldaber *et al.* 1991), and have not been shown to predict later neurologic morbidity better than, or as well as, Apgar scores (Ruth and Raivio 1988; Dennis *et al.* 1989).

Although only serious deviations from the norm of pH and of Apgar score relate to cerebral palsy risk, most interventions in labor have been tested by looking at their relationship to mild deviations in these neonatal measures, or to degrees of neonatal illness that are not themselves good predictors of later status. It seems that newer measures, such as umbilical artery Doppler velocitometry and fetal electrocardiography in labor, are being evaluated in a similar approach. It is therefore likely they will produce the same erroneous conclusions, and lead to unnecessary increases in the already high cesarean section rate.

Severe depressions of Apgar score or pH are rare, and it is not known at what point intervention is no longer useful. If 10 per cent or less of cerebral palsy is due to asphyxia during birth, then the effort is to prevent an outcome that is likely to be present in only one or two births per 10 000; few clinical trials can have a big enough sample size to allow the use of cerebral palsy as an outcome measure.

Furthermore, the positive predictive value of a test is related to the frequency of a condition in the population; with very uncommon outcomes, most positive tests will be erroneous. Indeed, all the prebirth measures for which information is available suffer from extremely high false-positive rates. For meconium in the amniotic fluid, severe fetal bradycardia, delayed first cry, and low Apgar scores, the false-positive rate for prediction of later cerebral palsy is at least 95 per cent (Nelson and Ellenberg 1986). This means that if these findings are used as a basis for undertaking an intervention, any risk or expense of that intervention will not benefit most of the mothers and infants for whom it is applied. If the interventions were entirely safe and fairly inexpensive, the problem would be slight, but often they are not. Apart from administering oxygen and turning the laboring woman on her side, interventions consist chiefly of surgical delivery. As Chanoine *et al.* (1988) point out, 'The message from the trials of continuous fetal heart rate monitoring, that "more information" may lead to harmful as well as beneficial effects, should not be forgotten when new techniques are developed.'

Assessing preventive measures

So there are many difficulties in attempting to establish that any measure or intervention to prevent cerebral palsy is effective. Yet to introduce new interventions without such demonstration means that we cannot tell whether we are doing more good than harm. Medical science has a lengthy history of causing unanticipated harm. Half the medications marketed prove to have unanticipated deleterious effects. Even the antiseptic solution used to clean the maternal abdomen for a cesarean section can suppress the baby's thyroid gland, confusing the mandatory screening tests for congenital hypothyroidism (Meyer *et al.* 1992), and leading to needless treatment and parental distress. Good intentions are no guarantee of a good result.

Considerations of medical costs and many patients' preferences might dictate a detechnologizing of the process of birth unless there is clear evidence that technology can prevent bad outcome. For long-term neurologic disability, proof of efficacy is scarce. Physicians face a real dilemma in determining how to avoid interventions that add to discomfort, risks, and costs and have not been shown to be beneficial for outcome and yet protect themselves from legal action if outcome is not good.

In modern industrialized countries, most cerebral palsy is probably not preventable by further interventions directed at labor and delivery factors and there is no reason to think that other neurologic disorders such as mental handicap, epilepsy, or autism are.

We do not know whether it is possible, without real threat of increasing risks to a far larger number of babies, to introduce innovations that might prevent brain injury in the few babies now at risk by virtue of asphyxial complications of birth.

Medico-legal aspects: an American perspective

The presence of cerebral palsy in a person is not a good tool for assessing the quality of medical care he or she has been given. Errors of nature appear to predominate over errors of medical attendants as determinants of cerebral palsy. This does not mean that human errors or negligent acts never cause cerebal palsy, but that bad actions cannot be assumed from the occurrence of bad outcomes. There is no evidence that much of the small fraction of cerebral palsy that is due to birth asphyxia is preventible through increasing interventions in the intrapartum period.

If we understand the causes of an outcome, we can predict that outcome. As already discussed, however, it is not possible to identify the cause of cerebral palsy from the facts about a case that are presented in courtrooms to indicate that action should have been taken earlier than it was. Since we probably do not know the cause of most cases of cerebral palsy, what is the purpose of asking the cause in an individual, as is required in litigation?

To judge causation requires a balancing of the probabilities to which many elements may contribute and no systematic approach has yet been agreed upon. Fenichel *et al.* (1989) used a Bayesian method to assess the probability that immunization procedures caused neurologic injury. Unless some such approach is accepted in the assessment of causation in cerebral palsy (or even cancer), it is unlikely that a confident assessment of causation can be made in most affected individuals.

Expert testimony that takes into account the circumstances of the individual case may be inferior to epidemiologic information in predicting outcome and therefore in recognizing causal relationship (Faust and Ziskin 1988). Bertrand Russell observed many years ago that people tend to draw general conclusions from just a few instances they happen to witness, based on 'the emotional interest of the instances, not on their number', nor on their legitimate generalizability. It is likely that this tendency is relevant to perceptions about obstetric factors and cerebral palsy. The emotional impact of instances in which obstetric calamity is followed by neurologic disaster is great and may be part of the reason why people who know of such instances, including those who provide expert testimony in courts, assume that such events are the usual cause of cerebral palsy. Piattelli-Palmarini (1991), of the Massachusetts Institute of Technology Center for Cognitive Science, has pointed out that such an emotional association leads to 'overconfident overgeneralization', a strong although irrational feeling of certainty about the connection of events that are not necessarily related according to other evidence. Piattelli-Palmarini comments, 'This should alarm us vastly more than it does'. It should alarm us especially when we base action upon such a fallible foundation, as when an expert witness uses such impressions rather than valid evidence.

Electronic fetal monitoring has been basis for legal judgments in a substantial majority of suits against obstetricians for neurologic injury of the fetus. Yet, as currently performed and interpreted, it has not been shown to predict long-term neurologic outcome. Courts have learned to examine the scientific validity of some kinds of scientific evidence, such as lie detector testing and DNA fingerprinting. It is curious that this logic has not been applied to fetal monitoring evidence.

The medico-legal climate in the USA (Chalmers 1986; Black 1988), and perhaps elsewhere has probably increased the pressure for more interventions, since litigation is much more likely to punish obstetric inaction than action. Few suits are brought for unnecessary cesarean sections, yet a high rate of cesarean sections and other interventions poses risks to mothers and babies and increases costs.

Solutions

1. Let us do better at preventing what we know how to prevent. Rubella causes some cases of cerebral palsy and can be controlled by effective programs of immunization. Yet, in some areas at least, programs are not as effective as they should be (Lee *et al.* 1992). Use of cocaine can cause of abruption of the placenta, preterm birth, and birth asphyxia.

2. Let us learn what we need to know to do better. The explosion of information in developmental neurobiology will have great relevance to understanding the causes of congenital neurologic impairment and some of it will have practical implications. For example, among therapies being considered for birth asphyxia are medications that may pose threats to the plasticity of the fetal and neonatal nervous system and the effects of agents used in this period will not be fully predictable from animal experimentation. Consultation across disciplinary lines will be required in an effort to anticipate problems. Randomized trials will be of the greatest importance in judging the balance between real risks and benefits once new agents are introduced into clinical use. As Chalmers (1986) has stressed, if we are to have innovation and progress, the choice is not between experimentation and non-experimentation, but between controlled and uncontrolled experimentation.

But there are, as already acknowledged, serious problems with using the rate of cerebral palsy as an outcome measure for studies. What surrogate measures are feasible? Candidates could be cited and validation studies are needed. Clearly it is not adequate to use intermediate ranges of pH or Apgar scores as outcome measures by which to evaluate interventions, as continues in the current literature.

New research, basic and clinical, will expand information on causes of cerebral palsy and suggest new strategies for prevention. The development and application of this information will require bidirectional communication between neuroscientistists and obstetric and perinatal clinicians.

3. Let us find ways to stop doing what is not helpful. In both developed and developing nations, it has often been assumed that, even in the absence of specific indications, cesarean sections result in better neurologic health for the infant. This assumption, not supported by available evidence, leads to additional expenses and risks but produces no known benefits, and uses resources that could better be deployed in other ways.

4. Let us seek a more rational approach to resolution of medico-legal disputes. In the USA, the threat of legal action against birth attendants in cases of poor neurologic outcome in the infant has influenced thought and driven many obstetric decisions. Of the many aspects of this topic that need public discussion, I raise only one: the quality of the evidence upon which legal decisions are based (Black 1988; Neufeld and Colman 1990).

Just as there are standards of evidence in the law, so there are standards of evidence in science. Epidemiology provides an approach to the orderly and objective evaluation of the quality of many kinds of biomedical evidence. This type of evaluation could be made available to the courts on a systematic basis. Dialogue between the medical and legal professions about the feasibility of objective assessment of biomedical evidence and evidentiary standards and admissability, could have wide application to obstetric brain injury cases and to other problems at the interface between medicine and the law as well.

I urge the establishment of a working group on medical evidence and the law.

Summary

Obstetric care in industrialized societies is now good in most hands, as measured by low rates of maternal mortality and morbidity, of birth injuries to mother and child, of survival of tiny infants, and of perinatal mortality and eventual neurologic morbidity in large babies. The obligation is great not to worsen care by the introduction of unproven interventions that, despite our best intentions, may not benefit the health of women and babies. Among the challenges that face us in the next medical, social, and legal decisions relating to obstetrics and neurologic outcome are such questions as: what constitutes appropriate testing for diagnostic and therapeutic interventions and how can it be assured? Are there risks too small or with predisposing factors and trade-offs too poorly understood, to justify generally applied efforts to avoid them? And can existing approaches to evaluation of the scientific quality of evidence contribute to the fair and rational resolution of medico-legal disputes concerning obstetrics and the neurologically impaired child?

Epilogue: medicolegal aspects: a British perspective

by Sir Donald Acheson (Adapted from the William Power Lecture of December 1990, published in *Midwives Chronicle and Nursing Notes*, June 1991)

In the UK, there has been a rapid, well-recognized upward trend in litigation for negligence in connection with the management of labor in women who give birth to babies with cerebral palsy. From 50 cases a year in 1983 and 1984, the number of cases filed against members of the Medical Defence Union in 1989 had risen by slightly more than 200 per cent to 157. As the Medical Defence Union insures about two-thirds of all the doctors practicing obstetrics in England, it is reasonable to estimate that the total number of cases brought in 1989 was on the order of 200. The recent change in the rules for legal aid, which bases the assessment not on the income of the parents but the disabled child, will mean that the figure for 1990 and for subsequent years is likely to be much higher.

According to one firm of solicitors which specializes in medical litigation (Capstick and Edwards 1990), twice as many cases were filed in 1990 as was the average in previous years. But in addition to the remarkable upward trend in the number of cases, there has also been a substantial increase in the sums of money awarded by the courts in these cases. At present, the average settlement is £700 000, which is almost three times as much as 7 years ago (*British Medical Journal* 1990). Awards exceeding £1000 000 are now being made and these figures do not include the legal costs. If we remember that there are slightly fewer than 200 District Health Authorities within the National Health Service, it must be clear that if the costs in this area of litigation continue to increase, they will soon become unaffordable.

Another disturbing feature of claims made for cerebral palsy is that of 713 cases filed between 1983 and 1989, only 514 (72 per cent) were commenced within 5 years of birth. A substantial number of the cases did not begin until after a considerably greater interval: no fewer than 105 cases (15 per cent) were commenced after the elapse of 10 or more years and of these, 13 were commenced more than 20 years after the birth. This suggests that not only are more cases being brought each year, more are also being brought many years after the event. Of the 13 cases brought 20 years after birth, eight were brought in 1989.

How likely are the facts concerning a delivery which took place 20 years ago (or even 10 years ago) to be elicited correctly? How likely is it that anyone who gives evidence today will be able to speak authoritatively about the climate of opinion and the practices regarded as acceptable at the time of such a birth? What is likely to be the effect on the decisions obstetricians make during a delivery if they are aware they may be sued for negligence up to 21 years after the event? How will these issues affect the career choices of young doctors considering obstetrics as a career?

Almost 30 per cent of all the costs and damages paid for the whole of the medical profession between 1985 and 1988 were in respect of actions against obstetricians and gynecologists (Medical Protection Society 1988), who represent only a tiny fraction of all medical practitioners. Of a total of some 60 000 medical practitioners, only about 1 500 (2.5 per cent) are engaged in obstetrics and this figure includes both fully trained and trainee obstetricians.

It is often said that what is happening in the USA now will happen in the UK in 5 years' time. If this is true, it is of concern that not only are claims for negligence against obstetricians in respect of cerebral palsy even more frequent there than in Britain, but it is also evident that the situation is having serious consequences for obstetric practice and for accessibility to women of skilled help during pregnancy and labour. According to a survey in 1987 (American College of Obstetricians and Gynecologists 1988), 71 per cent of their members had been sued for negligence at least once and 26 per cent had experienced three or more claims. No fewer than 69 per cent of those surveyed indicated that the fear of litigation had affected the way they conducted their clinical practice. Twenty-seven per cent had reduced the number of high-risk cases in their practices, 13 per cent had reduced the number of deliveries they conducted, and 12 per cent no longer practiced obstetrics at all. Surveys also show that a similar trend away from obstetrics among family practitioners in the USA, who undertake many deliveries as part of their general practice.

There are other indications of the unfortunate influence of litigation on obstetric practice in the USA. For example, in Georgia in 1987, there were 70 countries without a practising obstetrician. In Michigan, two-thirds of the obstetricians asked said that litigation was their most serious professional problem and, in California, two-thirds of the obstetricians said that the fear of litigation was causing them to do more cesarean sections. According to the United States Public Health Service, a particular area of concern is the reduced availability of obstetric care in rural areas. One study found the number of obstetric providers in non-metropolitan areas to have fallen by 20 per cent in the past 5 years.

According to a recent report by the US National Institute of Medicine (1988), the impact of these changes falls disproportionately on poorer women amongst whom, of course, unfavorable risks of pregnancy and delivery are more common. The Institute of Medicine notes that there are particular shortages of obstetricians in areas of high need, particularly in inner-city and some rural areas.

Thanks to the British Perinatal Mortality Survey of 1958 and the British Birth Survey of 1970, it is possible to make fairly precise comparisons between various indicators of labor and the perinatal care of mothers and babies during those 2 years (Peters *et al*. 1983). Between 1958 and 1970, the proportion of women who had labors lasting more than 24 h fell from 8 to 4 per cent and the proportion in whom the second stage of labor was in excess of 1 hour declined from 21 to 12 per cent. Perinatal deaths ascribed to damage to the brain during delivery fell from three per 1000 in 1958 to 0.4 per 1000 (a reduction by a factor of nearly eight) in 1970 (Northern Regional Health Authority 1984) and brain damage during delivery is now a very rare cause of perinatal death.

During the same period, electronic fetal monitoring came into general use. The rate of cesarean delivery increased, as did induction of labor. In terms not only of accepted indicators but also of the actual outcome the safety of both mother and baby during delivery steadily improved. These improvements have continued up to the present time. Yet it is a curious, sad, and chastening fact that in spite of all the improvements and attention to care of mother and baby, the prevalence of cerebral palsy today (about one case in 400 births, or 1500 cases each year) is unchanged from when the first reliable measurements were made 30 years ago. Close scrutiny of the data shows that in children of normal birth weight the rate is unchanged or has risen; in children of low birth weight, it has risen (Jarvis *et al*. 1985; Pharoah *et al*. 1987*a*,*b*; Dowding and Barry 1988; Stanley and Watson 1988; Hagberg *et al*. 1989; Pharoah *et al*. 1990).

It seems likely that in the great majority of cases, cerebral palsy has nothing to do with decisions made by the obstetrician concerning the care of the patient during the passage of the baby through the birth canal. As far as the scientific evidence is concerned, it is clear that perhaps as few as 10 per cent of cases of cerebral palsy are due to asphyxia during delivery and that in an even smaller proprotion could actions of commission or omission by the attendant have altered the outcome. Under these circumstances, the balance of probabilities must start in favor of the obstetrician and against the plaintiff. It also follows that, in future, cases where negligence is proved should be distinctly uncommon and should represent only a small fraction of the number being brought forward at present.

Yet the number and cost of such cases brought for negligence is rising steeply and we can expect a further escalation not only in respect of future cases of cerebral palsy but from the backlog of cases from 10, 20, and more years ago. We can also expect further increases in the damages awarded. But if a substantial proportion of the 1500 babies each year born with cerebral palsy are to be the subject of litigation—and why not, if the State pays the costs and the possible result is a large capital sum paid in one installment whether the child subsequently survives or not?—then the introduction of crown indemnity (which came into force in 1990 to meet the breakdown of our medical insurance system) will prove to have been only a temporary solution, because the State will be facing a contingent liability in relation to this disability of hundreds of millions of pounds.

One of the wider implications of large court awards for cerebral palsy is that the parents of a small proportion of the children with this disability receive a large sum of compensation when the great majority get no compensation. There is also the curious fact that in no case of personal injury, whether there is an issue of medical negligence or not, is the Court permitted to take account when determining the reasonableness of expenses the possibility of avoiding them by taking advantage of the National Health Service. In other words, of two children with identical disabilities, in the case where negligence is proven full 24 h care is provided on a private basis at home as if the NHS did not exist, while the other case depends exclusively on the NHS and social services. There is also the issue of whether structured settlements (that is, settlements where compensation is paid for a period of years and reviewed according to need) are more sensible than the payment of a once and for all capital sum as is currently the practice. Finally, there is the issue of the very extended time limits within which a claim can be made on behalf of a child who has been injured. I have already indicated the inherent improbability of reaching a valid judgment concerning events which occurred 20 years earlier. For the physically handicapped child, the current law permits claims up to the age of 21—in other words, 3 years after majority. When mental handicap is of such a degree that majority is never attained, a claim can be brought later—at any time during the life of such a disabled person.

Cerebral palsy also raises large issues of social justice and radical law reform. Some of the most important and difficult legal questions of our time include those regarding systems of arbitration and compensation by 'no-fault' schemes. In the USA, the State of Virginia recently introduced no-fault compensation to deal with the problem of cerebral palsy where causality can be proved. Under an Act which became law in 1988 (Code of Virginia 1987), compensation for medical and support services is offered up to the age of 18, with recompense after that date for loss of earnings. The cost of the system is met jointly by the State, the profession, and the hospitals. The system does not allow single lump-sum payments. As in the case of other no-fault schemes, it is limited to medical accidents where causality has been proved—which is rarely possible with cerebral palsy.

But because the great majority of cases of cerebral palsy have nothing to do with events during the passage of the baby through the birth canal, the introduction of a no-fault compensation scheme (whether for all medical accidents or, as in Virginia, a limited scheme for cerebral palsy only) would not be helpful. As the UK charity Spastics Society (1992) pointed out in a recent discussion paper, by providing support only for the very small number of cases where causality could be proved, the scheme would discriminate unfairly against the vast majority with similar needs who were ineligible. The Spastics Society is therefore continuing its campaign for a comprehensive disability income scheme for all disabled children regardless of cause.

Following a debate in the House of Commons on a motion on no-fault compensation, the Government published a consultation paper which proposed a number of measures to streamline medical litigation. Prime among these was the suggestion that with the agreement of both parties, cases brought for negligence under the tort system could be dealt with by an arbitrator (a lawyer) aided by two medical experts on the basis of the records alone. This would not only speed the process but remove the adversarial element which consumes so much time and energy.

The upward trend of litigation for cases of cerebral palsy is both unjustifiable in the face of present evidence, and unacceptable in terms of its potential consequences to the quality of the care available to pregnant women. If the small number of cases of negligence are to be identified correctly, it will be essential to ensure that up-to-date arguments about causation are brought to bear at all stages of the litigation. If not and if the current trend continues unstemmed and unreversed, there is not the slightest doubt that the same baleful consequences to the care of women in pregnancy and labor will occur in the UK as have already happened in the USA.

It is clear that the current slow, costly, and chancy system is under severe and increasing strain on both sides of the Atlantic and that change of one sort or another ought urgently to be considered.

As for research into this tragic affliction, the time is overdue for the emphasis to move from labor itself to events in the uterus before labor begins which determine whether damage to the fetal brain occurs.

For the future, it is to be hoped that new techniques such as infrared spectroscopy and magnetic resonance imaging will make it easier to determine with certainty whether cerebral palsy has resulted from a period of hypoxia (whether preventable or not). In the mean time, causality should not be accepted by the courts unless there is clear evidence of neonatal encephalopathy in the first 2–3 days of life. If not, many cases will continue to be decided incorrectly and inequitably, the morale of obstetricians will continue to fall to the detriment of their standards of care, and tens of millions of pounds will be diverted from health care to the compensation of a few cases of cerebral palsy on evidence that is usually fallacious.

References

Acheson, D. (1991). Are obstetrics and midwifery doomed? *Journal of the Royal Society of Medicine*, **64**, 158–66.

Alexander, G. R., Weiss, J., Hulsey, T. C., and Papiernik, E. (1991). Preterm birth prevention: an evaluation of programs in the United States. *Birth* **18**, 160–9.

Benda, G. I., Hiller, J. L., and Reynolds, J. W. (1986). Benzyl alcohol toxicity: impact on neurologic handicaps among surviving very low birthweight infants. *Pediatrics*, **77**, 507–12.

Black, B. (1988). Evolving legal standards for the admissibility of scientific evidence. *Science*, **239**, 1508–12.

Blair, E. and Stanley, C. J. (1988). Intrapartum asphyxia: a rare cause of cerebral palsy. *Journal of Pediatrics*, **112**, 515–9.

Brenneman, D. E., Schultzberg, M., Bartfai, T., and Gozes, I. (1992). Cytokine regulation of neuronal survival. *Journal of Neurochemistry*, **58**, 454–60.

California Birth Defects Monitoring Program (1992). *The cost of birth defects*. CBDMP,

Chalmers, I. (1986). Minimizing harm and maximizing benefit during innovation in health care: controlled or uncontrolled experimentation? *Birth*, **13**, 155–64.

Chanoine, I. P., Boulvain, M., Bourdoux, P., Pardou, A., van Thi, H. V., Ermans, A. M., *et al.* (1988). Increased recall rate at screening for congenital hypothyroidism in breast fed infants born to iodine overloaded mothers. *Archives of Diseases of Childhood*, **63**, 1207–10.

Cummins, S. K., Nelson, K. S., Grether, I. K., and Velie, E. M. Cerebral palsy in four northern California counties, births 1983 through 1985, (in press).

Dennis, J., Johnson, M. A., Mutch, L. M. M., Yudkin, P. Johnson, P. *et al.* (1989). Acid–base status at birth in term infants and outcome at 4.5 years. *American Journal of Obstetrics and Gynecology*, **161**, 213–20.

Ellenberg, J. H. and Nelson, K. B. (1988). Cluster of perinatal events identifying infants at high risk for death or disability. *International Pediatrics*, **113**, 546–52.

Emond, A., Golding, J., and Peckham, C. (1989). Cerebral palsy in two national cohort studies. *Archives of Diseases of Childhood*, **64**, 848–52.

Evans, P. M., Evans, S. J. W., and Alberman, E. (1990). Cerebral palsy: why we must plan for survival. *Archives of Diseases of Childhood*, **65**, 1329–33.

Eyman, R. K., Grossman, H. I., Chaney, R. H., and Call, T. L. (1990). The life expectancy of profoundly handicapped people with mental retardation. *New England Journal of Medicine*, **323**, 584.

Faust, D., and Ziskin, J. (1988). The expert witness in psychology and psychiatry. *Science*, **239**, 31–5.

Fenichel, G. M., Lane, D. A., Livengood, J. R. Horwtz, S. J., Merkes, J. H., Schwartz, J. F. (1989). Adverse events following immunization: assessing probability of causation. *Pediatric Neurology*, **5**, 287–90.

Freud, S. (1968). *Infantile Cerebral Paralysis*, University of Miami Press, Coral Gables.

Gibbs, R. S., Romero, R., Hillier, S. L., Eschenbach, D. A., and Sweet, R. L. (1992). A review of premature birth and subclinical infection. *American Journal of Obstetrics and Gynaecology*, **166**, 1515–28.

Goldaber, K. G., Gilstrap, L. E., III, Leveno, K. I., Dax, J. S., and McIntire, D. D. (1991). Pathologic fetal acidemia. *Obstetrics and Gynecology*, **78**, 1103–7.

Grant, A., O'Brien, N., Joy, M. T., Hennessy, E., and MacDonald, D. (1989). Cerebral palsy among children born during the Dublin randomised trial of intrapartum monitoring. *Lancet*, **ii**, 1233–6.

Grether, J. K., Cummins, S. K., and Nelson, K. B. (1992). The California Cerebral Palsy Project. *Paediatric and Perinatal Epidemiology*, **6**, 339–51.

Keith, L. G., Papiernik, E., and Luke, B. (1991). The costs of multiple Pregnancy. *International Journal of Gynecology and Obstetrics*, **36**, 109–14.

Lancet (1989). Cerebral palsy, intrapartum care, and a shot in the foot. *Lancet*, **ii**, 1251–2.

Landy, H. I., Weiner, S., Corson, S. L., Batzer, F. R., and Bolognese, R. I. (1986). The 'vanishing twin': ultrasonographic assessment of fetal disappearance in the first trimester. *American Journal of Obstetrics Gynecology*, **155**, 14–19.

Langendoerfer, S., Haverkamp, A. D., Murphy, I., *et al.* (1980). Pediatric follow-up of a randomized controlled trial of intrapartum fetal moniting techniques. *Journal of Pediatrics*, **97**, 103–7 (1980).

Lee, S. H., Ewert, D. P., Frederick, P. D., and Mascola, L. (1992). Resurgence of congenital rubella syndrome in the 1990s. *Journal of the American Medical Association*, **267**, 2616–20.

Little, W. J. (1861). On the influence of abnormal parturition, difficult labour, premature birth, and asphyxia neonatorum on the mental and physical condition of the child, especially in relation to deformities. *Lancet*, **ii**, 378–9.

Meyer, B. A., Dickinson, I. E, Chambers, C., and Parisi, V. M. (1992). The effect of fetal sepsis on umbilical cord blood gases. *American Journal of Obstetrics and Gynecology*, **166**, 612–7.

Mutch, L., Alberman, A., Hagberg, B., Kodama, K., and Perat, M. L. (1992). Cerebral palsy epidemiology: where are we now and where are we going? *Developmental and Medical Child Neurology*, **34**, 547–55.

Nelson, K. S. (1989). Perspective on the role of perinatal asphyxia in neurologic outcome. *Canadian Medical Association Journal*, Suppl, 3–10.

Nelson, K. B. and Ellenberg, J. H. (1981). Apgar scores as predictors of chronic neurologic disability. *Pediatrics*, **68**, 36–44.

Nelson, K. B. and Ellenberg, J. H. (1985*a*). Antecedents of cerebral palsy: univariate analysis of risks. *American Journal of Diseases of Childhood*, **139**, 1031–8.

Nelson, K. B. and Ellenberg, J. H. (1985*b*). Predictors of low and very low birthweight and the relation of these to cerebral palsy. *Journal of the American Medical Association*, **254**, 1473–9.

Nelson, K. B. and Ellenberg, J. H. (1986). Antecedents of cerebral palsy: multivariate analysis of risk. *New England Journal of Medicine*, **315**, 81–6.

Nelson, K. B. and Leviton, A. (1991). How much of neonatal encephalopathy is due to birth asphyxia? *American Journal of Diseases of Childhood*, **145**, 1325–31.

Neufeld, P. J. and Colman, N. (1990). When science takes the witness stand. *Scientific American*, **262**, 46–53.

Newton, E. R., Prihoda, T. J., Gibbs, R. S. (1989). Logistic regression analysis of risk factors for intra-amniotic infection. *Obstetrics and Gynecology*, **73**, 571–5.

Paludetto, R. (1991). Neonatal complications specific to twin (multiple) births (twin transfusion syndrome, intrauterine death of cotwin). *Journal of Perinatal Medicine*, **19** (Suppl. 1), 246–51.

Petterson, B., Stanley, F., and Henderson, D. (1990). Cerebral palsy in multiple births in Western Australia: genetic aspects. *American Journal of Medical Genetics*, **37**, 346–351.

Piattelli-Palmarini, M. (1991). Probability blindness. *Bostonia* March–April, pp. 28–35.

Ruth, V. I. and Raivio, K. O. (1988). Perinatal brain damage: predictive value of metabolic acidosis and the Apgar score. *British Medical Journal*, **297**, 24–7.

Romero, R., Mazor, M., Sepulveda, W., Avila, C., Copeland, D., and Williams, I. (1992). Tumor necrosis factor in preterm and term labor. *American Journal of Obstetrics and Gynecology*, **166**, 1576–87.

Rostow, V. P., Osterweis, M., and Bulger, R. J. (1989). Medical professional liability and the delivery of obstetrical care. *New England Journal of Medicine*, **321**, 1057–60.

Seidman, D. S., Paz, I., Laor, A., Gale, R., Stevenson, D. K., and Danon, Y. L. (1991). Apgar scores and cognitive performance at 7 years of age. *Obstetrics and Gynecology*, **77**, 875–8.

Selmaj, K. W. and Raine, C. S. (1988). Tumor necrosis factor mediates myelin and oligodendrocyte damage in vitro. *Annals of Neurology*, **23**, 339–346.

Shy, K. K., Luthy, D. A., Bennett, F. C., *et al.* (1990). Effects of electronic fetal heart rate monitoring, as compared with periodic auscultation, on the neurologic development of premature infants. *New England Journal of Medicine*, **322**, 588–93.

Soper, D. E., Mayhall, C. G., and Dalton, H. P. (1989). Risk factors for intraamniotic infection: a prospective epidemiologicstudy. *American Journal of Obstetrics and Gynecology*, **161**, 562–8.

Stanley, F. I. and Blair, E. (1991). Why have we failed to reduce the frequency of cerebral palsy. *Medical Journal of Australia*, **154**, 623–6.

Steer, P. I. (1991). Premature labour. *Archives of Diseases of Childhood*, **66**, 1167–70.

Steer, P. H., Eigbe, F., Lissauer, T. I., and Beard, R. W. (1989). Interrelationships among abnormal cardiotocograms in labor, meconium staining of the amniotic fluid, arterial cord blood pH, and Apgar scores. *Obstetrics and Gynecology*, **74**, 715–21.

Szymonowicz, W., Preston, H., and Yu, V. Y. H. (1986). The surviving monozygotic twin. *Archives of Diseases of Childhood*, **61**, 454–8.

Torfs, C. P., van den Berg, B. I., Oechsli, F. W., and Cummins, S. (1990). Prenatal and perinatal factors in the etiology of cerebral palsy. *Journal of Pediatrics*, **116**, 615–9.

Truwit, C. L., Barkovich, A. J., Koch, T. K., and Ferriero, D. M. (1992). *American Journal of Neuroradiology*, **13**, 67–78.

References—Sir Donald Acheson

American College of Obstetricians and Gynecologists (1987). *Professional liability and its effects: report of a 1987 survey of ACOG's membership*. ACOG, Washington DC.

British Medical Journal (1990). Obstetric claims boom (leading article). *British Medical Journal*, **301**, 947.

Capstick, B. and Edwards, P. (1990). Trends in obstetric malpractice claims. *Lancet* **336**, 931–2.

Code of Virginia (1987). Ss 65 1–164 to 65 1–179.

Dowding, V. and Barry, C. (1988). Cerebral palsy: changing patterns of birthweight and gestational age (1976–81). *Irish Medical Journal*, **81**, 25–29.

Hagberg, B., Hagberg, G., Olow, I., and von Wendt, L. (1989). The changing panorama of cerebral palsy in Sweden. V: The birth year period 1979–82. *Acta Paediatrica Scandinavica*, **78**, 283–90.

Jarvis, S. N., Holloway, J. S., and Hey, E. N. (1985). Increase in cerebral palsy in normal birthweight babies. *Archives of Diseases of Childhood*, **60**, 1113–21.

Medical Protection Society. (1988). *Medical negligence: addressing the issues: proceedings of the Medical Protection Society Symposium, 13 December 1988*. Medical Protection Society, London.

Northern Regional Health Authority Coordinating Group (1984). Perinatal mortality: a continuing collaborative regional survey. *British Medical Journal*, **288**, 1717–20.

Peters, T. J., Golding, J., Butler, N. R., Fryer, J. G., Lawrence, C. J., and Chamberlain, G. V. P. (1983). Plus ça change: predictors of birthweight in two national studies. *British Journal of Obstetrics and Gynaecology*, **90**, 1040–5.

Pharoah, P. O. D., Cooke, I., Rosenbloom, L. *et al.* (1987*a*). Effects of birthweight, gestational age, and maternal obstetric history on birth prevalence of cerebral palsy. *Archives of Diseases in Childhood*, **62**, 1035–40.

Pharoah, P. O. D., Cooke, T., Cooke, T. W. I., and Rosenbloom, L. (1987*b*). Birthweight specific trends in cerebral palsy. *Archives of Diseases of Childhood*, **62**, 379–89.

Pharoah, P. O. D., Cooke, T., Cooke, T. W. I., and Rosenbloom, L. (1990). Birthweight specific trends in cerebral palsy. *Archives of Diseases of Childhood*, **65**, 602–6.

Spastics Society (1992). *Paying for disability: no fault compensation—panacea or Pandora's Box*. The Spastics Society for People with Cerebral Palsy, London.

Stanley, F. J., and Watson, L. (1988). The cerebral palsies in Western Australia: trends, 1968–1981. *American Journal of Obstetrics and Gynecology*, **158**, 89–93.

US National Institute of Medicine (1988). *Medical Professional Liability and the Delivery of Obstetrical Care*, Vol. 1. Institute of Medicine National Academy Press, Washington DC.

25 Neonatal intensive care

Shoo K. Lee

Introduction

In many ways, neonatal intensive care represents the epitome of modern medicine. It practices at the leading edge of technology and medical knowledge and challenges the limits of viability of life itself. Through the regionalization of perinatal care, it revolutionized the health service delivery system and incorporated concepts of preventive medicine. And by establishing neonatal care as a discipline, it trained a new generation of health care providers and inspired medical research to reach new heights.

Indeed, the results have been remarkable. Since 1950, the neonatal mortality rate in the USA has dropped from 20.5 per 1000 live births to 7.5 per 1000 live births in 1985 (Wegman 1992). In other industrialized countries, the results are even more impressive. In Japan and Sweden in 1979, the neonatal mortality rates were 5.2 per 1000 and 5.3 per 1000 live births, respectively (WHO 1981). Even more remarkably, the limit of viability, considered by many authorities to be about 3 lb (about 1350 g) in the 1940s, has now been reduced to less than 1 lb (about 450g).

Yet, today, despite its many achievements, neonatal intensive care today is increasingly criticized by some as being a wasteful use of scarce health resources. Is this really true? What are the policy issues in neonatal intensive care? And what lies ahead? In this chapter, I will examine these issues by looking at the development and results of neonatal intensive care, its consequences, costs and implications, and its future.

Development of neonatal intensive care

Even in the nineteenth century, physicians realized that premature babies required different care than term babies. Indeed, interest in these babies led Heinrich Finkelstein and others to establish the early special programs for their care towards the end of the century (Taeusch *et al.* 1991), and to pay particular attention to the problems of feeding and temperature control. However, it was not until after the Second World War that significant gains were made in lowering the neonatal mortality rate. This was made possible largely through advances in technology and medical knowledge, regionalization of perinatal care, and the training of skilled health personnel.

The role of technology and medical knowledge

In few other areas of medicine has technology, combined with medical knowledge, been so instrumental in improving patients' outlook as in neonatal intensive care. At first, the technology consisted of relatively simple measures like heating cribs with hot water bottles, aseptic techniques, and using feeding tubes in babies who were unable to suck and swallow. Gradually, this gave way to more sophisticated equipment. Enclosed boxes replaced cribs, electrical heating was used, humidity was controlled, and thermostats regulated temperatures more effectively. By the 1960s, incubators began to resemble their modern counterparts.

The use of oxygen was soon followed by yet another milestone—the mechanical ventilator—and with it came improved methods of regulating the pressure, volume, and composition of gases being administered to babies unable to breathe on their own. More recently, high frequency ventilation and extra-corporeal membrane oxygenation have made it possible to treat an even wider range of respiratory disorders. In the 1970s, miniaturization of monitoring and measuring methods enabled accurate monitoring of babies without excessive blood loss, and improved material technology enabled catheters and instruments to be made small enough for use in very tiny babies. Imaging technology such as ultrasound, computerized axial tomography scanning and magnetic resonance imaging dramatically improved diagnostic abilities, and parenteral nutrition permitted babies to be adequately sustained without the limitations of oral feeding.

By the 1980s, research into cellular and molecular biology yielded artificial surfactant made by genetic engineering to treat lung disease of premature babies (hyaline membrane disease), one of the most important factors determining their survival. The result was a significant reduction in mortality and virtually all related morbidity, including air leaks in the lungs, intraventricular hemorrhages in the brain, and chronic lung disease (broncho-pulmonary dysplasia). The prophylactic use of glucocorticoids prenatally further improved the survival of premature babies, by reducing the incidence and severity of hyaline membrane disease and chronic lung disease, patent ductus arteriosus (a cardiac condition which can result in heart failure), necrotizing enterocolitis (severe illness of the intestines, often with infection), and intraventricular hemorrhage in the brain.

Thus, neonatal intensive care is very technology intensive. Indeed, milestones in neonatal intensive care can be measured by advances in technology and that pattern appears likely to be repeated in the future.

Organization and regionalization of perinatal care

With advances in technology and patient care came the recognition that services needed to be highly organized and available on a regional basis if the best use of resources was to be made (Sunshine 1974). The concept was introduced in the early 1970s and involved a team approach, designed to permit optimal use of both facilities and personnel.

In each region of the USA, six types of facilities—organized in pyramid fashion—provided for maternity patients and their babies. Primary care was provided through physicians' offices and clinics. Community hospitals (level 1 facilities) then cared for maternal and neonatal patients with no complications. Level 2 facilities were located in suburban hospitals and provided care for those with limited complications. Level 3 facilities provided services for a full range of maternal and neonatal complications, with the possible exception of specialized services like complex cardiac surgery. Regional perinatal centers were level 3 facilities charged with the responsibility of coordinating specialized services within each region. The last level consisted of specialized units such as children's hospitals and cardiac centers.

Institutions delivered care up to the limit of their abilities, but since 60–80 per cent of high-risk pregnancies can be detected in advance (Fanaroff and Martin 1992), these patients could be transferred to an institution with the appropriate level of care as close to their homes as possible and at minimum cost to the community. An efficient transport system is therefore essential to the smooth operation of this system. In addition, a public health nursing system provided an added dimension of care through home visits and follow-up programs provided continuing care and surveillance for at-risk babies.

The development of neonatal intensive care units and regionalization programs resulted in a marked decrease in neonatal mortality rates, as well as in the frequency of neurologic sequelae. In Toronto, Canada, for instance, the introduction of a neonatal intensive care unit resulted in a reduction of the neonatal mortality rate by over 50 per cent over a 10 year period (Ontario Perinatal Mortality study 1967, Segal 1972). Another study estimated that the effect of total access to neonatal intensive care in Nova Scotia, Canada, produced a saving of C$370 000 per year of survival, per annual birth cohort (Fuchs and Stubblefield 1972).

Manpower and training

As neonatal units were established, skilled personnel were required to staff them. Neonatal–perinatal medicine was recognized as a specialty and programs were developed to train not only neonatologists, but also neonatal nurses and nurse practitioners, respiratory therapists, technicians, and developmental therapists. Quality assurance guidelines were introduced by organizations such as the Joint Commission on Accreditation of Hospitals in the USA, and some states formed regulatory bodies to control the supply and distribution of neonatal facilities and manpower.

It is clear then that neonatal intensive care units, together with their supporting organizations, have significantly contributed to reducing the neonatal mortality rate in many developed countries. In less-developed countries, however, lack of resources often means that neonatal care is limited and consequently, neonatal mortality rates may be much higher. It is sobering to note that poor countries with infant mortality rates greater than 15 per 1000 live births comprise more than 85 per cent of the world's population and more than 90 per cent of the world's babies (Wegman 1992).

The effect of assisted reproductive technologies

In recent years, assisted reproduction techniques, such as fertility drugs and *in vitro* fertilization techniques have gained in popularity. Women impregnated by these methods, however, are more likely to have multiple conceptions and are therefore also at higher risk of delivering premature babies who may require neonatal intensive care. Levene *et al.* (1992) pointed out that there were four times as many higher order multiple births in the UK between 1971 and 1985, as between 1956 and 1970, largely as a result of the use of fertility drugs. Further, in the UK in 1989, only 47 per cent of higher order multiple births were conceived naturally. These data indicate that while assisted reproductive technologies are bringing hope to many infertile couples, they may also be contributing to the need for neonatal intensive care. Thus, public policies in support of these technologies must also take account of the need to devote resources to neonatal intensive care and follow-up services.

Adverse consequences of neonatal intensive care

The rise of neonatal intensive care has also been associated with an increasing number of previously uncommon problems. Among the first to appear was retinopathy of prematurity. Attributed largely to excessive exposure of the eyes of premature babies to excessive concentrations of oxygen, this vascular disease of the retina affected 12–54 per cent of premature survivors (Phelps 1981), and could result in a wide range of visual problems, ranging from myopia to blindness. However, through careful oxygen monitoring and early screening, blindness has largely disappeared among babies over 1500 g and now affects only 1.8–4 per cent of those under 1500 g (Phelps 1981).

Broncho-pulmonary dysplasia is a chronic disease of the lung occurring in babies with respiratory distress who require prolonged assisted ventilation, with consequent barotrauma. If often leads to oxygen dependency in later life and in the early months of life can cause many respiratory difficulties that may last for months. Babies suffering from this condition require prolonged hospitalization, have poor growth, and are especially susceptible to respiratory infections. In addition, their families may have to cope with managing oxygen therapy at home. Fortunately, the incidence of broncho-pulmonary dysplasia has been dramatically reduced by the advent of prophylactic use of steroids by the mother before birth, surfactant replacement therapy in the first few days after birth, and less damaging modes of assisted ventilation such as high-frequency ventilation.

Premature babies are at particular risk of intraventricular hemorrhage in the brain. Depending on the severity of hemorrhage and on whether hydrocephalus (fluid accumulation in the ventricles in the brain) and periventricular leukomalacia (cystic degeneration of the brain) subsequently develop, these babies are at risk of long-term neurologic sequelae, ranging from behavioral difficulties to developmental delay and cerebral palsy. It is estimated that approximately 20 per cent of babies born under 1000 g suffer a major disability (Yu *et al.* 1986). In addition, small premature babies may develop minor problems such as learning difficulties and clumsiness.

Apart from these major problems, babies requiring neonatal intensive care may suffer other afflictions. Many have residual scars resulting from procedures required for blood sampling, intravenous infusions, and chest tube insertions, and some may require plastic surgery. Hearing difficulties may result from prolonged intubation and antibiotic administration, infections and thromboses may occur at catheter sites, and colostomies may be necessary when bowel is resected in intestinal infections (necrotizing enterocolitis).

Thus, while neonatal intensive care has resulted in the survival of many babies, it has also resulted in significant short- and long-term morbidity, with substantial financial and emotional costs to the families of these babies, as well as to society.

Costs of neonatal intensive care

Today, there is an increasing awareness that since resources are limited, any therapy must be measured both by its benefits and its costs. These costs are both financial and emotional and affect not only the individual, but also the family, care givers, and society at large.

Financial costs

Neonatal intensive care is particularly expensive because it is not only technology and labor intensive, but also often prolonged. The Office of Technology Assessment (1987) in the USA reports that, in general, babies weighing less than 1000 g at birth spend an average of 45–50 days in hospital before initial discharge and cost US$45 000–$50 000 each. This rises to $150 000 for the very small and sick infant, who may stay 90 days or more in the hospital before initial discharge. In addition to these direct hospital costs, the babies' families often incur out-of-pocket costs arising from loss of work, hospital visits, transportation, and child care costs for siblings.

Costs are also incurred even after initial discharge from hospital. Up to half of these babies may require subsequent hospitalization for various illnesses during the first 3 years of life and many require substantially more ambulatory care than normal term babies. Shankaran *et al.* (1988) estimate that these babies incur between $60 and $1200 monthly in direct medical costs during the first 3 years of life, compared with $22–$26 monthly for normal term babies. In addition, parents incur time costs of caring for these babies. Finally, follow-up programs, early intervention programs, and special education programs also involve extra cost. Raphael *et al.* (1985) estimated that the average annual expenditure per student with special needs was $7026, almost twice that for regular education students.

However, these costs do not take into account the subsequent quality of life of the infant. Neither do they consider the potential economic benefits of the child to society. Using the concept of QALY (quality-adjusted life years), Boyle *et al.* (1983) found that for babies weighing less than 1000 g at birth, neonatal intensive care increased survival rates, but at a cost of C$102 500 per additional survivor, C$9300 per life year gained, and C$22 400 per quality-adjusted life year gained.

Thus, neonatal intensive care is an expensive proposition even for the most wealthy countries and its potential benefits must be weighed against its costs. When considering public policy options, however, these high costs must be considered in the context of the costs of other therapies. Indeed, Chance (1988) pointed out that while neonatal intensive care is expensive, it compares favorably with many other accepted therapies like hemodialysis, coronary artery bypass surgery, and even screening for hypertension in 40 year old men.

Non-financial costs

Neonatal intensive care results in other less commonly considered, but no less important costs. These include the suffering of the infant, the emotional and mental strain endured by the parents, the stress on the medical staff caring for the infant, and the financial burden placed on society at large (Murray and Caplan 1985).

Pain and suffering of the infant

The pain and suffering of infants who require prolonged hospitalization, and who often need assisted ventilation and multiple procedures, is frequently overlooked. It is also considered by some that since babies have no subsequent recollection of events in the neonatal intensive care unit, pain and suffering during that time is irrelevant. Yet babies feel pain and must surely suffer as a result. Today, few would challenge this proposition and, in fact, much attention is given to minimizing pain and suffering. For instance, babies are routinely sedated when they are critically ill, analgesics are administered for painful procedures, handling is minimized, and cuddling and bodily contact by both staff and parents is encouraged.

Emotional costs to parents

Perhaps the most emotional distress is suffered by parents. Having a seriously ill infant is totally unexpected for most parents. Apart from the shock of the event and the anxiety and concern for the infant's well-being, parents may also be overwhelmed by feelings of guilt and helplessness. They may feel anger towards the child for causing them distress and dislocation in their lives and marital breakdowns may occur. Bringing home a handicapped child is also extremely stressful and disruptive to family life. Fortunately, most families seem to eventually cope with their situation and families with babies who required neonatal intensive care but were eventually developmentally normal have even reported that the experience resulted in a net positive impact on the family (Lee *et al.* 1991*a*).

Stress on care givers

Neonatal intensive care unit staff also suffer significant stress in caring for babies who are very ill and who sometimes die despite their best efforts. Watching a baby die is probably much more emotionally difficult than watching an old person die and this emotional strain may account for the high turnover rates among nurses. In some units, this turnover rate is as high as 40 per cent. It may also account for the report by Lee *et al.* (1991*b*) that pediatricians and neonatal intensive care unit nurses tended to be unduly pessimistic about neonatal outcomes, and were less likely to advocate active treatment of very low birth weight babies than the parents of these babies.

Burden on society

The survival of a group of handicapped children resulting from improved care of preterm babies requires that society balance their needs with those of other children. Many countries have welfare, health, and educational systems that take these needs into consideration. In this era of cost constraint, however, potential conflicts arise because these children require a redistribution of resources away from normal healthy children. The issue of social priorities and equity, for instance, becomes contentious when parents of healthy children complain that school boards spend too much of their resources on handicapped children, to the detriment of educationally normal children. Thus, the burden on society is not only economic, but also moral, ethical, and social.

The costs of neonatal intensive care are therefore not insignificant, from either a financial or a non-financial viewpoint. This raises many questions about how neonatal intensive care should be employed and leads to many ethical dilemmas.

Ethical dilemmas and medico-legal implications

The ethical dilemmas raised by neonatal intensive care can be broadly classified into the substantive issues (what is right) and the procedural issues (who should decide) (Lee *et al.* 1991*b*) and they reflect many of the issues and conflicts surrounding other areas of medicine.

The most visible and controversial issue concerns the justification for treating babies at high risk of either mortality or subsequent handicap. As may be expected, there are differing views. One view contends that, in addition to being not cost-effective, treating such babies causes the family much unnecessary pain and suffering, particularly if it results in a severely handicapped child requiring long-term care. Some even advocate active euthanasia of such severely ill babies and countries like The Netherlands quietly condone this (Sauer 1992). Opponents point out, however, that it is not possible to predict which babies will have severe handicap and therefore selective treatment is not possible with any degree of accuracy. Some also advocate the sanctity of life and object to the use of quality of life measures to determine treatment.

The issue becomes particularly emotionally charged when parents and care givers disagree on whether active treatment should be provided. In some cases, legal action has resulted. In the USA, the 'Baby Doe' case proceeded to court when the parents refused life-saving treatment for their infant with spina bifida. It initially resulted in the State imposing penalties on care givers who failed to provide treatment to all babies, but this legislation was subsequently rescinded (Murray 1984). Today, the practice varies from country to country. In the USA, the President's Commission for the Study of Ethical Problems in Medicine (1983) advocated a 'best interest' of the child standard and treatment is therefore generally given when the infant is judged to be viable. When viability is in doubt, the wishes of the parents are generally considered paramount in determining treatment decisions. However, much public discussion and debate continues, particularly in this era of concern about costs and quality of life.

The ability to give informed consent to treatment or research practices is another ethical dilemma. Since babies are unable to give informed consent, parents are the usual accepted surrogates. Difficulties arise, however, when parents refuse consent for therapies that care givers feel are definitely in the interest of the child. For instance, members of the Jehovah's Witness sect commonly refuse blood transfusions for their babies. In these cases, the courts generally rule in the infant's favor and mandate the procedure. Alternatively, parents may not wish care givers to provide supportive therapy to a baby, yet those care givers have, in their view, a moral obligation to continue treatment.

Informed consent for clinical trials and dangerous treatments is another difficult area. Since babies are incompetent to give consent, the President's Commission for the Study of Ethical Problems in Medicine and Biomedical and Behavioral Research (1983), recommended that decisions made on such patients' behalf must protect the best interest of the patient and, therefore, limits may be placed on the range of acceptable decisions that surrogates may make. Institutional ethics committees therefore adopt much stricter ethical guidelines for clinical trials and research in babies than in adults.

An even more difficult issue, however, arises in maternal–fetal conflicts. While most people would agree that a pregnant woman has a moral obligation to accept reasonable, non-experimental medical treatment for the sake of her fetus, there is also compelling argument against coercing a pregnant woman to accept medical treatment against her will (Murray 1987). In many instances, a woman may decide to accept or reject such treatment because of personal considerations such as concern for her own health and mental well-being, responsibilities to her other children, husband and other loved ones, and religion. Thus, coercion of a pregnant woman would represent unacceptable social instrusion upon the private life of an individual in most instances. In practice, the woman's wishes are usually respected. In some cases, however, the courts have disagreed, and even ordered cesarean sections against the mother's wishes (Annas 1982).

Finally, society has an ethical responsibility to help provide for babies who survive, but need chronic care. Families of these babies suffer tremendous stress and financial hardships and it would be inconsistent for society to expend scarce health resources to save these babies and then not help provide for their subsequent care.

The future

The challenges that lie ahead for neonatal intensive care, then, are closely interlinked and relate to its many facets—technological, organizational, economic, ethical, or social. In the final analysis, however, they are all medical and human in nature.

Technology and medical knowledge promise even more advances in neonatal care. Already, research into liquid ventilation hints at the possibility of extending the viability of babies below 23 weeks' gestation and fetal surgery may allow treatment of conditions now considered fatal. Near infra-red imaging techniques and positron emission tomography scans promise to extend the visualization of physical structures to visualization of function. Gene therapy may become a reality, opening the door to new frontiers of therapy. Research is therefore of fundamental importance to the continued improvement of neonatal intensive care.

The constraints on whether we can exploit these technological advances are mostly economic. Escalating costs of health care have forced many countries to take drastic measures to contain them. In Canada, health care expenditure is now subject to a predetermined budget. In the USA, health care reform promises to rein in health expenditures. New technologies, therefore, have to be justified not only on medical but also on economic grounds and some will undoubtedly be judged too expensive to use on a large scale. Means of evaluating these technologies, therefore, have to be developed and refined and will gain in importance. It should also be remembered, however, that parental views are equally important. Indeed, Lee *et al.* (1991*b*) found that the overwhelming majority (more than 95 per cent) of parents felt they should be the principal decision makers in treatment decisions.

In addition to the current ethical issues, new technologies and cost considerations will introduce new ethical dilemmas. For instance, gene therapy will raise new questions about how we might ethically employ it. Questions about social equity and justice also arise if these new therapies are too expensive and can only be afforded by the wealthy. Efforts to ration health care as outlined in the Oregon proposal (Klevit *et al.* 1991), necessarily mean that questions about the justification of treating potentially impaired babies will gain in urgency. Thus, the ethical dilemmas are likely to increase rather than decrease and it will be prudent to anticipate the problems and encourage public debate before it becomes necessary to introduce them into the policy arena.

Finally, it is crucial that we continue to seek ways of preventing and treating high-risk pregnancies. A multi disciplinary approach is required since the problem is multi faceted and as much social in origin as it is medical. Thus, while scientists seek to find ways of preventing preterm labor and health services researchers seek to deliver prenatal care in more effective ways, it is necessary too that society find means of reducing teenage pregnancies, improving the health and economic well-being of mothers, and reducing the incidence of substance abuse.

The model of perinatal care might also need re-examination. Perhaps we need to extend the concept of perinatal care to include the preconceptional and interconceptional (between pregnancy) periods, and to include socio-cultural perspectives into its delivery, to improve compliance. Ultimately, neonatal intensive care can claim to be truly successful only when we have removed the need for it, because the only relevant measure of success is the health of the babies.

In conclusion, as neonatal intensive care continues to evolve, it remains fundamentally important that we continue to maintain a humane, caring, and compassionate approach and to remember that care for babies equally involves care and compassion for their families.

References

Annas, G. J. (1982). Forced cesarians: the most unkind cut of all. *Hastings Center Report*, **12**, 16–7.

Boyle, M. H., Torrance, G. W., Sinclair, J. G., and Horwood, S. P. (1983). Economic evaluation of neonatal intensive care of very low birth weight. *New England Journal of Medicine*, **308**, 1330–7.

Chance, G. W. (1988). Neonatal intensive care and cost-effectiveness. *Canadian Medical Association Journal*, **139**, 943–6.

Fanaroff, A. and Martin, R. J. (1992). *Neonatal–perinatal medicine*. Year Book, St Louis.

Fuchs, F., and Stubblefield, P. G. (1984). *Preterm birth: causes, prevention and management*. Macmillan, New York.

Klevit, H. D., Bates, A. C., Castanares, T., *et al.* (1991). Prioritization of health care services: a progress report by the Oregon Health Services Commission. *Archives of Internal Medicine*, **151**, 912–6.

Lee, S. K., Penner, P. L., and Cox, M. (1991*a*). The impact of very low birth weight infants on the family and its relationship to parental attitudes. *Pediatrics*, **88**, 105–9.

Lee, S. K., Penner, P. L., Cox, M. (1991*b*). A comparison of the attitudes of health care professionals and parents towards active treatment of very low birth weight infants. *Pediatrics*, **88**, 110–4.

Levene, M. I., Wild, J., and Steer, P. (1992). Higher multiple births and the modern management of infertility in Britain. *British Journal of Obstetrics and Gynaecology*, **99**, 607–13.

Murray, T. H. (1984). At last, final rules on Baby Doe. *Hastings Center Report*, **14**, 10.

Murray, T. H. (1987). Moral obligations to the not-yet-born: the fetus as patient. *Clinics in Perinatology*, **14**, 329.

Murray, T. H. and Caplan, A. L. (1985). *Which babies shall live*? Humana Press, Clifton.

Office of Technology Assessment (1987). *Neonatal intensive care for low birth weight infants: costs and effectiveness* (Health Technology Case Study 38, OTA-HCS-38). US Congress, Washington DC.

Ontario Perinatal Mortality Study Committee (1967). *Second report of the perinatal mortality study in ten university teaching hospitals in Ontario, Canada*. Ontario Department of Health.

Phelps, D. L. (1981). Retinopathy of prematurity: an estimate of vision loss in the U. S.—1979. *Pediatrics*, **67**, 924–6.

President's Commission for the Study of Ethical Problems in Medicine and Biomedical and Behavioral Research (1983). *Deciding to forgo life-sustaining treatment*. US Government Printing Office, Washington DC.

Raphael, E. S., Singer, J. D., and Walker, D. K. (1985). Per pupil expenditures on special education in three metropolitan school districts. *Journal of Education Finance*, **11**, 69–88.

Sauer, P. J. (1992) Ethical decisions in neonatal intensive care units: the Dutch experience. *Pediatrics*, **90**, 729–32.

Segal, E. S., ed. (1972). *Transport of high risk newborn infants, Toronto*. The Fetus and Newborn Committee of the Canadian Pediatric Society.

Shankaran, S., Cohen, S. N., Linver, and Zonia, S. (1988). Medical care costs of high risk infants after neonatal intensive care: a controlled study. *Pediatrics*, **81**, 372–8.

Sunshine, P. (1974). *Regionalization of perinatal care: report of the sixty-sixth Ross conference on pediatric research*. Laboratories, Columbus.

Taeusch, H. W., Ballard, R. A. and Avery, M. E. (1991). *Shaeffer's and Avery's diseases of the newborn*. W. B. Saunders, Philadelphia.

Yu, V. Y. H., Loke, H. L., Bajuk, B., Szymonowicz, W. Orgill, A. A., and Astbury, J. (1986). Prognosis for infants born 23–28 weeks' gestation. *British Medical Journal*, **293**, 1200.

Wegman, M. E. (1992). Annual summary of vital statistics—1991. *Pediatrics*, **90**, 835–45.

WHO (1981). *World health statistics annual, 1980–81: vital statistics and causes of death*. WHO, Geneva.

VI Obstetrics and Public Policy

26 Human genome project: implications for practicing obstetricians

Benjamin P. Sachs and Bruce Korf

The human genome project is an international effort to discern the complete genetic make-up of human beings. The human genome is estimated to consist of 50 000–100 000 genes encoded in 3 billion base pairs of DNA; these base pairs in turn are packaged into 23 pairs of chromosomes. It is likely that new technologies will be developed while the project is under way, making it difficult to predict how quickly the work will proceed. There is a debate about the best technical methods for mapping and cloning the human genome. It is clear, however, that a coordinated effort is needed to identify at least that subset of the human genome which encodes genes responsible for disease.

It is safe to say that the knowledge gained will revolutionize medicine, because a better understanding of the ways in which genes control the body will make it possible to develop new methods for diagnosis, treatment, and prevention. Genetics is already an important part of clinical practice for the obstetrician. The introduction, approximately 25 years ago, of amniocentesis and more recently of chorionic villus sampling, has provided the tools to screen for a few genetic disorders, the most common being trisomy 21 (Down's syndrome).

But the near future holds the possibility for dramatic advances in genetic research and the introduction of new techniques for prenatal screening. There have been reports of gene therapy in humans and, more recently, fetal gene therapy. However, gene therapy or gene replacement will lag behind our ability to detect genetic disorders and because of this, society will face some very difficult ethical and social challenges. This chapter will focus on these challenges. There is an urgent need for debate in the obstetrical community on the implications of the human genome project. The advances in genetic research and prenatal diagnosis will significantly affect our specialty in a more profound way than many other areas of medicine. During the period when we will be able to screen for increasing numbers of genetic disorders but be unable to offer therapy other than termination of pregnancy, the obstetrician will be under increased pressures.

History

In 1953, James Watson and Francis Crick described the double helix structure of DNA; in 1962, they received a Nobel prize for this work. However, not until the 1970s did development of gene splicing techniques give scientists the ability to understand the structure and function of genes. The concept of a national project to map all 46 chromosomes arose in a meeting held in Alta, Utah in 1984 by the US Department of Energy. The subject of this meeting was how to monitor the health effects of exposure to low doses of radiation and other environmental hazards. As a result of this meeting and the opportunity presented by rapid advances in chromosome mapping and DNA techniques, the National Institutes of Health established the National Center for Human Genome Research on 1 October, 1989. In Europe, the initiative is spearheaded by the Human Genome Organization, founded in 1988.

The first congressional appropriation specifically for this project was in 1988 for $17.2 million. In fiscal year 1991, approximately $87 million was made available. It is estimated now that work on the project in the USA will require $200 million a year for the next 10–15 years. Similar research is being funded by other US agencies, including the Department of Energy. However today the goal of the Genome project is also being met by many individual efforts. In many countries researches funded by industry and Governments are defining genomes. This process is accelerating the initiative both in the US and Europe.

Why the human genome project?

Genetic diseases and congenital malformations occur in approximately 3–5 per cent of all live births. They account for one-third of pediatric admissions to hospitals and between 40–50 per cent of deaths in childhood. Today, the best estimate is that 10 per cent of chronic adult diseases have a genetic component (WHO 1986); however, this is probably a gross underestimate, because almost monthly there are announcements of discoveries of genes associated with specific disorders. Increasingly, the role of genetic factors in common illnesses such as cancer, diabetes, neurophyschiatric disorders, cardiovascular disease, developmental defects, and atherosclerosis is being recognized. In fact, the almost 40 000 recognized genetic defects contribute to some of the most devastating diseases affecting humans. Many of these diseases probably result from the interaction of genes and environmental factors such as food, drugs, and pollutants. Discovery of the responsible genes will permit physicians to study these interactions.

Advances in genetic research will permit the introduction of more efficient screening programs for populations considered to be at risk. For example, today in the USA we recommend that all women over the age of 40 undergo annual mammography. If we can could identify the subset of the population at greatest risk, a more intense screening program could be introduced. Furthermore, if we understood the interaction between genes and the environment, the environmental factors could be manipulated early on. The next step would be to use this genetic knowledge to offer advice and counseling to individuals who are known to be carriers for genetic disorders. Presently, for most autosomal recessive disorders, prenatal testing can only be offered if there is a prior history. Screening for the heterozygous or carrier state could identify couples for whom prenatal diagnosis should be carried out. Such a program is already available for Tay–Sachs disease and is being considered for cystic fibrosis (CF).

One in 25 Caucasians carries a mutant CF gene and most of these do not have a family history of the disorder. The gene for CF has been cloned; approximately 90 per cent of the mutations responsible for the disorder can be detected with molecular testing. This makes it possible to identify approximately 80 per cent of couples at risk of having an affected child and to offer they prenatal diagnosis (Wilfond and Fost 1990). The technical feasibility of population testing has sparked a vigorous debate on the social and ethical implications of population screening. The intensity of the debate surrounding CF screening is merely a harbinger of what we will see in the future. It has been estimated that if a national screening program were introduced, it would cost $2.2 million for each case of cystic fibrosis avoided. Furthermore, with a test sensitivity of 90 per cent, a person with a negative test result may still have an approximately one in 480 chance of being a carrier (Wilfoud and Fost 1990). These and other complex clinical issues will place a tremendous additional burden on existing genetic services. There are approximately 450 certified genetic counselors and 500 clinical geneticists in the USA. Just dealing with the issue of cystic fibrosis counseling, would take approximately 17 weeks per counselor each year. This need could only be met if the number of counselors were increased and if obstetricians became familiar with the issues and counseled their own patients. These issues will have to be resolved if the potential benefits of the new information are to be realized.

Another important benefit of the human genome project will be a better understanding of human embryology. The development of a complete being from a fertilized egg involves the orchestration of a large number of genes that must be turned on or off at the right time and place. The more we understand of these developmental genes, the better our chances of learning to prevent birth defects.

How the project is being conducted

The ability to map the human genome and characterize the genes has evolved from advances in molecular genetics during the past two decades. These advances made it possible to purify segments of the genome corresponding to particular genes and determine their precise structure, both in normal people and in people with genetic diseases. The pace of advances has been accelerating steadily, especially as the effort to map the entire genome has demanded the development of approaches of great efficiency and low cost.

Central to the effort is the ability to splice segments of the human genome to 'vector' DNA, allowing the segments of human DNA to be purified and grown in large quantities and subjected to further study. This cloning process begins with cleavage of human DNA into fragments using an enzyme (called a restriction endonuclease) which recognizes a specific sequence of four to eight DNA bases. The fragments can then be enzymatically ligated to a piece of vector DNA, which is a bacterial plasmid, a virus, or a specially engineered yeast artificial chromosome. These vectors accommodate progressively larger fragments of inserted DNA but have in common the ability to replicate within a bacterial or yeast cell. Each cell incorporates a different recombinant molecule and can be isolated and grown in quantity. Purification of the vector DNA thus results in the isolation of a large quantity of the inserted human DNA.

Through recombinant DNA methodology it is possible to generate 'libraries' of cloned human DNA fragments (genetic libraries). It is also possible to isolate messenger RNA (mRNA) from a cell, copy the mRNA molecules into DNA (cDNA), and clone these cDNA molecules in bacteria. This results in the formation of a cDNA library, in which only genes transcribed in a particular cell type are cloned.

It is relatively easy to determine the base sequence and location in the genome of cloned DNA. A number of sequencing strategies have been developed and automated processes now make it possible to sequence upwards of several thousand base pairs per day in a single laboratory. Mapping technologies include the powerful technique of fluorescence *in situ* hybridization. The cloned DNA is tagged with a fluorescent label, separated into single strands, and allowed to bind to its complement in preparations of human mitotic chromosomes on a glass slide. The site of binding of the cloned DNA can be visualized with a fluorescence microscope and marks the location of the DNA on the chromosome.

More difficult challenges are to determine the function of cloned DNA and to identify the genes responsible for specific diseases. Genes which encode known proteins can be cloned by taking advantage of prior knowledge of the structure or function of the protein. For example, bacterial cells can be made to express the cloned human DNA, and antibodies can be used to detect bacterial colonies which make the product of interest. If a portion of the amino acid sequence of the protein is known, bacterial colonies can be screened for those which contain a segment of DNA which would encode that set of amino acids. In this manner, a large number of genes important in human disorders have been cloned, such as the α and β globin genes (mutations in which are responsible for sickle cell disease and thalassemia) and the hexosaminidase A gene (Tay– Sachs disease). Knowledge of the structure of these genes has shed light on the molecular pathogenesis of the diseases and has provided powerful diagnostic tools which can be applied to any nucleated cell, including those obtained by amniocentesis and chorionic villus biopsy.

The crowning achievement of molecular genetics in the past decade, however, has been the development of an approach to clone genes responsible for diseases where the gene product is unknown. The approach, referred to as positional cloning, is based on first establishing the location of the disease gene in relation to other cloned 'marker' sequences, usually by a process called linkage analysis. The region surrounding these marker sequences is then systematically cloned until the disease gene itself is found. Cloned marker sequences now exist which are located at regular intervals along the human genome, and can be used for linkage analysis. It has been found that there are commonly slight variations in base sequence for most segments of DNA from person to person in the population. These variations are called DNA polymorphisms. If the two copies of a DNA segment in an individual happen to differ in base sequence, this DNA polymorphism can be used to track the transmission of that segment from generation to generation in a family. Genetic linkage between a polymorphic sequence and a disease trait can be established by looking for instances in which the disease consistently tracks with a particular marker allele in a family. If the disease is transmitted independently of the marker allele, then the two are unlinked; if they segregate together, they are linked and must reside near one another on the chromosome.

Progressing from closely linked markers to identification of a gene responsible for a disease involves meeting several criteria. DNA segments which encode functioning genes can be revealed by looking for regions which are conserved through evolution. Functioning genes are usually conserved, whereas non-coding sequences are not. Cloned genes can also be examined for expression in tissues known to be affected by the disease of interest. Final proof of the identity of a disease gene is the demonstration that affected individuals carry mutations in the sequence which disrupt the activity of the gene product.

Although this is a complex process, it may be the only way to define the basis of diseases for which decades of pathophysiological research has not revealed the identity of the abnormal protein. The positional cloning strategy has achieved brilliant success in recent years with the cloning of genes responsible for chronic granulomatous disease, Duchenne muscular dystrophy, cystic fibrosis, retinoblastoma, neurofibromatosis, fragile X syndrome, and myotonic dystrophy. All that is required is the availability of large families and a suitable panel of informative genetic markers. The cloning of these genes makes it possible to provide genetic diagnosis and to study basic disease mechanisms.

As the human genome becomes increasingly well characterized, another approach emerges for identifying genes responsible for disease—candidate gene approach. By this method, cloned genes from individuals with a specific genetic disorder are examined and evidence of mutation is sought. As the library of cloned genes expressed in particular tissues, or involved in specific developmental or physiological functions, increases, the candidate gene approach is likely to result in identification of an increasing number of disease genes. It may be the only way to reveal the basis for some disorders which do not affect many members of large families.

Clinical implications

Usually, the first clinical impact to result from cloning of a gene is improved means of diagnosis. In some cases, disease-causing mutations can be easily detected in a majority of patients. Such testing is highly accurate and usually can be done quickly and inexpensively. Genetic linkage analysis may be used to diagnose disorders which have been mapped by linkage to marker genes but not yet cloned or those in which the diversity of possible mutations is too large for direct DNA analysis to be efficient. Genetic analysis obviates the need to sample affected tissues and enables prenatal diagnosis using fetal cells obtained by chorionic villus biopsy or amniocentesis. Linkage-based testing, however, has the disadvantage of requiring sampling of several family members and is subject to inaccuracy due to genetic recombination or genetic heterogeneity (the existence of multiple loci which may be responsible for a type of genetic disorder).

Currently, genetic diagnosis is most often applied when there is a known disorder affecting some member of a family. As mutations responsible for relatively common disorders become increasingly well characterized, however, population screening for disease susceptibility or risk of transmission of a disorder to offspring is becoming a possibility. Technical advances, such as the polymerase chain reaction (which allows a DNA sequence, such as one which may harbor a mutation, to be rapidly and inexpensively amplified in large quantities), have increased the feasibility of population screening (Rose 1991). The pace of these technical advances threatens to outstrip the ability of society to use the new knowledge intelligently (WHO 1986; Watson 1990).

Controversy surrounding the project

The human genome project has its critics. Controversy surrounds the cost of the program, the question of whether it is necessary to sequence the complete human genome, and lastly, ethical questions. As indicated, it is estimated that the project will cost $200 million per year over the next 10–15 years (Watson 1990). Although there has been some reassurance from the National Institutes of Health and other organizations, it is feared that without significant additional appropriations by Congress these monies will be diverted from other biomedical research programs. Much of the human genome is little understood and may or may not have a function. Many scientists have argued that it would be far more appropriate to focus the endeavor on particular areas of chromosomes and specific diseases rather than on sequencing the complete genome. The advances in technology will markedly facilitate this project. The process is not very intellectually stimulating but because of the available funding laboratories may be forced to concentrate on this area of research. Last, but by no means least, there are some who argue that without first addressing the ethical challenges that would result from advances in genetic research it is inappropriate to perform the research. Some of the criticisms directed at the human genome project are appropriate. However, whether we like it or not, the project has begun and is being carried out in many parts of the world.

Advances in perinatal medicine

In the last few years, we have seen very significant advances in prenatal diagnosis that will permit us to use the products of the human genome research in a way that is almost unimaginable today.

Prenatal diagnosis is currently performed by either amniocentesis or chorionic villus sampling. Recently, sampling of fetal umbilical blood has become more widely used for both prenatal diagnosis and fetal therapy. It has been shown in both veterinary and human medicine that gamete biopsy is a possible technique for very early prenatal diagnosis. In the future, we may be able to isolate fetal cells from the maternal circulation and use them for diagnostic purposes. This would facilitate the offering of prenatal testing to every patient. The combination of universal prenatal testing plus advances in genetic research will create enormous possibilities.

Prenatal diagnosis is a technique which today only permits us the ability to offer the patient a termination of pregnancy. The goal in the future would be to routinely offer gene therapy as an alternative.

Gene therapy or more correctly gene supplementation, has become a reality (Weatherall 1989). In July 1990, the National Institute of Health approved gene therapy to treat children suffering from a rare immune disorder, adenosine deaminase deficiency (ADA). Fewer than 20 people world-wide suffer from this disorder: nevertheless the fact that gene therapy is possible offers great hope. A copy of the gene that produces the missing enzyme is inserted into blood cells isolated from the patient; the modified blood cells are then reintroduced into the child.

Gene therapy at the fetal stage offers many theoretical advantages. In some diseases, by the time the baby is born, the damage caused by the genetic defect is so widespread that gene therapy could not play a role. Examples are lipid storage diseases and Lesch–Nyhan syndrome. In some disorders, such as hemoglobinopathies, bone marrow transplantation has been attempted to correct the disorder. However, the bone marrow recipient must be immune suppressed and there is a risk of graft rejection. For the fetus, neither of these considerations holds. The technique of percutaneous umbilical blood sampling in the second trimester offers the possibility of gene therapy as advances in genetic research permit.

Ethical considerations

The ethical questions raised by the genome project fall into two categories. The first is the question of privacy and the second is the broader implications of prenatal diagnosis and gene therapy.

Recognizing the enormity of the ethical and social questions presented by the genetic research, the US National Institutes of Health and the Department of Energy have established the Ethical, Legal and Social Issues Joint Working Group (ELSI). Currently, 4 per cent of the genome project's budget is allotted to ELSI (Watson 1990).

It is common practice today that someone applying for health or life insurance is required to undergo a complete physical examination in addition to a number of laboratory tests. Sometimes, this may include an assessment of HIV status. Through this process, the insurance companies screen out people who are at risk because of past medical history, family history, social behavior, or positive laboratory tests. One of the primary objectives of the human genome project is to identify individuals who are carriers of genes that put them at risk of serious diseases. If one assumes that our ability to correct the genes will not develop for many decades, then these individuals are also at risk for being rejected for insurance. It could be argued that this fact alone will require a change in the way that health care is paid for and provided.

The first legislative attempt to prevent the creation of a biological underclass was passed in September 1991 by the California state legislature. Bill AB1888 amends the California State Civil Rights Act to add genetic characteristics to the list of traits protected from discrimination by employers. A provision was also added with respect to health insurance (which will remain in effect until 1 January 2000), which prohibits health insurers from either not enrolling or charging higher rates to people carrying disease genes. Similarly, life and disability insurance firms cannot refuse to accept an application on the basis of a person's genetic characteristics. Life insurers are also prohibited from mandating genetic testing. Although many of the genes to be identified may indicate that a person is at risk, he or she will not necessarily develop the disease because many conditions result from the interaction between the environment and the gene. Nancy Wexler, who is the president of the Heredity Disease Foundation and Chair of the ELSI, noted that she would not have been eligible for health or life insurance because her mother had Huntington's chorea. It is hoped that ELSI will recommend model laws that could be enacted by states in order to prevent insurance discrimination.

In 1989, a survey conducted by the Office of Technological Assessment, entitled 'Medical Monitoring and Screening in the Workplace' found that less than 10 per cent of surveyed Fortune 500 companies currently use genetic testing to detect susceptibility to workplace hazards and to assess health insurance risk. However, 36 per cent of health officers surveyed assessed the health insurance risk of job applicants. This information did affect their decision whether to hire an individual. Clearly, genetic information could be used to discriminate against individuals in the area of employment. To address this question, ELSI urged the Equal Employment Opportunities Commission to include language to protect individuals, otherwise healthy, who are at risk based on genetic susceptibility. The EEOC declined, stating, 'The American and Disability Act [which came into effect in 1992] does not protect individuals, who are not otherwise impaired, from discrimination based on genotype alone.'

A major opponent of federally funded genetic research has been Jeremy Rifkin, President of the Foundation on Economic Trends. One of his main concerns is that despite ongoing genetic research, such as the National Institutes of Health pilot project on cystic fibrosis screening, it is unlikely that ELSI will present any recommendations for several years.

A more fundamental and perhaps philosophical question is the one related to genetic diversity of human beings. There is an analogy with advances in genetic research in agriculture and animal husbandry. In the last decade, new superstrains of food products have lead to a 'green revolution'; similar progress has been made in animal husbandry. The result has been that in agriculture there is less genetic diversity than in the past. Many have argued that this leaves our food supply very vulnerable to diseases. Genetic diversity provides some protection from such a threat. It is similarly argued that genetic diversity among humans in some ways protects us against unknown diseases. An expanded role for prenatal diagnosis based on new knowledge of genetic related disorders may result, at least theoretically, in a decrease in genetic diversity of mankind.

Today we offer prenatal diagnosis for such conditions as Down's syndrome Tay–Sachs disease, cystic fibrosis, and other major medical disorders. At this time, abortion is fairly widely available up to approximately 22 weeks' gestation. Today, obstetricians can be confronted by a couple seeking to choose the sex of their child and requesting prenatal diagnosis and selective abortion; the advent of chorionic villus sampling and earlier prenatal diagnosis may have increased this possibility. How are we going to respond in the future to pressures for prenatal diagnosis and possibly the termination of pregnancy for diseases such as diabetes, which are not characterized as being as serious as cystic fibrosis? Or how will we respond to the issue of screening for genes that only increase the risk of an individual's risk of developing cancer or heart disease later in life, but do not mean that the disease will definitely occur? Many of these ethical dilemmas will eventually decrease in importance as the potential for gene therapy increases. However, over the next few decades it is very likely that we will have to face these very difficult questions.

John F. Kennedy once suggested that, 'life on other planets is extinct because scientists were more advanced than ours'. It is our contention that this is an overly pessimistic perspective. We believe that there is an urgent need to include the obstetrical community in the ongoing national discussion. It is through an open debate in our society that we can address the social and ethical implications and at the same time take advantage of the tremendous opportunities presented to us by the human genome project.

Recommendations

In response to the challenges presented to the specialty of obstetrics and gynecology by the human genome project, we make the following recommendations:

1. *Education in genetics and genetic counseling* The story of cystic fibrosis screening and the expected increased requirement for genetic counseling is just the beginning with respect to clinical demands. It is clear that patient needs will not be adequately met by existing professionals in the USA and elsewhere. The obstetrical community is going to have to assume a greater responsibility for counselling patients on genetic issues. This can only be accomplished by increasing the content of genetics in residency training, as well as requiring of practitioners more postgraduate training in this field.

2. *Clinical standards* We urge the American College of Obstetricians and Gynecologists, and similar organizations in other countries, to consider establishing standards and acting as a resource for clinicians, the public, and legislatures.

3. *Legislative agenda* In the USA, the ethical and legal implications of the human genome project are being addressed through the Ethical, Legal and Social Issues Joint Working Group, as well as other organizations. Because so many of the questions deal with obstetrics, we urge ACOG to play a greater role in developing legislation and working with ethicists in the field.

4. *Computer-based interactive video programs* One possible solution to the burden of genetic counseling is the development of computer-based interactive video programs. The use of this type of technology in the field of genetic counseling has not yet been attempted. However, it offers tremendous possibilities, through its ease of use, the ability to add new information as it becomes available, and the opportunity to tailor presentations to specific patients on the basis of information provided by both patients and the clinician.

Conclusions

Some people have reacted very negatively to the human genome project. Muller-Hill in 1988 said, 'We should remember that it was scientists in pre-war Germany, the psychiatrists, geneticists, and anthropologists, just as much as the politicians who established the concepts and principals that came to represent the racial underpinning of the Nazi extermination programs.' Such thoughts are lurking in the background. In our opinion, the benefits to mankind offered by scientific advances in genetics far outweigh the possible social and ethical ills. This can only be true, though, if we work as a society together to ensure that the individual is safeguarded. It has been said that a more appropriate approach would be restructuring our social and political institutions to ensure that they do not have the opportunity to use the genetic information as a tool for injustice and inequity.

The human genome project is an inevitability. The obstetrical community needs to play a more active role in discussing and finding solutions to many of the problems it presents.

References

Rose, E. A. (1991). Applications of the polymerase chain reaction to genome analysis. *FASEB J*, **5**, 46–54.

Watson, J. D. (1990). The human genome project: past, present, and future. *Science*, **248**, 44–9.

Watson, J. D. and Crick, F. H. C. (1953). Molecular structure of mucleic acids: a structure for deoxyribose nucleic acid. *Nature*, **171**, 737–8.

Weatherall, D. J. (1989). Gene therapy. *British Medical Journal*, **298**, 691–2.

Wilfond, B. S. and Fost, N. (1990). The cystic fibrosis gene: medical and social implications for heterozygote detection. *Journal of the American Medical Association*, **263**, 2777–83.

World Health Organization (1986). Prevention of avoidable mutational disease. *Bulletin of the WHO*, **64**, 205–16.

27 Professional liability and the practice of obstetrics

Alan Pinshaw and Howard Hiatt

Overview

The first American medical malpractice suit was filed in Connecticut in 1794 (Stetler 1957) Even then, the issue of medical professional liability was not new, having had its humble beginnings in England over 400 earlier (Stetler 1957). Ever since, and particularly over the last 20 years, professional liability issues have gained momentum, having an impact on society, on physicians' clinical decision making, on physician–patient relationships, and even on the availability of health care itself. In 1970, one in 25 American physicians had been sued (Jacobs 1980). Twenty years later, in 1990, over 75 per cent of all obstetricians practicing in the USA had been sued. The percentage of obstetricians who had never been sued for medical liability fell from 33.1 per cent in 1983 to 22.4 per cent in 1990. During the same period, the number of obstetricians who had been sued three or more times rose from 20 to 36.6 per cent. (ACOG 1983, 1985, 1988, 1990)

Since the mid-1970s, medical professional liability has been of great concern to the National Institute of Medicine (NIM). In 1987, the NIM assembled an interdisciplinary committee of 15 experts in obstetrics, pediatrics, family and general medicine, law, medical ethics, health services research, insurance, economics, nursing, and public health policy. The committee's scope of inquiry was to be the effects of medical professional liability on delivery of and access to obstetrical health care.

The NIM committee commissioned more than 20 papers by experts in various fields as well as three surveys to garner new data. In addition, it reviewed more than 50 surveys bearing on medical malpractice problems in obstetrics. Their efforts culminated in the publication of *Medical professional liability and the delivery of obstetrical care: Vol 1 and 2: interdisciplinary review*.

This chapter will highlight the impact of professional liability considerations on the demographics and habits of obstetrical care providers and on the availability of obstetrical services.

Demographics and clinical practices of obstetrical care providers

Between April 1985 and March 1992, 90 obstetric and gynecology claims and suits were filed against all Harvard medical institutions. Of these, 32 (35.6 per cent) related to obstetrics only, accounting for 46.1 per cent of the financial pay-out. The average loss was $320 756 per claim. Data from CRICO, the insurer of all practitioners at hospitals affiliated with Harvard Medical School, reveal that the premium for insuring an obstetrician against professional liability risk increased from $15 817 in 1985–1986 to $39 000 in 1988–1989—an increase of almost 250 per cent in 3 years. Encouragingly, however, the premiums fell to $30 000 for 1991–1992 and 1992–1993; these are the lowest premium levels since about 1987 (personel communication).

In 1983, 1985, 1988, and 1990, the American College of Obstetricians and Gynecologists (ACOG) surveyed its fellowship and issued reports on professional liability and its effects. The reports detailed important trends over this 7-year period. (ACOG 1983, 1985, 1988, 1990)

In 1983, 68.2 per cent of obstetricians had not altered their practice habits; however, 17.2 per cent had decreased the level of high-risk obstetrical care, 10.1 per cent had decreased the number of deliveries they undertook, and 9.1 per cent no longer practiced obstetrics. By 1985, 62.9 per cent of obstetricians had made no change in their personal practice habits as a result of the risk of malpractice litigation. Those decreasing their practice of high-risk obstetrics had increased from 17.7 to 23.1 per cent and 54.2 per cent of obstetricians reported that they had stopped practicing clinical obstetrics before the age of 55. By 1990, 88 per cent of 55 year old obstetricians in Florida were no longer practicing clinical obstetrics.

Changes in obstetrics practice patterns were by no means limited to obstetricians. In 1987, the American Academy of Family Physicians (AAFP) reported that approximately 28 per cent of all family practitioners had either decreased their obstetric load or had discontinued the practice of obstetrics on account of liability insurance considerations. A further 36 per cent had discontinued obstetrics for other reasons.

Family practitioners had traditionally been important providers of obstetric services in rural areas. Their high rate of attrition in the practice of obstetrics began to generate significant access problems in certain parts of the country. Debra Lewis-Idema estimated, on the basis of data from the AAFP and ACOG, that the number of obstetric providers in non-metropolitan areas fell by about 20 per cent over the last 5 years, particularly affecting certain rural areas in Georgia, Nevada, Arizona, and West Virginia (Lewis-Idema 1989).

The difficulty of obtaining professional liability insurance coverage in many states has made it virtually impossible for nurse–midwives to continue clinical practice unless in the direct employment of physicians. Many would prefer to practice autonomously, consulting with physicians when necessary, but without insurance this autonomy is not possible. In addition, the current insurance situation occasionally presents difficulties for nurse–midwives who wish to practice in hospitals. Hospitals usually consider them to be non-employee professional staff and as such they must carry their own professional liability insurance. Because the insurance policies offered by the American College of Nurse–Midwives often do not provide the necessary level of coverage, nurse–midwives are often denied hospital privileges. Furthermore, many carriers who insure obstetricians place surcharges on premiums of obstetricians who employ or work with nurse–midwives. In 1987, 47 per cent of obstetricians who employed nurse–midwives had such surcharges imposed (ACOG 1988).

Available data indicate that professional liability considerations are affecting the clinical practice of nurse–midwives. In a 1988 survey, approximately 20 per cent indicated that they order more diagnostic tests, and 13 per cent that they were giving up nurse–midwifery practice. More than 30 per cent said that there were fewer job opportunities for them now than there had been before the costs of insurance rose and coverage decreased (Patch and Holaday 1988)

In addition to clear evidence that obstetricians are curtailing the clinical practice of obstetrics, reducing the frequency of their involvement in high-risk situations and reducing their obstetric load, there is also evidence that medical liability considerations affect clinical practice habits. Obstetricians who responded to an ACOG (1983) survey reported that they had begun to implement some of the following changes:

(1) increased use of testing and other diagnostic and monitoring procedures;

(2) increased use of informed consent;

(3) increased frequency of consultation with and referral to other physicians;

(4) increased attempts to provide written and tape-recorded information for patients.

More specifically, Benjamin Sachs has analyzed cesarean section rates in the USA, these rose dramatically (Sachs 1989) from less than 5 per cent of births in 1965 to 23.5 per cent in 1992 (Placek 1988; NCHS 1990). According to Sachs, this rise in the cesarean section rate is at least partly a result of the 'defensive medicine' being practiced in response to medical liability pressures. As evidence for this argument, he cites the following:

(1) the widespread use of fetal monitoring in low-risk patients—fetal monitoring, frequently employed because of medico-legal considerations, has a poor predictive value for detecting perinatal asphyxia and thus results in more cesarean sections;

(2) the lower incidence of forceps deliveries and vacuum extraction procedures;

(3) the virtual abandonment of vaginal breech deliveries;

(4) physicians' perception that the majority of allegations in obstetrical malpractice suits involved issues of fetal monitoring and failure to perform a timely cesarean section.

Further, the NIM committee concluded that the incidence of cerebral palsy (still popularly—and erroneously—believed to be a result of fetal asphyxia) had not been reduced by widespread use of electronic fetal heart rate monitors. Evidence did suggest, however, that professional liability concerns contributed to continued use of these monitors.

In an informal survey to determine whether the perceived risk of malpractice litigation was causing changes in clinical practices in departments of obstetrics at academic medical centers, letters were sent to 132 heads of departments, all members of the Association of Professors of Gynecology and Obstetrics. Many of those who responded indicated that current professional liability considerations were indeed having a significant effect on the teaching and training of obstetrical residents. Many also acknowledged that some of these changes had led to improved patient care, in particular better documentation and more liberal physician–patient discussion.

The survey also indicated further between 1984 and 1987, the percentage of graduating medical students choosing obstetrics as a career fell from 8.7 to 6.7 per cent. Fortunately, more recent statistics do not confirm this trend and many of the department heads surveyed by letter agreed that the great increase in the proportion of women entering the specialty (on the order of 50 per cent) had helped avoid what otherwise might have been a major drop in the number of physicians choosing obstetrics as a career.

Access to and delivery of obstetrical care

In 1986, the Robert Wood Johnson Foundation found that access to medical care among minority groups and uninsured individuals had deteriorated since 1982. (Robert Wood Johnson Foundation 1987). The study concluded further that this deterioration had occurred despite a nation-wide increase in the number of medical care providers.

Inadequate financing has always been one of the most significant barriers to obstetrical care for poor and indigent women in the USA. In an attempt to evaluate the relationships between professional liability issues, physician participation in Medicaid, and low-income women's access to Medicaid the NIM committee examined 39 studies conducted by state and national medical associations as well as consultant studies, research conducted by the National Governors' Association, and university-based research.

These studies generated voluminous and often imperfect data. None the less, the conclusion was that reductions in obstetrical practice among obstetricians, family physicians, and nurse–midwives, as reported in both state and national surveys, appear to have had a disproportionate effect on the availability of care for low-income women and women whose obstetric care is financed by Medicaid or provided by Community Health Centers and migrant health centers.

Indeed, 1988 data from a random sample of 208 center directors nation-wide indicates that the rise in malpractice premiums has had a major adverse impact on the number of medical care providers willing to serve low-income patients (Hughes *et al.* 1989). Many centers with adequate staff have been forced to reduce or curtail services on account of the cost of malpractice insurance coverage. Others have had problems with referral arrangements to specialists, as more and more obstetricians either left the specialty entirely or reduced their load of high-risk patients. Poor women are often perceived as being high risk on account of their poverty, insufficient food, poor nutrition, and histories of inadequate health care.

Testimony in the United States House of Representatives on the effect of medical malpractice insurance costs on access to obstetrical care (Rosenbaum and McNulty 1989) underscores the committee's perception that poor women are most likely to be affected by the declining availability of maternity health care providers. Sara Rosenbaum and Mouy McNulty of the Children's Defence Fund testified before the Senate House Committee on Small Business that a variety of forces are driving the startling rise in the costs of malpractice insurance, including the profit-seeking practices of insurance companies. Rosenbaum and McNulty believe, however, that poor patients are less likely to sue; these patients are often less aware of their rights and often have less time, money, and legal representation. They also believe that large awards in malpractice suits are unusual and have little to do with the astounding rise in obstetric premium rates.

Many physicians and other observers believe that the professional liability climate has been eroding patient–provider trust. This erosion is one of the consequences—and one of the causes—of the crisis that now exists. If indeed almost 80 per cent of all obstetricians expect to be sued at one time or another (ACOG 1990), it is clear that malpractice suits are not being filed only against the worst practitioners or worst health care institutions. The physician–patient relationship is disintegrating and the consequences are costly to physicians, patients, and ultimately to all who pay health care bills in this country.

A framework for solutions: the Harvard Medical Practice Study

Although anecdotes describing the problem abound, reform of the laws concerned with medical malpractice has been stymied by a paucity of data. In 1985 in the USA, a multidisciplinary group undertook a major investigation of medical injury and the legal system that deals with such injury. Five years later, with the encouragement and support of Dr David Axelrod, Commissioner of Health in the state of New York and one of the most visionary and effective public health figures of our time, this group completed the major components of what is known as the Harvard Medical Practice Study. The observations of this study are described in a series of articles (Hiatt *et al.* 1989; Brennan *et al.* 1990; Brennan *et al.* 1991*a*, *b*; Leape *et al.* 1991; Localio *et al.* 1991; Weiler *et al.* 1992; Johnson *et al.* 1992), and a book (Weiler *et al.* 1993).

The study attempted to answer the following four questions concerning all patients hospitalized in 1984 in New York state's acute-care, non-psychiatric hospitals.

1. How many were injured as a result of medical interventions and what fraction of injuries resulted from negligence?

2. How many of the injured patients brought claims and how many of those who brought claims were injured?
3. What were the costs of the injuries and how were those costs met?
4. Does the tort system serve to deter negligence on the part of providers and, if so, can its effects be quantified?

Following is a summary of this study's findings and their implications. Because the study required information about all patients in acute care hospitals, the data concerning any single group, such as obstetrical patients, are necessarily limited. However, many of the conclusions about physicians and patients in general are applicable to obstetricians and obstetrical patients.

The term adverse event was used to describe an injury that resulted from medical care rather than from the underlying medical problem and prolonged hospitalization or led to disability at the time of discharge. A negligent adverse event was one due to care beneath the standard of the average medical practitioner. In drawing conclusions, the study group made judgments not only of causation and negligence but also of the resultant disability.

Medical injuries

The study sample comprised 31 429 medical records in 51 hospitals. Identified among these were a total of 1133 adverse events that either resulted from medical management during the hospitalization under investigation or had occurred earlier but had precipitated that hospitalization under investigation. Of these, 280 were the result of negligent care. Based on these findings, the incidence of adverse events in New York in 1984 was 3.7 per cent. Of the adverse events, 27.6 per cent were due to negligence; thus, a negligent adverse event occurred in 1 per cent of all hospitalizations.

Projecting the findings of the study to the population as a whole reveals that of the 2.6 million people discharged from New York hospitals in 1984, 56 000 experienced injuries that led to minimal impairment from which they recovered within 1 month. Another 13 500 injuries led to moderate impairment with recovery in less than 6 months. Although more than 70 per cent of adverse events led to short-term disability, many individuals suffered more serious injuries. In 3800 cases, adverse events produced permanent impairment a rate of 2.6 per cent. More than 2500 patients had permanent and total disabilities as a result of adverse events. Finally, 13 400 adverse events caused death.

The overall adverse event rate for obstetrical patients was 1.7 per cent, and 26 per cent of these events were negligent. Projecting these figures to the state as a whole suggests that of the 2 318 282 births in New York in 1984 that were sampled, injuries occurred in about 3900, and rearly 1000 of these resulted from negligence.

To identify risk factors for the occurrence of adverse events and negligence, several socio-demographic attributes in the population as a whole were considered. (Again, it is not certain that these conclusions apply equally to obstetrical patients.) Blacks suffered more negligent care than Whites. However, this finding may have been confounded by the observation that uninsured patients experienced more negligent care and that more Blacks were without insurance. There was a nearly 16-fold variation in adverse event rates among hospitals and negligence rates varied from 10–70 per cent.

Adverse events were associated with severity of illness. Many adverse events took place in operating rooms or followed the use of potent medications. Moreover, large city hospitals and teaching centers, which receive large numbers of critically ill patients from other institutions and are the site of care for many very sick individuals, had higher adverse event rates.

The factors that promoted adverse events did not necessarily lead to substandard care. Indeed, negligence was not correlated with medical injury. For example, hospitals with little teaching activity had very high rates of substandard care, but not high adverse event rates. Moreover, the emergency room was infrequently the site of medical injury, but when such injury did occur there, it was quite often the result of negligence.

Malpractice claims rates

Many—if not most—physicians believe that patients and their attorneys file excessive numbers of malpractice claims and that the bulk are ill-founded. To assess the validity of those perceptions, the study group collected all tort claims filed by New York patients in and after 1984 and matched them with the study's findings of negligent injury.

On an aggregate basis, one malpractice tort claim was filed for every 7.5 negligently inflicted injuries. Because about one in two patient claims is ultimately paid, this means that the tort litigation–insurance system paid one claim for every 15 tort incidents. Even when one focuses only on those claims that are potentially more valuable for patients and their lawyers (serious injuries to patients under 70 years old), the ratios were one claim filed for every three negligent injuries and one claim paid for every six such injuries.

Matching tort claims filed, on the one hand, with an appraisal of hospital records, on the other, provided evidence of even greater inefficiency in the system. In only one-sixth of the claims was there persuasive evidence of negligent injury in the record. On the basis of its earlier work, the study group concluded that a modest number of cases of negligence might have occurred and yet not have been detected in the hospital record. A substantial majority of the tort claims filed, however, appeared not to have had a certain basis in provider carelessness or even in iatrogenic injury.

That fact has two implications. First, at least in its initial stages, the tort system is very error-prone. Even if the litigation process proves reasonably effective in screening the valid from the spurious claims—and this has not yet been shown by our study—physicians and their insurers suffer sizeable financial and emotional burdens simply from being caught up in lawsuits due to initial mistakes by patients' lawyers.

Second, the fact that a substantial proportion of tort claims were false positive, means that the number of false negatives (cases in which negligent injuries did not lead to tort claims), was even greater than first appears. Thus, although the tort system appears quite erratic, there is no basis for the charge that the amount of malpractice litigation is excessive. On the contrary, there seems to be a major deficit of litigation.

Patient losses

Malpractice law is supposed to compensate patients for past injuries and to prevent future ones. The survey of all injured patients was designed to measure the adequacy of compensation under the existing system and to provide information that would help estimate the feasibility of a no-fault alternative.

Attributing financial losses (for medical care, lost earnings, and lost household production) is far more complicated for medical injuries than for motor vehicle or workplace injuries, because most non-obstetrical patients who go to the hospital have a condition that would in its own right produce this kind (if not quantity) of financial loss. In contrast, the injured driver and worker are typically healthy. To deal with this problem, the study group surveyed patients who had been injured during a hospitalization 5 years previously. Subsequent episodes of disability were analyzed and estimates were made of the proportion of costs attributable to the injury on the one hand and to the underlying medical problem on the other. In addition, interviews were conducted with a group of control patients who had been hospitalized at the same time but who had not suffered injury. On the basis of this work, the losses caused by the injuries were found to be relatively modest when compared with those that resulted from the medical problems: typically the medical injury increased time taken off work by 20 per cent.

This finding suggested that the costs of compensating patients for all serious medical injuries might not be excessive. The Harvard study group verified that conclusion, however, by estimating the losses incurred by each patient. The amount required to compensate their losses would reveal the cost of a hypothetical no-fault plan. The key ingredients of this plan are payments only for:

(1) financial losses, thus excluding pain and suffering;

(2) more serious losses, that is, those occurring after a 6-month 'deductible' period had elapsed after hospitalization;

(3) net losses left uncompensated by broader programs of loss insurance (for medical cost or time lost from work).

This plan would provide more limited, but more sensible, insurance protection to all severely injured patients, whether or not the provider had been negligent. In contrast, the insurance offered by the present tort system guarantees full compensation, but only to those patients who are able to prove negligence to the satisfaction of the legal system.

The net financial losses of all injured patients within the study's parameters in New York could be compensated for about $870 million a year. Any such no-fault program would entail administrative costs of at least an additional 25 per cent, based on the workers' compensation experience. The total of those figures can be compared with the present cost of malpractice insurance in New York, which is now well over $1 billion a year, just to pay the claims of the relative handful of injured patients who are able to claim malpractice. And that tort figure might well increase sharply in the 1990s if the more litigation gap (serious medical injuries and financial compensation) begins to close again as it did in the 1970s and 1980s.

Injury prevention: deterrence

The study group concluded that a no-fault program appeared better than tort-fault as a vehicle for sensible and economical compensation of medical accident victims. A no-fault program would not, however, obviate the need for tough decisions concerning causation. For example, was a child's cerebral palsy the result of a difficult delivery? None the less, in the Harvard study it was possible to make decisions about causation of injury with much greater confidence than those about negligence. Five per cent in the former category were close calls compared with 20 per cent in the latter. In a no-fault setting, the 5 per cent figure would presumably still apply, and to a potentially much larger body of claimants than under the present fault-based schemes.

Such decisions could be avoided altogether, it is true, by a program of social insurance that would cover all medical expenses and some lost income, no matter their cause. However, an arrangement that places the legal and financial burden for disabling injury on the responsible actor or activity makes it possible to provide incentives for effective prevention of future injuries. Such a social policy objective is at least as important as compensation for past injuries. Injury prevention is usually asserted to be the major comparative advantage of tort law, which focuses liability on the person at fault for the accident and thus presumably in the best position to alter future behavior. But critics of malpractice law regularly assert that little preventive value can be secured from the prospect of such legal liability, either because so few cases are actually brought to light or because the cases that are lodged are often the wrong ones. Finally, even when negligent physicians are held legally liable, it is not they but their insurers who bear the greater financial burden of court judgments.

The study's surveys of physicians cast doubt on this assessment of the preventive effects of malpractice litigation. Although only a fraction of potentially litigable claims are filed, physicians systematically overestimate the risk of suit they face. Further, although they are insured for the cost of legal liability, physicians bear substantial uninsured costs as a result of being sued. Some of these are financial and others, often stronger, are psychological. Despite the considerable possibility of groundless litigation, the risk of suit is substantially greater if there is a valid basis for the claim. In any event, physicians do report substantial changes in their practice behavior as their perceived tort threat varies. Malpractice law litigation functions, then, somewhat like income tax audits. First, only a small portion of potential cases are singled out for scrutiny. Second, although the targets are too often innocent parties, the risk is much greater for error-prone parties. Finally, the costs imposed by the process seem so high as to motivate significant changes in behavior to avoid running foul of the law.

The acid test of the deterrent effect of the tort system, though, is whether it actually leads to fewer injuries. The most compelling answer to that question would be provided by a truly controlled experiment, one in which negligence is compared in environments with and without a tort system. Such an experiment is impossible, because the tort system alone operates in New York (and throughout the USA). Instead, the frequency of injury was examined at New York hospitals that were subject to varying threats of litigation. The results, while consistent with deterrence, were not close to statistical significance at conventional levels. Nevertheless, those results and several additional findings lead to the conclusion that the tort system exerts a deterrent effect. First, the self-reported behavior of New York physicians interviewed for this study is consistent. Second, the finding of increased negligent care of the elderly and the uninsured may be attributable, at least in part, to the fact that in these groups, injury results in lesser economic losses and therefore in a smaller likelihood of their bringing claims.

No-fault versus strict liability

The term no-fault understandably carries for some a negative connotation: whatever the cause of a bad outcome, nobody is assigned responsibility. In terms of patient compensation, however, the term has clearly positive implications: whatever the cause of a bad outcome, the patient will be reimbursed. Recall that almost three-quarters of the medical injuries found in New York were deemed not to have resulted from negligence. Although many patients with non-negligent injuries suffered losses as great as, or greater than, those of the victims of negligence, these individuals were entitled to nothing under the tort system.

Despite its conclusion that tort law is more likely than not to deter injury, the Harvard study group believes that fundamental changes should be made in our liability system. In particular, a shift is needed from our present fault-based system of liability, which focuses on the personal negligence of individual physicians, to a broader system of strict liability imposed on the hospital or other health care organization for all accidents befalling its patients, whether or not carelessness is demonstrated. This preference is based not simply on the evident advantage of no-fault systems as sensible and economic insurance for compensating the victims of accidents. At least as important, such an expansion of legal liability could materially improve the law's leverage on the health care system to develop more effective preventive measures against future patient injuries, both negligent and non-negligent.

Under a system of social insurance, the victims of medical injuries are compensated, whether or not there was negligence. With the proposed 'strict liability' arrangement, both groups would also be compensated; however, the institution with which the provider is affiliated would also be held legally and financially responsible for all injuries, whether negligent or not. Insurance premiums for institutions would be partially experience-rated; every institution would therefore have a powerful incentive not only to monitor itself for the carelessness, ignorance, or illness that generally underlies negligence, but also to mount prevention programs directed at non-negligent injuries as well.

References

American Academy of Family Physicians (1987). *Family physicians and obstetrics: a professional liability study*. American Academy of Family Physicians, Kansas City, MO.

ACOG (1983). *Professional liability insurance and its effects: report of a survey of ACOG's membership*. American College of Obstetrics and Gynecologists, Washington, DC.

ACOG (1985). *Professional liability insurance and its effects: report of a survey of ACOG's membership*. American College of Obstetrics and Gynecologists, Washington, DC.

ACOG (1988). *Professional liability insurance and its effects: report of a 1987 survey of ACOG's membership*. American College of Obstetrics and Gynecologists, Washington, DC.

ACOG (1990). *Professional liability insurance and its effects: report of a 1990 survey of ACOG's membership*. American College of Obstetrics and Gynecologists, Washington, DC.

Brennan, T. A., Localio, A. R., Leape, L. L., Laird, N. J., Hiatt, H. H., and Barnes, B. A. (1990). Identification of adverse events suffered by hospitalized patients: a cross-sectional study of litigation, quality assurance and medical records at two teaching hospitals. *Annals of Internal Medicine*, **112**, 221–6.

Brennan, T. A., Leape, L. L., Laird, N. M., Herbert, L. E., Localio, A. R., Lawther, A. G., *et al.* (1991*a*). Incidence of adverse events and negligence in hospitalized patients: results of the Harvard Medical Practice study I. *New England Journal of Medicine*, **324**, 370–6.

Brennan, T. A., Herbert, L. E., Laird, N. M., Lawthers, A. G., Thorpe, K. E., Leape, L. L., *et al.* (1991*b*). Hospital characteristics associated with adverse events and substandard care. *Journal of the American Medical Association*, **265**, 3265–9.

Hiatt, H. H., Barnes, B. A., Brennan, T. A., Laird, N. M., Lawthers, A. G., Leape, L. L. *et al.* (1989). A study of medical injury and medical malpractice: an overview. *New England Journal of Medicine*, **321**, 480–4.

Hughes, D., Rosenbaum, S., Smith, D., and Fader, C. (1989). Obstetrical care for low-income women: the effects of medical malpractice on community health centers. In *Medical professional liability and the delivery of obstetrical care*: Vol II, *an interdisciplinary review*. National Academy Press, Washington, DC.

Institute of Medicine (1989). *Medical Professional Liabrary and the Delivery of Obstetrical Care*, 1989 Vols. I and II. Institute of Medical National Academy Press, Washington, DC.

Jacobs, C. M. (1980). *Hospital risk management and malpractice liability control*. Interqual, Chicago.

Johnson, W. G., Brennan, T. A., Newhouse, J. P., Leape, L. L., Lawthers, A. G., Hiatt, H. H., and Weiler, P. C. (1992). The economic consequences of medical injuries. *Journal of the American Medical Association*, **267**, 2487–92.

Leape, L. L., Brennan, T. A., Laird, N., Lawthers, A. G., Localio, A. R., Barnes, B.

A., *et al.* (1991). The nature of adverse events in hospitalized patients: results of the Harvard Medical Practice study II. *New England Journal of Medicine*, **324**, 377–84.

Lewis-Idema, D. (1989). Medical professional liability and access to obstetrical care: is there a crisis? In *Medical professional liability and the delivery of obstetrical care*: Vol. II, *an interdisciplinary review*. National Academy Press, Washington, DC.

Localio, A. R., Lawthers, A. G., Brennan, T. A., Laird, N. M., Herbert, L. E., Peterson, L. M., *et al.* (1991). Relation between malpractice claims and adverse events due to negligence: results of the Harvard Medical Practice study III. *New England Journal of Medicine*, **325**, 245–51.

National Center for Health Statistics (1990). *National hospital discharge summary for 1990*. Government Printing Office.

Patch, F. B., and Holaday, S. (1988). Effects of changes in professional liability insurance on certified nurse–midwives. Paper presented at the *33rd ACNM Annual Convention research forum*, Detroit.

Placek, P. J., Taffel, S. M., and Moien, M. (1986). C-section rates rise; VBAC inch upward. *American Journal of Public Health*, **78(5)**, 562–3.

Robert Wood Johnson Foundation (1987). *Access to health care in the United States: results of a 1986 survey*. Robert Wood Johnson Foundation, Princeton, NJ.

Rosenbaum, S. and McNulty, M. (1989). *Testimony to the Committee on Small Business, Subcommittee on Regulation, Business Opportunities, and Energy*. US House of Representatives, 11 October.

Sachs, B. P. (1989). Is the rising rate of cesarian section a result of more defensive medicine? In *Medical professional liability and the delivery of obstetrical care*: Vol. II, *An interdisciplinary review*. National Academy Press, Washington, DC.

Stetler, C. J. (1957). The history of reported medical professional liability cases. *Temple Law Quarterly*, **30(4)**, 366.

Weiler, P. C., Newhouse, J. P., and Hiatt, H. H. (1992). Proposal for medical liability reform. *Journal of the American Medical Association*, **267**, 2355–8.

Weiler, P. C., Newhouse, J. P., Hiatt, H. H., Brennan, T. A., Leape, L. L., and Johnson, W. G. (1993). *A measure of malpractice*. Harvard University Press.

Index

DMU 0349694 01 1

WITHDRAWN
DE MONTFORT UNIVERSITY
LIBRARY

Normal loan Kimberlin

Please return this item at or before the date shown below.
Fines will be charged if the item is returned after this date.
Item issued subject to reservation recall see Library Guide for details
Renewals/loan information t 257 7043 Library information t 257 7042

16 JAN 2004
5 4 04
14 MAY 2004
15 APR 2005
19 DEC 2005
5 OCT 2007

DE MONTFORT UNIVERSITY
LEICESTER • BEDFORD

© De Montfort University Library all rights reserved
Kimberlin library www.library.dmu.ac.uk PC28
Library label series design/print The Printing Centre